D1179663

Hair Loss
and Restoration

Second Edition

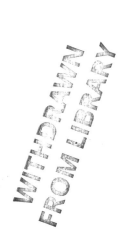

Hair Loss
and Restoration

Second Edition

Jerry Shapiro, MD, FRCPC

Professor, Disorders of Hair and Scalp
The Ronald O. Perelman Department of Dermatology
New York University Langone Medical Center
New York City, New York, USA

Nina Otberg, MD

Clinical Lead
Hair Clinic, Skin and Laser Center
Berlin, Germany

Clinical Lead
Hair Transplant Center
Otberg Medical Group
Berlin, Germany

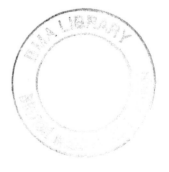

CRC Press
Taylor & Francis Group
Boca Raton London New York

CRC Press is an imprint of the
Taylor & Francis Group, an **informa** business

CRC Press
Taylor & Francis Group
6000 Broken Sound Parkway NW, Suite 300
Boca Raton, FL 33487-2742

© 2015 by Taylor & Francis Group, LLC
CRC Press is an imprint of Taylor & Francis Group, an Informa business

No claim to original U.S. Government works

Printed on acid-free paper
Version Date: 20150304

International Standard Book Number-13: 978-1-4822-3197-7 (Hardback)

Visit the Taylor & Francis Web site at
http://www.taylorandfrancis.com

and the CRC Press Web site at
http://www.crcpress.com

We dedicate this book to all our hair loss patients who have trusted us and given us the privilege of taking care of their hair.
It continues to be an honor for us.

Contents

Contents

Foreword

The fact that research and treatment of hair disorders have progressed so much in recent times makes the second edition of this book a necessity. The numbers of patients interested in hair care are increasing, and they expect results. They are bombarded and carried away by advertisements on the Internet and in magazines, never mind on their telephones.

In reality, hair disorders are complex and require accurate diagnosis for suitable treatment. The importance of listening to the patient and taking a full history is emphasized. The main purpose at the opening visit is to listen to patients voice their concerns and expectations. A hands-on examination with adequate look-and-see is stressed, in addition to appropriate testing. Biopsies have a place in many patients and make them feel that they are taken seriously. The differentiation between scarring and nonscarring alopecia is stressed.

Detailed descriptions of patterned hair loss and diffuse shedding allow the average caregiver to distinguish which is present. New developments in the diagnosis and treatment of alopecia areata are discussed in full.

The new worldwide player in scarring hair loss is frontal fibrosing alopecia, which is on the rise. It may exist as a single entity or be complicated by lichen planopilaris. It is well discussed here. Hair restoration procedures are described in detail.

All in all, the two authors are to be commended for a clear, concise, and up-to-date description of the diagnosis and treatment of hair disorders. It is compact, accessible, and easy to read. A copy of this book in the hair clinic will be valuable for both doctors and patients.

David Whiting

Acknowledgments

I express my greatest gratitude to the people who have helped and supported me throughout the process of writing this book and who have played an important role in my career.

First of all, I thank Jerry Shapiro who has been my friend and mentor for over 9 years. I am grateful for the opportunity to write this book together with him, for his trust in me, and for his ongoing advice and encouragement. A special thanks to my dear colleague and friend Tanja Fischer who helped me build up a hair clinic in Germany at the Skin and Laser Center in Potsdam and Berlin, who always supported my projects and ideas, and who helped and encouraged me to found my Hair Transplant Center in Berlin. I thank my hair transplant team Manuela Hampel, Senem Asurova, Steffi Fruhstorfer, Petra Visic, Martina Bialowons, and Michael Braun for their dedication, diligence, and empathy to our patients.

I thank Jürgen Lademann and Ulrike Blume-Peytavi, who were my first teachers in skin physiology and hair disorders, for the continuing exchange of thoughts and ideas. I thank Howard Maibach, Kevin McElwee, and David Whiting for allowing me to learn from them and to spend time in their clinics and laboratories. I thank my sister Mari Otberg and Marion Bernert-Thomann for the artwork and graphic design in Figures 1.9, 1.22, 2.2, 2.9, 2.11a, 2.20, 5.5, 7.2, 7.3, 7.7, 7.14a, 7.15, 7.16, 7.17, and 7.28. Last but not the least, I thank my family and friends who supported me and allowed me to take weekends, holidays, and evenings to finally accomplish this project.

Nina Otberg

I thank my parents Brajna Estrin Shapiro and Faivish Shraga Shapiro, who immigrated from small villages in Eastern Europe after World War II. It is their perseverance and risk-taking mentality in coming to North America that helped mold who I am and my drive to be a physician and dermatologist. I thank my sister Sarah Jesion and brother Haim Shapiro and their respective spouses Morris and Leona for all their advice over the years.

I also thank Brian Logan for encouraging me in my career and being my rock for over two decades. If not for Brian, I could not do what I am presently doing.

I further thank my coauthor Nina Otberg. Her hard work in the preparation of this book and her knowledge and friendship over the years have been very important in my life.

I thank all my previous fellows from all over the world who have shaped who I am with their questions and their knowledge.

I thank my "hair" colleagues David Whiting, Elise Olsen, Vera Price, and Wilma Bergfeld for their guidance.

I thank my nonhair dermatology colleagues David McLean, Harvey Lui from UBC, and Seth Orlow and David Cohen from NYU, who encouraged me and gave me the privilege to practice exclusively trichologic medicine.

I would like to thank Kevin McElwee for his immense knowledge of the basic science of hair.

I thank three important nurses who have helped shape my career: Nina MacDonald, Lucianna Zanet, and Heather McKie.

Last but not least, I thank my hair patients who have trusted me to take care of their hair disorders over the past 27 years.

Jerry Shapiro

1 How to diagnose the patient with hair loss

Hair loss (alopecia) and scalp problems are very common complaints in the everyday dermatological clinic. Hair loss of any kind frequently causes major distress for the patient and can lead to anxiety and depression. Patients who suffer from hair loss and scalp problems often see several physicians and frequently report that they were not taken seriously, nobody looked at their scalp, and they got the advice to just live with their problem.

Even though we do not fully understand the pathophysiology of many hair diseases, there are always treatment options available. The patient needs to understand that the treatment of hair loss takes time and patience.

Hair basics

The entire scalp contains around 100,000 pigmented, terminal hair follicles. Blonds tend to have more, at 120,000, and redheads fewer, at 80,000 hair follicles [1,2]. There is ethnic variation, with an average density of 250–310 hairs/cm² in people of European decent [3–6], approximately 150 hairs/cm² in African-American patients [6], and 120 hairs/cm² in Asian patients [7]. In Europeans, hair shafts usually show an oval cross section; diameters can range from approximately 50 to 120 μm. Very fine hair with diameters less than 50 μm is most frequently seen in the Scandinavian population and northwestern Europe [8,9]. Hair of people originating from east Asia (China, Korea, and Japan) is usually referred to as oriental or Asian hair. It generally shows the greatest diameter, ranging from 100 to 130 μm [9]. Asian hair shafts are straight with no or very few twists along the shaft and with a round cross section [10–12]. The hair of people from sub-Saharan Africa is highly characteristic in shape. African hair is considerably flattened and grooved and frequently varies in diameter along one single shaft [13].

Every hair follicle undergoes an individual recurring cycle with growing and resting periods. The growing period (anagen) persists for 2–8 years, and the hair grows approximately 1 cm/month or 0.35 mm/day during this time. During the hair cycle, the middle and upper portions of the hair follicle are the permanent segment, whereas the lower portion is nonpermanent (Figure 1.1). The root (bulb area) of an anagen terminal follicle reaches deep into subcutaneous fat tissue. The anagen phase is followed by a transition period (catagen) of 2 weeks, during which the hair follicle undergoes programmed apoptosis. This transitional state is followed by a resting period (telogen) that lasts around 3 months. During telogen, the hair does not grow longer; the shaft is anchored in the mid-deep dermis.

Unlike most fur-bearing animals, where the hair cycle is synchronous, on the human scalp there is an asynchronous mixture of hairs actively growing and resting. In a healthy scalp, 80%–90% of hair follicles are in anagen [14]. A normal anagen to telogen ratio

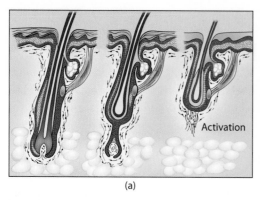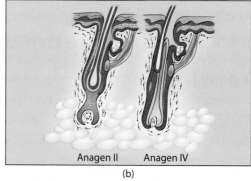

Figure 1.1

During the hair cycle, the middle and upper portions of the hair follicle are the permanent segments of the hair follicle, whereas the lower portion is nonpermanent. (a) The growing or anagen hairs are anchored deeply within the subcutaneous fat and cannot be pulled out easily. The telogen hairs are located higher up in the dermis and can be pulled out relatively easily. The scalp consists of almost 90% hairs in anagen, 1% in catagen, and 10% in telogen. Anagen may last up to 2–6 years, telogen 3 months, and catagen 3 weeks. This ratio is usually uniformly distributed over the entire scalp. The dermal papilla (dp) is pulled upward with each cycle and during telogen is closely associated with the stem cells of the bulge area. Communication signals between dp and stem cells of the bulge probably determine the length of anagen and the matrix girth of the next hair cycle. (b) The newly formed anagen hair pushes out the previous telogen hair.

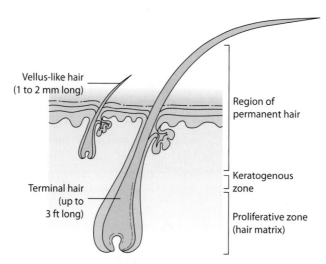

Figure 1.2

Vellus-like hairs are less than 0.03 mm in diameter and rarely grow more than 1–2 mm. Terminal hairs are coarse, over 0.06 mm in diameter, and can grow up to 1 m (3 ft).

for the scalp hair is 9:1, although seasonal variations can be found [15,16]. The scalp sheds around 100 telogen hairs per day. Normal scalp skin also shows a variable number of small vellus hair follicles. Vellus hair follicles cover our entire body, except for palms and soles, with variable densities in different body sites. Vellus hairs are anchored in the mid-upper dermis; the hair shaft is free of color and less than 30 μm thick [17] (Figure 1.2).

Basic trichologic anatomy

To appreciate an organized protocol for alopecia, it is important to review the basics of hair anatomy. Hair follicles are skin appendages that are formed in week 16 of the early fetal period. They can be divided into four parts (Figures 1.3 and 1.4):

1. Infundibulum, extending from the follicular orifice to the sebaceous gland
2. Isthmus, extending from the sebaceous gland to insertion of the arrector pili muscle
3. Suprabulbar area, insertion of the arrector pili muscle to matrix
4. Bulb, consisting of the dermal papilla and matrix intermixed with melanocytes (Figure 1.5)

The lower portion of the follicle consists of five major portions: (1) the dermal papilla; (2) the matrix; (3) the hair shaft, from the inside to the outside of medulla, cortex, and cuticle; (4) the inner root sheath (IRS), consisting of the IRS cuticle, Huxley's layer on the inside and Henle's layer on the outside; and (5) the outer root sheath (ORS) (Figures 1.6 and 1.7). The base of the follicle is invaginated by the dermal papilla, which contains highly vascularized connective tissue. Dermal papilla fibroblasts are inherently different from nonfollicular fibroblasts. There is a large amount of acid-mucopolysaccharides within the dermal papilla, staining positively for Alcian Blue and metachromatically for toluidine blue. The ground substance consists of not only nonsulfated polysaccharides such as hyaluronic acid, but also sulfated mucopolysaccharides such as chondroitin sulfate. Increased activity of alkaline phosphatase can be found in the anagen phase.

The hair matrix has large vesicular nuclei and deeply basophilic cytoplasm. DOPA-positive melanocytes are interspersed between

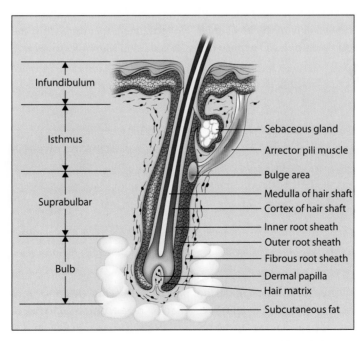

Figure 1.3
Diagrammatic representation of hair anatomy. The hair follicle is divided into four parts: bulb, suprabulbar area, isthmus, and infundibulum.

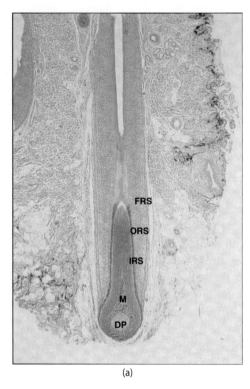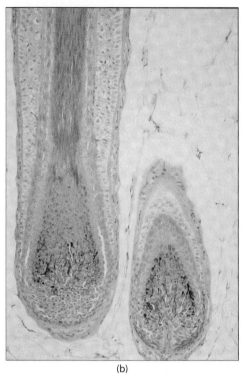

(a)   (b)

Figure 1.4
(a) Histology of the hair follicle on longitudinal section showing dermal papilla (DP), matrix (M), inner root sheath (IRS), outer root sheath (ORS), and fibrous root sheath (FRS). (b) Two anagen follicles side by side at the level of fat. Note the melanocytes within the matrix providing pigment to the hair. (Courtesy of Dr. Magdalena Martinka and Dr. David Shum.)

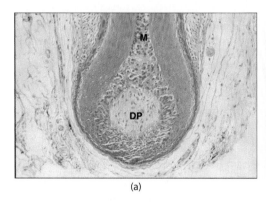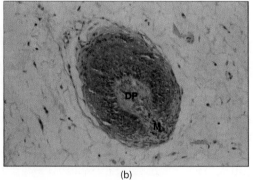

(a)   (b)

Figure 1.5
(a) Close-up of longitudinal section of dermal papilla (DP), which is an invagination of the dermis into the matrix (M). The DP allows capillaries to gain entrance to the cells of the matrix. It is the signal transduction and communication between the DP and the matrix that determines how long a hair will grow and how thick a shaft will be. Melanocytes fill the matrix and produce the pigment of the hair. (b) Cross section of the follicle at the level of DP. (Courtesy of Dr. Magdalena Martinka.)

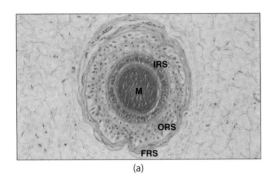

(a)

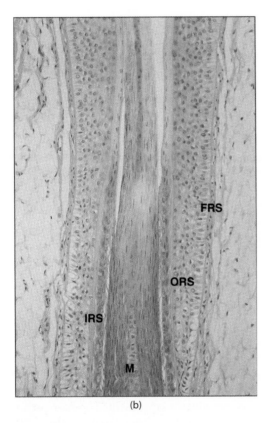

(b)

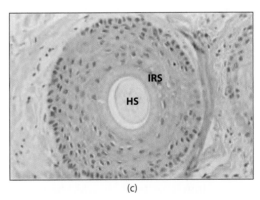

(c)

Figure 1.6
(a) Cross section and (b) longitudinal sections of the follicle at the suprabulbar level. In the central portion of the follicle, the matrix (M) is forming cortex, which is surrounded by the cuticle. This is subsequently invested by the cuticle of the inner root sheath (IRS), Huxley's layer with trichohyaline granules, and the already keratinized Henle's layer. The outer root sheath (ORS), hyaline membrane, and fibrous root sheath (FRS) surround the whole structure. (c) Cross section of the follicle just beneath the isthmus showing the eosinophilic completely keratinized IRS enclosing the hair shaft (HS). All of this is surrounded by the ORS, hyaline membrane, and FRS. Only anagen hairs have IRSs. (Courtesy of Dr. David Shum.)

the basal cells of the matrix. Melanocytes are dendritic neural crest–derived cells that migrate into the epidermis in the first trimester. Melanin is a complex quinone-/indole–quinone-derived mixture of biopolymers produced in melanocytes from tyrosine [18]. Melanin is incorporated into the future cells of the hair shaft through phagocytosis of the distal portion of the dendritic melanocyte (Figure 1.8). Melanosomes of the hair follicle are larger than those of the epidermis. They lie singly or within groups not within lysosomes. They are located usually in the interfibrillary matrix, within the cells and only rarely in the intercellular space in the hair cortex. Two different types of melanin can be distinguished: eumelanin is brown or black, and pheomelanin, which results from the incorporation of cysteine, is yellow or red [19–23]. In eumelanin-containing follicles, melanocytes contain ellipsoidal melanosomes with lamellar internal structure (eumelanosomes). Pheomelanogenesis is associated with melanocyte-containing spherical melanosomes, which have a less well-defined internal structure containing granules and vesicles. Eumelaninogenic and phaeomelanogenic melanosomes can coexist in the same melanocyte but are produced in different pathways [24–26]. A preponderance of eumelanin is associated with brown or black hair and a preponderance of phaeomelanin with red or blond hair. The absence or relative absence of both melanin types results in white hair.

Cells of the hair matrix differentiate into six different types of cells, each of which keratinizes at a different level. The outer layer, Henle's layer, of the IRS keratinizes first, establishing a firm coat around the soft central portion of the follicle. The two opposed cuticles covering the hair shaft and the inside portion of the IRS keratinize next, followed by the Huxley's layer. The hair cortex then follows, and the medulla is last.

The hair medulla appears amorphous because of its only partial keratinization. It

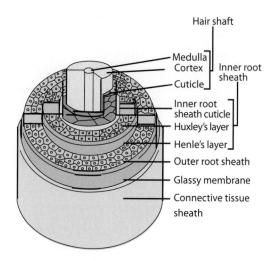

Figure 1.7
The different layers of the hair follicle.

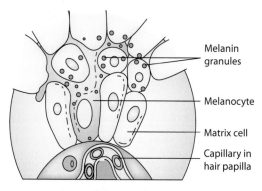

Figure 1.8
Melanosomes, either eumelanin or pheomelanin, during anagen are transferred from melanocytes to matrical cortex cells via dendritic ends.

may not always be present. The hair cortex during upward growth from the matrix cells keratinizes gradually by losing its nuclei and becoming filled with keratin fibrils. No-keratohyalin granules (i.e., keratinizing epidermis) or trichohyalin granules (i.e., keratinizing IRS) are formed during the keratinization of the cortex. Keratin of the cortex is hard keratin, in contrast to the IRS or epidermis, which is soft keratin. The hair cuticle is the outermost layer of the hair shaft. It consists of overlapping cells arranged like shingles and pointing upward with their peripheral portion. Up to the isthmus, the cells of the hair shaft cuticle are tightly interlocked with the cells of the IRS cuticle, resulting in the firm attachment of the hair to its IRS. The hair shaft and the IRS move upward in unison.

The IRS is composed of three layers (Figure 1.7). None of these layers contains melanin, and all keratinize with trichohyalin granule formation. These granules stain eosinophilic, in contrast to the basophilic keratohyalin granules of the epidermis. The cuticle of the IRS consists of one layer of flattened overlapping cells that point downward in the direction of the hair bulb. Because the cuticle cells of the hair shaft point upward, these two types of cells interlock tightly. Trichohyalin granules are few in the IRS cuticle. Huxley's layer is two cell layers thick and develops numerous trichohyalin granules. Henle's layer is only one cell layer thick and already shows numerous trichohyalin granules as it emerges from the matrix. Just before the isthmus, the IRS becomes fully keratinized. However, at the level of the isthmus the IRS disintegrates and loses its tight connection to the hair shaft cuticle. The IRS cuticle cells therefore do not contribute to emerging hair but serve as a hard molding scaffold up to the arrector pili muscle.

The ORS extends from the matrix cells to the entrance of the sebaceous duct, where it changes into the infundibular epidermis. The ORS is thinnest at the level of the hair bulb, gradually increasing in thickness, and is thickest in the middle portion of the hair follicle, the isthmus. In the lower portion below the isthmus, it is covered by IRS and does not undergo keratinization. The ORS is rich in vacuolated cytoplasm owing to its plentiful glycogen.

The point of insertion of the arrector pili muscle is referred to as the bulge area. The bulge area is where hair follicle stem cells are located [27]. Stem cells from the bulge area migrate to other portions of the follicle and differentiate into different specialized layers.

The isthmus is the segment that extends from the arrector pili muscle to the sebaceous gland duct entrance. No more IRS can be found here. The ORS undergoes trichilemmal keratinization, producing large homogeneous keratinized cells without the formation of keratohyalin granules.

The upper portion of the follicle above the entrance of the sebaceous duct is the infundibulum. It can be regarded as a funnel, filled with scaled-off keratinocytes and sebum. The sebum flow and the movement of the hair shaft push the dead keratinocytes toward the skin surface. The infundibular epidermis undergoes keratinization with the formation of keratohyalin granules similar to the interfollicular epidermis.

The glassy or vitreous membrane, which forms a homogeneous eosinophilic zone peripheral to the ORS, is periodic acid Schiff (PAS) positive and diastase resistant. It differs from the interfollicular basement membrane zone by being much thicker. It is thickest around the lower third of the hair follicle in the suprabulbar area. The fibrous root sheath is composed of thick collagen bundles.

Patient approach

It is most important for successful patient management and treatment to make the correct diagnoses. The following five steps (Figure 1.9) are key to making the right diagnosis, to proper treatment, and to patient satisfaction:

1. Listen
2. Look
3. Touch
4. Magnify
5. Sample

Many etiological factors can lead to clinical hair loss, including genetic predisposition, systemic illness, drugs, endocrine abnormalities, psychological distress, diet, trauma, infections, autoimmunity, and structural hair defects. Hair is one of the fastest growing tissues of the body; therefore, any metabolic and hormonal changes can result in shedding and alopecia. Because of the multiplicity of causes that can result in hair loss, a thorough history is of critical importance in developing the initial differential diagnosis.

Listen

The first task of a physician is to address the patient's concerns fully, exploring the impact of alopecia on the patient's psychosocial well-being. A simple questionnaire can help lead the conversation and can give first hints to possible underlying causes (Figure 1.9).

Important questions are as follows: When did you begin losing your hair? Are you shedding a lot of hair and do you find hair all over the place, or did you notice a more gradual thinning? Where are you losing your hair? How many hairs are you approximately losing per day? What percentage of your hair have you lost in what amount of time?

Moderate and massive shedding is frequently seen in telogen effluvium and alopecia areata. Gradual thinning can be seen in androgenetic alopecia and often in cicatricial alopecias. The pattern described by the patient can also give first hints. Patches of hair loss are suspicious for alopecia areata and cicatricial alopecia, generalized shedding is seen in telogen effluvium and sometimes alopecia areata, and frontoparietal or vertex thinning is most commonly seen in androgenetic alopecia.

Further questions should comprise present and past physical and mental health conditions and a full list of current and past medication. How is your general health? Have you had any severe diseases in the past? Are you or have you been taking any medication? Do

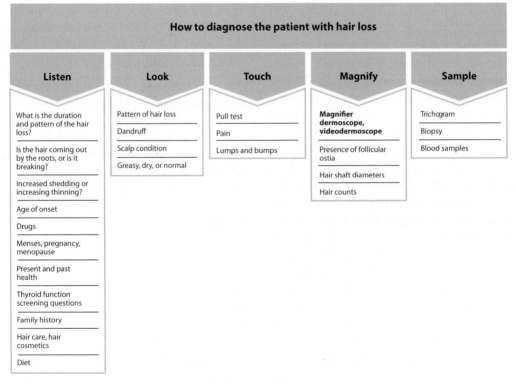

Figure 1.9
Patient approach.

you have any thyroid problems? What happened in your life 3–6 months prior to the onset of your hair loss (pregnancy, high fever, operations/general anesthesia, crash diets, accidents/trauma, or psychological stress)?

It is also important to ask about the diet in general (well balanced/vegetarian, vegan or pescetarian), family history of hair loss, and hair care practices. Unbalanced and restrictive diets or strict vegetarian or vegan diets can implicate iron deficiency or other deficiencies (zinc, selenium, vitamin B12, etc.). A positive family history of alopecia areata or androgenetic alopecia may point to a genetic predisposition for hair loss. Some hair care practices (e.g., bleaching, back combing, permanent waving, hot combs, hot blow drying, and straightening) may result in structural defects and hair breakage. Furthermore, heavy extensions, dreadlocks, cornrows, tight ponytails, and braids can lead to traction alopecia.

Questions should also be asked about the loss of axillary and pubic hair, eyelashes, eyebrows, and other body hairs, as any hair-bearing area may be affected by alopecia areata or trichotillomania.

Female patients should be asked about the regularity of their menstrual cycle; intake, duration, and change of oral contraceptives; use of other hormonal contraceptives; and/or onset of menopause. It is also important to know if a woman already has children or has recently given birth or if there is an unfulfilled desire to have children. Excessive growth of body hair, irregularity in menstrual cycle, and unwanted childlessness are often indicators of hormonal imbalance. These patients need a thorough endocrinological workup with a gynecologist and/or endocrinologist.

The age of the patient is also very important to make the first differential diagnosis. Certain conditions are more common in childhood compared to adulthood. The two most common forms of hair loss in children are tinea capitis and alopecia areata.

Finally, the physician should ask if the patient has tried any treatments for hair loss. The patients will often answer this question by stating that they have already tried everything. Because most medications for hair loss take at least 3 to 4 months to start working, it is crucial to exactly find out what the patient had been taking, how regularly, and for how long. It is also important to know if the patient noticed any effects or side effects from the treatment.

The patient's expectations should be acknowledged and fully explored. Many patients with hair and scalp problems become frustrated when their worries are either ignored or dismissed as insignificant. Explanation and discussion will oftentimes relieve the distress or may even resolve the problem without specific intervention. Occasionally, an underlying depression or dysmorphophobia (pathologically focused fixation on body image) may be present. It is important that these psychological and psychiatric conditions are recognized and carefully addressed and if possible discussed with the patient. Body dysmorphophobic patients are a challenge for every physician. These patients will often question diagnosis, treatment, and treatment results. This can be frustrating for the treating physician. Nonetheless, it is very important to take the patient's concerns seriously, confront the patient with the problem, and carefully lead the patient to an appropriate psychological or psychiatric treatment.

Look and touch

A thorough inspection of the entire scalp is the first step of the clinical examination. The clinical examination should be performed in three steps. First, examine the pattern of density and distribution of hair. Certain patterns are characteristic for certain diseases. Bald patches are seen in alopecia areata and cicatricial alopecia (Figure 1.10). Diffuse thinning and shorter, thinner hair in the front and vertex are characteristic for androgenetic

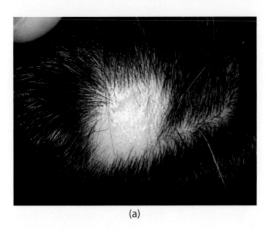

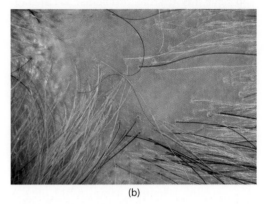

(a)

(b)

Figure 1.10
Presence or absence of follicular ostia is crucial in the differential diagnosis. (a) Follicular ostia in a nonscarring alopecia, such as alopecia areata. (b) Absence of follicular ostia in a scarring alopecia.

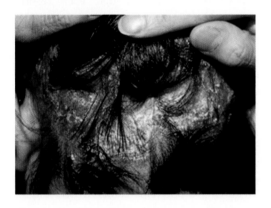

Figure 1.11
Severe scaling and erythema in a patient with lupus erythematosus of the scalp.

alopecia, and diffuse reduction in hair density and thinning in the temporal area are often seen in telogen effluvium. Second, inspect for scales and erythema (Figure 1.11). It is important to determine if the hair loss is associated with signs of inflammation or scarring. Scarring can be caused by trauma or can lead to the diagnosis of primary or secondary cicatricial alopecias. Scaling and dandruff can also be part of cicatricial alopecias or can point to a concomitant scalp disorder like psoriasis, seborrheic dermatitis, or pityriasis amiantacea. Third, use simple methods to determine the activity of hair loss and regrowth.

Pull test

A pull test should be conducted in every hair patient on different areas of the scalp. The patient should always be informed about the test and about the fact that any pulled hair would fall out anyway during that day. Approximately 60 hairs are grasped between the thumb and index and middle fingers from the base of the hair near the scalp and firmly, but not too forcefully, tugged away from the scalp. If more than 5%–10% or three to six hairs are pulled away from the scalp, this constitutes a positive pull test and indicates active hair shedding. Less than three hairs are considered normal physiological shedding. The patient must not shampoo at least 1 day prior to the pull test. The pull test helps to determine the localization and severity of hair loss (Figure 1.12).

Contrast paper

The contrast paper method should be part of every hair examination. A contrast paper (white in patients with dark hair and black in patients with light or white hair) is simply placed vertically against the hair near the scalp. The amount of regrowing hair (tapered tips) and hair breakage (blunt tips) can be easily detected.

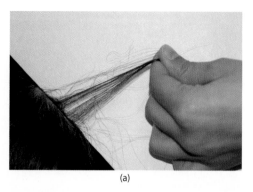
(a)

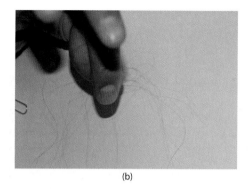
(b)

Figure 1.12
Pull test: (a) approximately 60 hairs are grasped from the proximal portion of the hair shafts at the level of the scalp. The hairs are then tugged from proximal to distal end. (b) The number of hairs extracted is counted. It is normal to pull up to 6/60 (<10%) hairs. More than 6/60 hairs indicates a positive pull test and implies pathology. This is a 57-year-old female with diffuse alopecia areata displaying a positive pull test.

Hair counts

It is normal to lose 100–150 hairs per day. Daily scalp hair counts can sometimes be useful to the physician to help quantify how much the patient is losing. The patient is asked to collect all the hairs shed in 1 day, count them, and place them in plastic sandwich bags. All hairs shed in the shower, sink or brush, counter, or pillow are collected. Shampoo days are labeled separately. The patient is instructed to do this for 7 days. If the patient is losing less than 100 hairs per day, it can be suspected that there is no active shedding. However, the physiological loss of 100–150 hairs per day is only an approximate value. It is impossible for the physician to know how much hair the patient was shedding prior to the onset of the hair problem. Performing a hair count is tedious and time consuming for the patient, but it is something that the patients can do on their own to follow their progress. A hair count should be reserved for exceptional cases, because it can also trigger fears about the hair loss and aggravate a fixation on the hair problem (Figure 1.13).

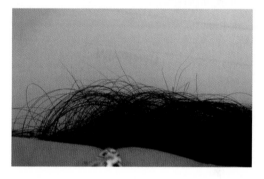

Figure 1.13
A contrast paper positioned at an involved area of the scalp will help determine the length, size, and overall caliber of the hair shafts. This alopecia areata patient showed 1 month of spontaneous regrowth in a bald patch without any treatment.

Bag sign

Sometimes, patients present with a bag of hair to show the physician how much they have lost. This so-called bag sign frequently points to the diagnosis of telogen effluvium. It is important to closely look at the hair and the roots to determine if the hairs are telogen hairs and to ask the patient over how many days the hair has been collected (Figure 1.14).

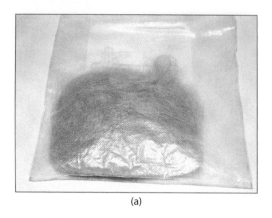

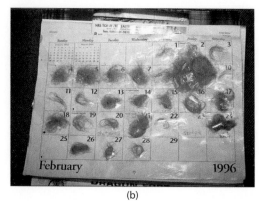

(a)   (b)

Figure 1.14
(a) Patients with telogen effluvium frequently present with bag of hair to show the physician. This is unusual with androgenetic alopecia. (b) A 28-year-old female with telogen effluvium who kept a diary of hair loss for 5 years. This amount of hair loss would not be seen in androgenetic alopecia.

Global photography

Global photography is an essential tool in the everyday hair clinic. It easily allows the physician as well as the patient to assess scalp coverage in general and certain areas of thinning or bald spots.

Standardized or semistandardized scalp pictures should be taken of every hair patient at their first visit or before the start of a new therapy. Disease progression or success of therapy can be tracked when photographs are taken at a later time point [28] (Figure 1.15).

Magnify

The second step of the clinical examination should involve magnifying devices for a better detection of the presence or absence of follicular ostia; the evaluation of signs of inflammation; and the assessment of hair thickness, hair density, and differences in hair caliber.

Dermoscopy

A dermatoscope is used in every dermatological skin examination for the examination of different skin lesions and early detection of melanoma and nonmelanoma skin

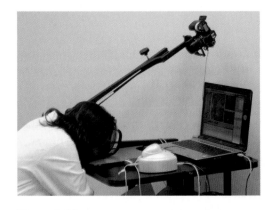

Figure 1.15
Setup for standardized global scalp photography.

cancer. Traditional dermatoscopes consist of a magnifier (typically 10-fold), a nonpolarized light source, a transparent plate, and a liquid medium between the instrument and the skin. This allows inspection of skin lesions unobstructed by skin surface reflections. Modern dermatoscopes dispense with the use of the liquid medium and instead use polarized light to cancel out skin surface reflections. A dermatoscope with polarized light should preferably be used for the examination of the scalp, as the liquid medium of the traditional dermatoscope leaves an oily film on the scalp.

Videodermoscopy

When dermatoscopic images or videos are digitally captured or processed, the instrument can be referred to as a "videodermatoscope." In the past years, this noninvasive technique has revealed novel features of scalp and hair disorders and has become more and more popular for clinical and research use [29,30].

A videomicroscope can be equipped with various objective lenses. The usual working magnifications are 20-fold to 100-fold. All digital images may be stored for further controls. Several reports have shown the usefulness of this technique in diagnosing hair and scalp disorders, such as microsporiasis [31], androgenic alopecia [32], alopecia areata [33,34], lipedematous alopecia [35], pediculosis [36], or inherited hair shaft abnormalities [37,38].

Videodermoscopy in combination with analyzing software allows the determination of hair density and thickness without the need to remove hair for diagnostic purposes. The measurement of thickness and density at the first visit or before the start of a new treatment and at a later time point allows one to track disease progression and therapy success (Figure 1.16). It can be used in a semistandardized way, by marking an area on the scalp, for example, 12 cm from the glabella to the frontal scalp (Figure 1.17). The same area can then be measured again at subsequent visits.

Videodermoscopy also allows in vivo visualization of the epidermal portion of hair follicles and perifollicular epidermis [39,40]. It is useful for the differential diagnosis between cicatricial alopecia and noncicatricial alopecia by visualizing follicular ostia and between alopecia areata (yellow dots) and trichotillomania (broken hairs at different distances from the scalp). In addition, one may study the vascular pattern of the scalp [30].

Dermoscopy and videodermoscopy of hair and scalp are also referred to as trichoscopy.

Phototrichogram

The phototrichogram is a noninvasive method for follow-up diagnostic of hair growth parameters. Saitoh et al. [41] first described this macrophotographic technique for long-term observation of hair growth on different body sites [41]. The term phototrichogram was first used by Bouhanna et al. [42,43]. Phototrichograms are mainly used for the evaluation of scalp hair [44].

The basic principle of the phototrichogram is taking close-up photographs of a certain defined scalp area. Before taking the first photograph, the hair in the area is cut close or short to a defined length (usually 1 mm). To increase the contrast of hair and scalp, the hair has to be dyed with dark hair dye to make vellus hair and light or white hair visible against the background. After certain periods, repeated photographs are taken. Different image analysis techniques allow the determination of hair growth rates, anagen to telogen ratio, scalp coverage, hair density, and vellus to terminal hair ratio.

Several variants of phototrichograms have become popular for evaluating hair in the clinic and in clinical research trials. Modern techniques use automated digital image analysis. Figure 1.18 shows an example of the TrichoScan® technique. Depending on the type of image analysis, the following parameters can be determined:

1. Total number of hairs per area (hairs/cm^2)
2. Vellus to terminal hair ratio
3. Anagen to telogen ratio
4. Linear hair growth rate (millimeters per day) (measured by the change in length of renewable hair on the subsequent picture)
5. Hair thickness

The phototrichogram, especially when combined with automated digital image analysis, is a reliable, reproducible, noninvasive technique. It can be used to support

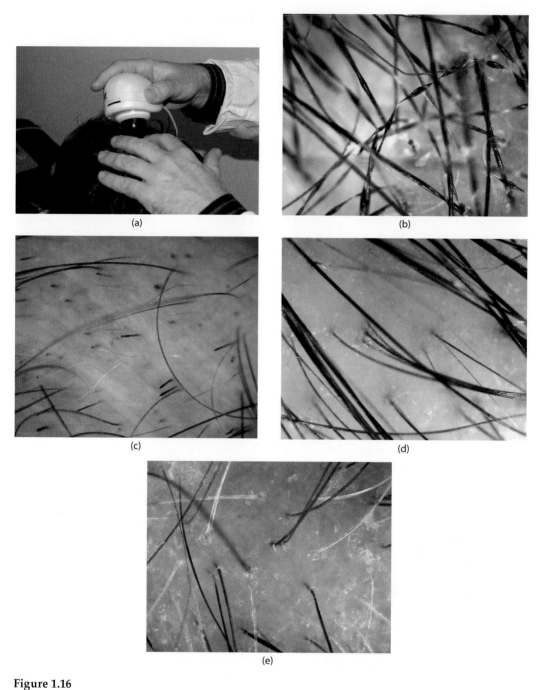

Figure 1.16
(a) Videodermoscope (Folliscope®); (b) monilethrix characteristic strands of hair with a beaded appearance; (c) exclamation point hair in alopecia areata; (d) differences in hair shaft caliber in androgenetic alopecia; (e) early cicatricial alopecia with mild follicular hyperkeratosis.

the diagnosis. Early changes in androgenetic alopecia can be detected well. It can also be used to track disease progression and success of therapy and is therefore frequently used in clinical trials (Figure 1.18).

However, most hair patients are concerned about the clipped, bald area on the scalp. Automated techniques are usually not suitable for dark skin types because of the lack of contrast. Patients with allergies to hair dye are excluded from this technique.

Sample

If the diagnosis is in doubt or the physician finds signs of inflammation and scarring, it becomes necessary to take hair and/or skin samples.

Light-microscopic examination

Hairs extracted by slow pull can be examined under a light microscope. Hair shafts are mounted in parallel between two glass

Folliscope® – HAIR DENSITY AND THICKNESS IN WOMEN

DATE _____

PATIENT _____

Measurements	Hair/cm²	Hair thickness in µm
1.		
2.		
3.		
Mean		

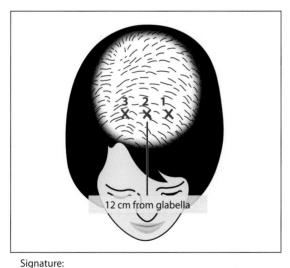

12 cm from glabella

Signature:

(a)

Figure 1.17
Documentation sheets for videodermoscopy: (a) for women.   (*Continued*)

Folliscope® – HAIR DENSITY AND THICKNESS IN MEN

DATE _____

PATIENT _____

Measurements	Hair/cm²	Hair thickness in μm
1.		
2.		
3.		
Mean		

Measurements	Hair/cm²	Hair thickness in μm
4.		
5.		
6.		
Mean		

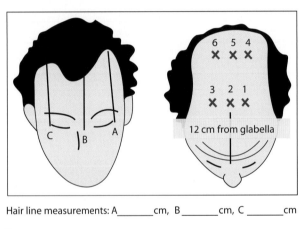

Hair line measurements: A_____cm, B_____cm, C_____cm

Signature:

(b)

Figure 1.17 (Continued)
Documentation sheets for videodermoscopy: (b) for men.

slides taped together. A drop of cyanoacrylate glue placed on the slide will give greater contrast under the microscope compared to dry mount. Roots should be examined to determine the stage of the hair cycle and for the presence of dystrophy. Hair shaft abnormalities (which can increase hair fragility and cause hair loss) can be diagnosed with this method. The hair shafts need to be examined to detect fractures, irregularities in coiling and twisting, and extraneous matter (Figure 1.19). The free ends of the hair should be checked to see whether they are tapered, cut, fractured, or weathered. If fungal diseases are suspected, hairs should be placed on a glass slide with 20% potassium hydroxide added to demonstrate fungal spores and hyphae.

Trichogram

A trichogram is the traditional method for the morphological, microscopic examination

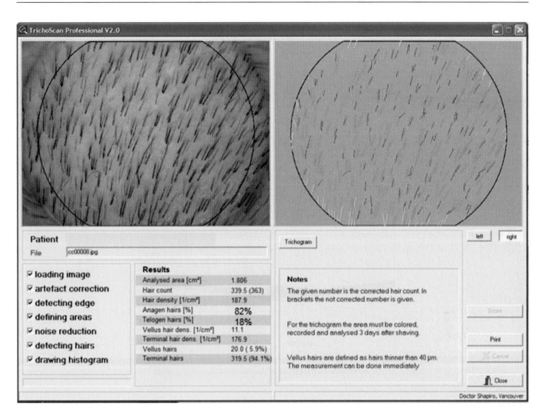

Figure 1.18
Phototrichogram (TrichoScan).

of hair roots. It was first developed by van Scott in 1957 [45], and the term "trichogram" was first used by Pecoraro in 1964 [46]. The trichogram quantifies hair follicles in their different growth phases and allows the examination of shaft diameter, root patterns, and anagen to telogen rate [47].

In general, the technique involves the examination of two different scalp areas. If androgenetic alopecia or telogen effluvium is the tentative diagnosis, hair is plugged from the frontoparietal and occipital scalp. If alopecia areata of traction alopecia is suspected, the hair is plugged from an active area and an inactive area [48,49]. The hair should not be washed and should only be combed gently 5 days prior to epilation to avoid premature plugging of telogen hairs.

Using a rubber-coated medical clamp, 50–70 hairs are plucked at two specific scalp locations depending on the hair disorder. The instrument is closed tightly over the hairs close to the scalp surface. Then, the hairs are plugged with one quick, forceful pull in the direction of hair growth. For optimal evaluation results, hair bulbs are immediately embedded with their roots on a glass slide in an embedding medium, which allows microscopic evaluation later. If mounted on a glass slide in water or on adhesive tape, the trichogram must be examined immediately by microscopy. The microscopic evaluation is done by low-power microscopy (not more than 40-fold magnification). The following types of hair roots can be distinguished:

1. Normal anagen hair
2. Dysplastic hair (anagen hair without a root sheath)
3. Catagen hair

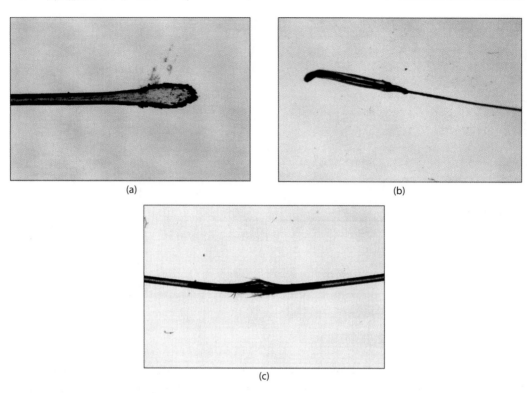

Figure 1.19
Light-microscopic examination of hairs: (a) telogen hair with characteristic club; (b) anagen hair with inner root sheath; (c) hair shaft abnormality—trichorrhexis nodosa secondary to trauma. (Courtesy of Dr. David Shum.)

4.   Telogen hair
5.   Dystrophic hair (hair with a tapered proximal end instead of a real root)
6.   Broken hair (with a sharp horizontal proximal end)

Normal values for adult scalp hair are >80% for anagen hair, <20% for telogen hair, <5% for dystrophic hair, <3% for catagen hair, and <10% for broken hair.

An increase in dysplastic hair can be found in children with loose anagen syndrome and when the hair is plugged too slowly. An increase in telogen hair in both the frontoparietal and occipital areas is found in an active diffuse telogen effluvium. If the increase of telogen hair is higher in the frontoparietal area in combination with variation in hair shaft diameter, androgenetic alopecia

can be suspected. An increase in dystrophic hair may indicate a stronger toxic agent such as thallium, cytotoxic drugs, or high doses of vitamin A-acid, or can be found in active alopecia areata.

Unit Area Trichogram

The unit area trichogram is an advanced trichogram technique that was developed mainly for clinical trials [46]. The unit area trichogram is based on plucking hair in a defined area (usually >30 mm^2) and allows the determination of hair density (Figure 1.20).

Because anagen to telogen ratio, hair density, and thickness can be easily determined by videodermoscopy and phototrichogram, trichograms should be reserved for special cases like loose anagen syndrome or diffuse

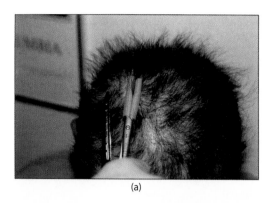

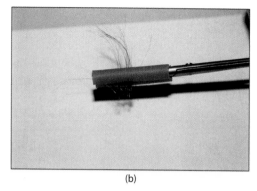

(a)   (b)

Figure 1.20

The trichogram/pluck test is another method of assessing hair loss. On the fifth day after the last shampoo, hairs are taken from specified sites. (a) The surrounding hair is fixed with clips, and 60–80 hairs are grasped with a hemostat covered with rubber and plucked, twisting and lifting the hair shafts rapidly in the direction of emergence from the scalp. (b) Anagen hairs are distinguished from telogen hairs, and anagen to telogen ratios are calculated.

alopecia areata. The hair plucking causes discomfort to the patient and leaves a small bald patch that can last for weeks. Moreover, many patients find it unpleasant not to shampoo for 5 days.

Biopsy

A scalp biopsy is the ultimate tool for diagnosis of hair and scalp disorders. Scalp biopsies are indicated in all cases of cicatrizing alopecias and in all cases of unexplained non-cicatrizing alopecias [50]. It involves, following local anesthesia, removal of one or two small 4-mm punches down to the level of subcutaneous fat to remove the entire follicular unit; the skin is subsequently sutured (Figure 1.21). Horizontally cut punches can be examined for number of hair follicles, follicular units, hair diameter, integrity of sebaceous glands, and growth parameters (terminal to vellus hair ratio, anagen to telogen ratio, and catagen hair) [51]. A punch biopsy can be trisected at two levels, and subsequently horizontal sections are read from the base of the follicle to the papillary dermis.

Normally, a 4-mm punch of the scalp has 35–40 hairs at the upper level in the papillary dermis. At the level of the reticular dermis near the base of the infundibulum, the number is reduced to 35; at deeper levels near subcutaneous fat, the numbers are even lower, at around 30. The upper levels contain telogen and anagen terminal hair, as well as vellus and vellus-like miniaturized hairs. The mid-level consists of telogen and anagen terminal hairs. The deeper levels contain anagen terminal hair, as only the roots of thick anagen follicles reach down to the subcutaneous fat. The difference between the upper levels and the mid-levels is usually the number of vellus or vellus-like hairs. The difference between the mid-levels and the lower levels is the number of terminal telogen hairs. Anagen to telogen hair ratios as well as terminal to vellus ratios and the total number of hairs per square centimeter can easily be calculated on the bases of the aforementioned factors and the morphology of the follicles. The presence, type, and localization (peri-, intra-, or interfollicular) of inflammatory cells can also be detected at all levels of the biopsy.

For cicatrizing alopecias, the following recommendations were developed at a consensus meeting in February 2001 [52]: One 4-mm punch biopsy including subcutaneous tissue should be taken from a clinically active area, processed for horizontal sections, and stained with hematoxylin and eosin. Elastin (acid alcoholic orcein), mucin, and PAS stains may provide additional diagnosis-defining information. A second 4-mm punch biopsy

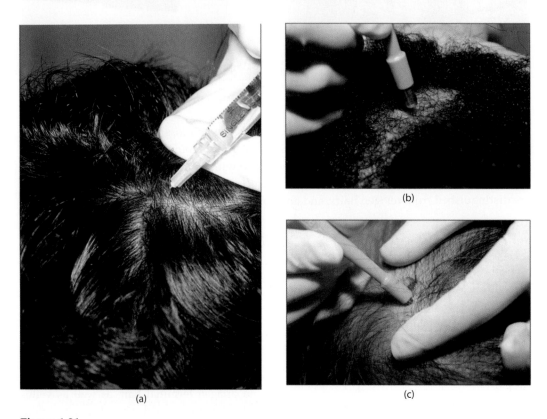

(a)

(b)

(c)

Figure 1.21

How to perform a scalp biopsy. (a) To obtain sufficient histopathologic information, the scalp biopsy should be taken from an active inflammatory area containing hair follicles or active hair destruction. In noninflammatory conditions, a biopsy in a representative area is sufficient. If possible, the biopsy should be taken from a cosmetically less-apparent area of the scalp. Staying away from hair parts or the frontal portion of the scalp is recommended. The area to be biopsied is marked with a red China marker. For local anesthesia, lidocaine 1% with epinephrine in a concentration of 1:100,000 is injected with a 30-gauge needle into the scalp. Epinephrine causes vasoconstriction, which has a hemostatic effect in a highly vascular site such as the scalp. In addition, a mandatory waiting period of at least 10 minutes is suggested following the anesthetic injection. This allows the vasoconstrictive effect of epinephrine to take effect and maximize the hemostasis. (b) A 4.0-mm punch biopsy is placed parallel to follow the direction of the hair. In patients who have curly hair as in the figure, insert the punch perpendicular to the scalp. (c) Direct vertical pressure is applied along with the rotation of the punch. Penetration of the punch to a depth of approximately 3.5–4.0 mm is sufficient to obtain a full scalp thickness. The typical punch should be pushed right through to the hub.

(Continued)

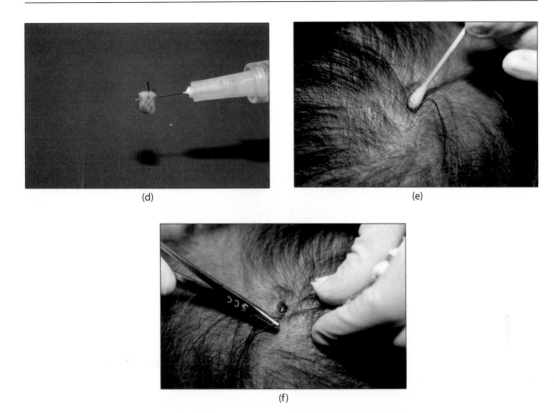

(d)

(e)

(f)

Figure 1.21 (*Continued*)
(d) The same needle for the anesthesia can be used to hook the tissue beneath the hair bulbs.
(e) Aluminum chloride 20% solution on a Q-tip can be used for hemostasis after the biopsy
has been removed. (f) The biopsy defect is closed with a blue-colored monofilament suture,
which helps to identify the suture on the hairy scalp, particularly with pigmented hairs.
The suture needle is passed through the upper dermis, preventing damage to the hair bulbs
located in the deep dermis. Wound dressings are not necessary for the scalp.

from a clinically active disease-affected area should be cut vertically into two equal pieces. One half provides tissue for transversely cut routine histological sections, and the other half can be used for direct immunofluorescence studies [50,52]. The characteristic histologic features of the most common non-cicatrizing and cicatrizing alopecias are discussed in subsequent chapters.

Biopsies are an excellent tool for the diagnosis of hair and scalp disorders (Figure 1.22), but they are difficult to reproduce because the one area of interest has been removed; therefore, they are less suitable for the evaluation of therapy success and disease progression. However, in cicatricial alopecia, subsequent biopsies may be useful to document burnt out stages. A scalp biopsy is an invasive technique and results in discomfort for the patient and leaves a small scar. The horizontal preparation and evaluation of the punch biopsy requires an experienced pathology technician and dermatopathologist.

Laboratory tests

Laboratory tests should be performed in every patient with hair loss. Every patient should be checked for iron deficiency and thyroid dysfunction. Especially in patients

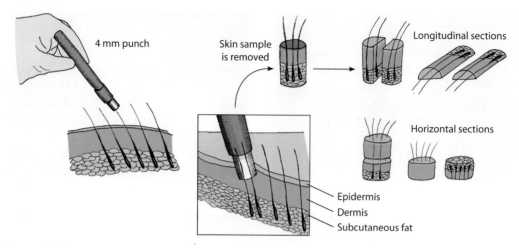

Figure 1.22
Scalp biopsy and horizontal sectioning.

with telogen effluvium, it is important to find out underlying causes. Low serum ferritin levels (<70 ng/mL) can indicate a lack of iron storage and can be the cause or aggravating factor for hair loss. Thyroid dysfunctions are often seen in patients with telogen effluvium, most frequently hypothyroidism; slight fatigue and mild depression are often the only symptoms along with hair loss. Hashimoto thyroiditis is often accompanied by alopecia areata. A thyroid-stimulating hormone level should be investigated. Vitamin D deficiency can also be associated with hair loss. Furthermore, the patient can be checked for low vitamin B12, selenium, and zinc levels as aggravating factors.

In women with androgenetic alopecia who complain about irregular menses, hirsutism, acne, and the inability to have children, levels of free testosterone and dehydroepiandrosterone sulfate (DHEA-S) should be determined to rule out hyperandrogenism. Additionally, women with the aforementioned complaints should be sent to an endocrinologist and/or gynecologist for further workup. In cases of confirmed scarring alopecia due to discoid lupus erythematosus, an antinuclear antibodies examination is necessary.

Differential diagnosis of nonscarring versus scarring alopecias

In noncicatricial alopecias, there is preservation of follicles on clinical and histological examination, although they can sometimes be difficult to appreciate when miniaturized. The three most common forms of noncicatrizing alopecias are androgenetic alopecia, telogen effluvium, and alopecia areata. Table 1.1 compares the key clinical features that distinguish these three conditions from each other. Each condition is discussed separately in Chapters 2, 3, and 5.

Cicatricial alopecias result in the destruction of hair follicles and the loss of regrowth potential. Scarring of localized areas of the scalp may result from trauma; burns; or fungal, viral, or bacterial infections. The destruction of the follicles in these cases

Table 1.1
Common nonscarring alopecias

	Androgenetic alopecia	Telogen effluvium	Alopecia areata
Hair loss distribution	Focal balding pattern: Norwood–Hamilton (men) Ludwig (women)	Generalized	Usually patchy, but can be generalized
Course	Gradual onset with progression	Onset abrupt/trigger factor	Onset abrupt; often waxes and wanes with relapses
Appearance	Thinning with or without bare patches. Bare patches are gradual, not abrupt	Thinning with no bare patches	Thinning with abrupt bare patches; exclamation mark hairs
Shedding	Minimal	Prominent	Prominent
Age onset	Onset at puberty or older	Onset at any age, but usually not childhood	Onset at any age; majority have their first patch before the age of 20
Pull test	Usually negative	Positive; telogen hairs	Positive; dystrophic anagen and telogen hairs

Table 1.2
Differential diagnosis

Hair coming out by roots	Hair breaking
• Telogen effluvium	• Tinea capitis
• Androgenetic alopecia	• Structural hair shaft abnormalities
• Alopecia areata	• Breakage due to improper use of hair care cosmetics
• Drugs (anagen or telogen effluvium)	• Anagen arrest

Table 1.3
Causes of alopecia

Noncicatricial	Cicatricial
• Androgenetic alopecia	• Discoid lupus erythematosus
• Telogen effluvium	• Lichen planopilaris
• Alopecia areata	• Severe fungal, viral, or bacterial infection
• Traction alopecia	• Injury or burn

is a secondary, nonfollicular process that eventually encroaches on the follicle and ultimately destroys it.

In primary cicatricial alopecia, the hair follicle is the prime target of destruction. The most common causes of cicatricial alopecia are lichen planopilaris and discoid lupus erythematosus. A biopsy is necessary to establish the acute diagnosis. Evidence of cutaneous disease elsewhere on the body, oral or genital mucous membranes, and nails should be looked at carefully. Scarring alopecias are considered true trichologic emergencies, as they result in irreversible hair loss. The importance of prompt and appropriate therapy is crucial. Diagnosis and management of the most common cicatricial alopecias are discussed in Chapter 6 and Tables 1.2 and 1.3.

Conclusion

Most hair and scalp disorders can easily be diagnosed in the physician's office through the recognition of the characteristic differential features of each disorder. The first task of the physician is to acknowledge the patient's concerns and have an empathetic approach to the hair loss problem. The diagnosis depends on a combination of findings obtained from meticulous history, a thorough scalp examination, and any necessary investigation. An organized approach will help to quickly find the correct diagnoses and direct the patient to appropriate management and therapy.

REFERENCES

1. Tobin DJ, The biogenesis and growth of human hair. In *Hair in Toxicology—An Important Bio-Monitor*, Tobin DJ, Editor. 2005. Cambridge: RSC Publishing.
2. Szabo G, The regional frequency and distribution of follicles in human skin. In *The Biology of Hair Growth*, Montagna W and Ellis RA, Editors. 1958. New York: Academic Press, Inc. p. 33–8.
3. Whiting DA, Diagnostic and predictive value of horizontal sections of scalp biopsy specimens in male pattern androgenetic alopecia. *J Am Acad Dermatol*, 1993. **28**: 755–63.
4. Aslani FS, Dastgheib L, and Banihashemi BM, Hair counts in scalp biopsy of males and females with androgenetic alopecia compared with normal subjects. *J Cutan Pathol*, 2009. **36**(7): 734–9.
5. Templeton SF, Santa Cruz DJ, and Solomon AR, Alopecia: Histologic diagnosis by transverse sections. *Semin Diagn Pathol*, 1996. **13**: 2–18.
6. Sperling LC, Hair density in African Americans. *Arch Dermatol*, 1999. **135**: 656–8.
7. Lee HJ, et al., Hair counts from scalp biopsy specimens in Asians. *J Am Acad Dermatol*, 2002. **46**(2): 218–21.
8. Hutchinson PE and Thompson JR, The cross-sectional size and shape of human terminal scalp hair. *Br J Dermatol*, 1997. **136**(2): 159–65.
9. Gray J, *Human Hair Diversity*. Vol. 1. 2000. Oxford: Blackwell Science.
10. Hrdy D, Quantitative hair form variation in several populations. *Am J Phys Anthropol*, 1973. **39**: 7–8.
11. Steggerda M and Seiber HC, Size and shape of head hairs from six racial groups. *J Hered*, 1942. **32**: 315–8.
12. Wilborn WS, Disorders of hair growth in African Americans. In *Disorders of Hair Growth—Diagnosis and Treatment*, Olsen EA, Editor. 2003, Barcelona: McGraw-Hill. p. 497–517.
13. Lindelöf B, et al., Human hair form: Morphology revealed by light and scanning electron microscopy and computer-aided three-dimensional reconstruction. *Arch Dermatol*, 1988. **124**(9): 1359–63.
14. Kligman AM, The human hair cycle. *J Invest Dermatol*, 1959. Dec;**33**: 307–16.
15. Courtois M et al., Periodicity in the growth and shedding of hair. *Br J Dermatol*, 1996. Jan;**134**(1): 47–54.
16. Randall VA and Ebling FJ, Seasonal changes in human hair growth. *Br J Dermatol*, 1991. **12**(2): 146–51.
17. Otberg N et al., Variations of hair follicle size and distribution in different body sites. *J Invest Dermatol*, 2004. Jan;**122**(1): 14–9.
18. Ito S, Ozeki H, and Wakamatsu K, Spectrophotometric and HPLC characterization of hair melanins. In *Melanogenesis and Malignant Melanoma: Biochemistry, Cell Biology, Molecular Biology, Pathophysiology, Diagnosis and Treatment*, K Hori, VJ Hearing, and J Nakayama, Editors. 2000, Oxford: Oxford University Press. p. 63–72.
19. Rees JL, Genetics of hair and skin color. *Annu Rev Genet*, 2003. **37**: 67–90. Review.
20. Nordlund JJ et al., *The Pigmentary System: Physiology and Pathophysiology*. 1998. New York: Oxford University Press.
21. Wakamatsu K and Ito S, Advanced chemical methods in melanin determination. *Pigment Cell Res*, 2002. **15**: 174–83.
22. Wakamatsu K, Ito S, and Rees JL, Usefulness of 4-amino-3-hydroxyphenylalanine as a specific marker of pheomelanin. *Pigment Cell Res*, 2002. **15**: 225–32.

23. Tobin DJ, *Pigmentation of Human Hair, in Hair in Toxicology—An Important Bio-Monitor*, Tobin DJ, Editor. 2005. Cambridge: RSC Publishing.

24. Oyehaug L et al., The regulatory basis of melanogenic switching. *J Theor Biol*, 2002. **215**(4): 449–68.

25. Inazu M and Mishima Y, Detection of eumelanogenic and pheomelanogenic melanosomes in the same normal human melanocyte. *J Invest Dermatol*, 1993. **100**(2 Suppl): 172S–5S.

26. Rochat A, Kobayashi K, and Barrandon Y, Location of stem cells of human hair follicles by clonal analysis. *Cell*, 1994. **76**(6): 1063–73.

27. Canfield D, Photographic documentation of hair growth in androgenetic alopecia. *Dermatol Clin*, 1996. **14**(4): 713–21.

28. Tosti A and Gray J, Assessment of hair and scalp disorders. *J Investig Dermatol Symp Proc*, 2007. **12**(2): 23–7.

29. Ross EK, Vincenzi C, and Tosti A, Videodermoscopy in the evaluation of hair and scalp disorders. *J Am Acad Dermatol*, 2006. **55**(5): 799–806.

30. Slowinska M et al., Comma hairs: A dermatoscopic marker for tinea capitis. A rapid diagnostic method. *J Am Acad Dermatol*, 2008. **59**(5 Suppl): S77–9.

31. Olszewska M and Rudnicka L, Effective treatment of female androgenic alopecia with dutasteride. *J Drugs Dermatol*, 2005. **4**: 637–40.

32. Inui S, Nakajima T, and Itami S, Dry dermoscopy in clinical treatment of alopecia areata. *J Dermatol*, 2007. **34**: 635–9.

33. Tosti A et al., The role of scalp dermoscopy in the diagnosis of alopecia areata incognita. *J Am Acad Dermatol*, 2008. **59**: 64–7.

34. Piraccini BM et al., Lipedematous alopecia of the scalp. *Dermatol Online J*, 2006. **12**: 6.

35. Di Stefani A, Hofmann-Wellenhof R, and Zalaudek I, Dermoscopy for diagnosis and treatment monitoring of pediculosis capitis. *J Am Acad Dermatol*, 2006. **54**: 909–11.

36. Rakowska A et al., Dermoscopy as a tool for rapid diagnosis of monilethrix. *J Drugs Dermatol*, 2007. **6**: 222–4.

37. Rakowska A et al., Trichoscopy in genetic hair shaft abnormalities. *J Dermatol Case Rep*, 2008. **2**: 14–20.

38. Lacarrubba F et al., Videodermatoscopy enhances diagnostic capability in some forms of hair loss. *Am J Clin Dermatol*, 2004. **5**: 205–8.

39. Ross EK, Vincenzi C, and Tosti A, Videodermoscopy in the evaluation of hair and scalp disorders. *J Am Acad Dermatol*, 2006. **55**: 799–806.

40. Saitoh M, Uzuka M, and Sakamoto M, Human hair cycle. *J Invest Dermatol*, 1970. **54**(1): 65–81.

41. Bouhanna P, The tractiophototrichogram, an objective method for evaluating hair loss. *Ann Dermatol Venereol*, 1988. **115**(6–7): 759–64.

42. Bouhanna P, The phototrichogram, a macrophotographic study of the scalp. *Bioengineer Skin*, 1985. **3**: 265.

43. Friedel J, Will F, and Grosshans E, Phototrichogram: Adaptation, standardization and applications. *Ann Dermatol Venereol*, 1989. **116**(9): 629–36.

44. Van Scott EJ, Reinertson RP, and Steinmuller R, The growing hair roots of the human scalp and morphologic changes therein following amethopterin therapy. *J Invest Dermatol*, 1957. **29**(3): 197–204.

45. Pecoraro V et al., The normal trichogram in the child before the age of puberty. *J Invest Dermatol*, 1964. **42**: 427–30.

46. Blume-Peytavi U and Orfanos CE, Microscopy of the hair—The trichogram. In *Handbook of Non-Invasive Methods and the Skin*. 2 ed. Serup J et al., Editors. 2006. Boca Raton: CRC Press. p. 875–81.

47. Blume-Peytavi U and Orfanos CE, Microscopy of the hair. In *Non-Invasive Methods and the Skin*. Vol. 1. Serup J and Jemec GBE, Editors. 1995. Ann Arbor: CRP Press. p. 549–54.

48. Maguire HC and Kligman AM, Hair plucking as a diagnostic tool. *J Invest Dermatol*, 1964. **43**: 77–9.

49. Olsen EA et al., Summary of North American Hair Research Society (NAHRS)-sponsored Workshop on Cicatricial Alopecia, Duke University Medical Center. Workshop on Cicatricial Alopecia. *J Am Acad Dermatol*, 2003. **48**(1): 103–10.

50. Whiting DA, Diagnostic and predictive value of horizontal sections of scalp biopsy specimens in male pattern androgenetic alopecia. *J Am Acad Dermatol*, 1993. **28**(5 Pt 1): 755–63.

51. Olsen EA et al., Summary of North American Hair Research Society (NAHRS)-sponsored Workshop on Cicatricial Alopecia, Duke University Medical Center, February 10 and 11, 2001. *J Am Acad Dermatol*, 2003. **48**(1): 103–10.

52. Olsen EA, Disorders of hair growth: Diagnosis and treatment. In *Cicatricial Alopecia*. 2 ed. Bergfeld WF, Editor. 2003. New York: McGraw-Hill Companies. p. 363–98.

2 Pattern hair loss: Pathogenesis, clinical features, diagnosis, and management

Androgenetic alopecia (AGA) or pattern hair loss is by far the most common form of alopecia in men and women. The development and occurrence of AGA depends on genetic predisposition and an interaction of endocrine factors [1]. Although it is a medically benign condition, it can have a significant psychosocial impact for patients. Hair plays an important role in human social and sexual communication. Patients with visible hair loss are perceived as older and less physically and socially attractive [1–12]. Although AGA can be seen as a physiological process, millions of dollars are spent every year on hair restoration products [13].

Hair has been of social and psychological importance throughout the centuries. A 4000-year-old Egyptian papyrus states that ancient Egyptians were afraid of losing their hair and contains recipes for different formulations for the treatment of hair loss [13,14]. The first medical description of AGA goes back to the ancient Greek physician Aristotle (384–322 BC). He recognized that baldness does not occur in eunuchs or before sexual maturity and drew the conclusion that libido and the degree of hair loss are related [15].

The modern understanding of AGA started with the studies of Hamilton in 1942, who established that pattern hair loss is a physiological process induced in genetically predisposed hair follicles under the influence of androgens [16]. Animal studies by Montagna and Uno confirmed Hamilton's findings in 1968 [17].

This chapter highlights the pathogenesis, clinical features, and state-of-the-art medical management of male pattern hair loss (MPHL) and female pattern hair loss (FPHL).

Pathogenesis

Changes in hair cycle in androgenetic alopecia

Knowledge of the pathophysiology of AGA is essential in understanding the mechanism of action of current therapeutic agents. The following is a summary of the current knowledge on AGA pathogenesis.

AGA involves both genetic and hormonal factors [1]. Different gene loci have been linked to the development of AGA in past years. Genetics determines both the density and the location of androgen-sensitive hair follicles on site-specific areas of the scalp. After puberty, androgens trigger a series of events within these genetically programmed hair follicles, predominantly in the frontoparietal scalp, that transform terminal to miniaturized follicles [18–27]. The progression of patterned hair loss is the result of a gradual transformation of pigmented, thick scalp hair (terminal hair) into fine colorless, almost invisible vellus-like hair follicles [28].

A normal hair cycle for scalp hair involves a long growing period (anagen) with an average length of 2–6 years, a short transitory period of approximately 2–3 weeks (catagen), and a resting period (telogen) of around 12 weeks [29]. A normal anagen to telogen ratio for the scalp hair is 9:1, although seasonal variations can be found [30,31].

In AGA, hair cycle dynamics change. With each passage through the hair cycle, the duration of the anagen phase decreases. Because the duration of the anagen phase is the main determination of hair length, the maximum length of the new anagen hair is shorter than that of its predecessor [31]. The proportion of telogen hair increases, which can already be seen before balding becomes visible. With every hair cycle, the affected follicle produces a thinner, finer hair [32,33]. These finer, small, vellus-like hairs of varying lengths and diameters are the hallmark of AGA (Figure 2.1). Moreover, the time between shedding of the hair and anagen regrowth becomes longer, leading to a reduction of present hair on the scalp [34].

Genetics

The development of AGA shows a strong genetic involvement. The risk of AGA increases significantly with a positive family history [35]. Bergfeld and Carey et al. suggested an autosomal dominant inheritance [36,37]. However, Kuester and Happle had already presented in 1984 that a polygenic inheritance of the trait is far more likely [38]. A variation of the *CYP17* gene on chromosome 10q24.3 was suggested to be responsible for the development of polycystic ovary syndrome and female pattern hair loss [37,39].

The expression of insulin-like growth factor (IGF)-1 in the dermal papilla is discussed to play an important role in the development of

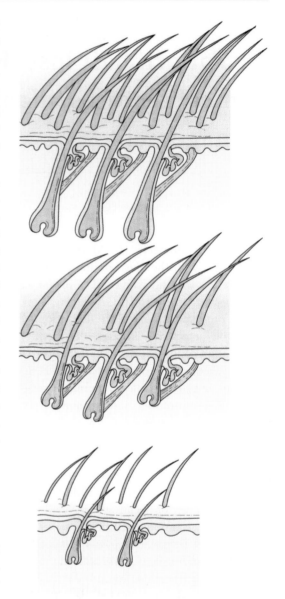

Figure 2.1
In androgenetic alopecia, there is miniaturization of coarse terminal hairs into small vellus-like hairs with each subsequent cycle.

pattern balding. Older men with vertex balding showed higher plasma levels of IGF-1 and lower circulating levels of IGF binding protein 3. A decreased expression of IGF-1 was found in the balding scalp tissue. The gene locus for IGF-1 can be found on chromosome 12 (12q22-q23) [40,41].

The observation that patients with pseudohermaphroditism who showed a 5α-reductase-2 deficiency did not develop MPHL presumed an involvement of the genes *SRD5A1* on chromosome 5 and *SRD5A2* on chromosome 2. Ellis et al. conducted genetic association studies of the 5α-reductase enzyme gene and its two isoenzymes in balding and nonbalding men. The results showed no association of the 5α-reductase isoenzymes with male pattern baldness [42,43].

Garton et al. reported a possible association of a polymorphism in the ornithine decarboxylase gene in 2005. Ornithine decarboxylase is a regulatory enzyme in polyamine biosynthesis and is known to play an important role in the regulation of the hair cycle. In humans, there are two functionally distinct alleles of ornithine decarboxylase [44,45]. Konig et al. [46] found that an X-linked adrenoleukodystrophy mutation can be taken into consideration as gene locus within the polygenic spectrum of genes responsible for AGA. More recently, it was shown that 20p11 confers risk for AGA and that a specific genetic locus, chromosome 17q21.31, which is associated with Parkinson's disease, is also a susceptibility locus for early-onset AGA [47–49].

Androgen response is attenuated by the androgen receptor. Therefore, it was suggested that a polymorphism in the androgen receptor gene may be responsible for the development and extent of AGA. The androgen receptor gene is located at band q12 in the X chromosome. In the balding scalp, a higher expression of the androgen receptor gene was found [19,24]. Ellis et al. [50] found that a functional mutation in or near the androgen receptor may explain these higher levels of gene expression in the balding scalp. Hillmer et al. [51] demonstrated that genetic variability in the androgen receptor gene is the cardinal prerequisite for the development of early-onset AGA.

The involvement of the X chromosome in the development of AGA stresses the importance of the maternal line in the inheritance. However, several other autosomal gene loci are associated with the development of AGA.

Hormonal factors

The first recognition of a correlation between MPHL and male hormones goes back to the fourth century BC, when Aristotle observed that baldness does not occur in eunuchs. More than 2000 years later, Hamilton demonstrated the role of androgens on hair growth and on the development of male pattern baldness. He observed that baldness did not develop in 10 eunuchoids, 10 men castrated at puberty, and 34 men castrated during adolescence. After the administration of testosterone, baldness developed in predisposed individuals. When testosterone was discontinued, the baldness did not progress, although it did not reverse [52].

Another interesting finding was that castration before puberty prevented the development of a beard, whereas between 16 and 20 years of age it partly prevented the full development of the beard and after 20 years it had no effect on beard development [53]. However, neither a correlation between baldness and testosterone levels nor a correlation between libido and testosterone levels could be found [54]. An Australian study, investigating 1390 men aged 40–69, showed that the average ejaculation frequency did not differ between men with and without different grades of AGA [55].

The skin is an endocrine target tissue for androgen hormone action, similar to the ovaries, testes, and adrenal glands [56]. The circulating androgens dehydroepiandrosterone sulfate (DHEA-S) and androstenedione are predominantly produced in the adrenal glands, and testosterone and 5α-dihydrotestosterone are mainly synthesized in the gonads [57]. DHEA-S and androstenedione have a relatively weak androgen potential. They can be metabolized to more potent androgens such as testosterone and DHT.

Basically, six enzymes are involved in androgen metabolism in the skin: (1) steroid sulfatase, (2) 3β-hydroxysteroid dehydrogenase/Δ5-4-isomerase (Δ5-3βHSD), (3) 17β-hydroxysteroid dehydrogenase (17βHSD), (4) 5α-reductase, (5) 3α-hydroxysteroid dehydrogenase (3αHSD), and (6) aromatase. Steroid sulfatase metabolizes DHEA-S to dehydroepiandrosterone (DHEA). Isoenzyme 1 of Δ5-3βHSD converts DHEA to androstenedione in human skin [58]. Androstenedione can be activated by 17βHSD to testosterone. Eight isoforms of 17βHSD are known [59]. In hair follicles, 17βHSD is found in the outer root sheath cells. Anagen hair mainly expresses high levels of isotype 2, leading to an inactivation of potent sex steroids and moderate levels of isotype 1, which supports the formation of active androgens [60].

5α-Reductase seems to play the key role in AGA. Two isoenzymes of 5α-reductase are found in dermal papilla cells of beard and scalp follicles [61,62]. In the balding scalp a predominance of 5α-reductase isotype 1 over isotype 2 can be found, whereas in the prostate the two enzymes are present in equal proportions [63]. 5α-Reductase irreversibly converts testosterone to DHT, the most potent naturally occurring androgen in the skin [64].

3αHSD exists in three isoforms. It catabolizes active androgens to compounds that do not bind the intercellular androgen receptor [57]. Finally, aromatase can convert testosterone and androstenedione to estradiol and estrone [56]. Aromatase is localized in the inner and outer root sheaths as well as in the sebaceous gland and may play a "detoxifying" role by removing excess androgens [59]. It has been shown that the concentration of aromatase is five times higher in female scalp skin compared to male scalp skin. These findings could explain the differences in male and female patterns of balding and the sparing of the frontal hairline.

All enzymes can be localized in the sebaceous glands and different parts of the hair follicle of scalp skin [65,66]. Therefore, the pilosebaceous unit has the potential to mediate androgen action without relying on elevated systemic levels or production of testosterone or DHT [67–69].

Androgen activation and deactivation are mainly intercellular events. Their effects are mediated by binding to a single nuclear receptor, the androgen receptor. The androgen receptor, as a polymeric complex that includes the heat shock proteins hsp90, hsp70, and hsp56, is initially located in the cytoplasm [57,70].

Complex enzyme mechanisms such as phosphorylation and sulfhydryl reduction of the androgen receptor are necessary for the activation of the ligand–receptor complex. The androgen–androgen receptor complex is now transported into the nucleus and ligates to promoter DNA sequences of androgen-regulated genes [57]. The following signaling cascade can lead to either an inhibition or a stimulation of messenger proteins or receptors. These messengers again alter cellular processes mediating hair growth or miniaturization [56,71–75].

Role of androgens in female pattern hair loss

The role of androgen hypersecretion, in situ enzyme activity, and androgen receptors in FPHL is still not completely understood. Androgens in women come from three different sources: (1) adrenal gland, usually as a by-product of cortisol biosynthesis (zona fasciculate) and not from zona reticularis, because these cells seem to mature during puberty [76]; (2) ovaries; and (3) peripheral compartment. The skin and especially the pilosebaceous unit, composed of the sebaceous gland and hair follicle, can synthesize androgens either de novo from cholesterol or by local conversion of circulating weaker androgens to more potent ones [59].

Sex hormone–binding globulin (SHBG) is the main transport protein for circulating testosterone and estradiol. SHBG is produced in liver cells and to some degree in the brain, uterus, placenta, and vagina. SHBG levels are regulated by a delicate balance of inhibiting and enhancing factors. High androgen levels decrease the production of SHBG, whereas estrogen and thyroxine increase SHBG. Moreover, IGF can suppress SHBG. Only unbound testosterone and estradiol are biologically active; therefore, the lower the SHBG blood levels, the higher the bioavailability of androgens. Conditions in which low SHBG occurs include polycystic ovary syndrome, diabetes, and hypothyroidism. Vexiau et al. [77] were able to show that SHBG levels are inversely correlated to the degree of hair loss in women with FPHL.

It has been shown that hyperandrogenemia can lead to patterned hair loss in susceptible women. Women with marked androgen excess often develop a more male pattern alopecia with deep bitemporal recession and vertex thinning [78–80]. Irregular hormone profiles and hyperandrogenemia were shown in 82%–87% of women with FPHL and hirsutism or oligomenorrhea [77,79]. However, the majority of women with FPHL show no clinical signs of hyperandrogenism and several studies showed normal testosterone and DHEA-S levels in this group of patients [79–81].

Vexiau et al. [77] found abnormal hormone profiles in 67% of women with FPHL and no clinical signs of hyperandrogenism after implementation of β-1-24 corticotropin stimulation test. Especially, 5α-androstane-3α,17β-diol glucuronide levels were found to be elevated in this patient group. 5α-androstane-3α,17β-diol glucuronide is a C19 steroid and reflects the transformation of androgen precursors, mainly of adrenal origin, in women

[82]. Increased levels of 5α-androstane-3α,17β-diol glucuronide indicate both splanchnic and extrasplanchnic 5α-reductase hyperactivity [77,83,84].

These findings indicate the importance of androgen secretion and enzyme activity in the development of FPHL. Testosterone and DHEA-S may not be the sufficient markers to recognize slight hormonal irregularities that possibly lead to FPHL.

Risk factors and association with other diseases

An increased risk of coronary heart disease and insulin resistance has been correlated with early vertex balding. Early-onset vertex balding appears to be a marker for early-onset severe coronary heart disease, especially in young men with hypertension or higher cholesterol levels [85–87]. Matilainen et al. [88] in 2000 showed that men aged 19–50 years who developed AGA earlier in life (<35 years of age) showed an increased incidence of hyperinsulinemia and disorders associated with insulin resistance, such as obesity, hypertension, and dyslipidemia. Moreover, a higher incidence of prostate cancer was found in men with male pattern baldness compared with men without AGA. An association of early-onset vertex balding with the incidence of prostate cancer, but no correlation of prostate cancer and frontal AGA, was noted [89,90]. The pathophysiology of these findings is unknown. Further studies will be necessary to investigate the role of shared androgen pathways in coronary heart disease, insulin resistance, and prostate cancer.

Male pattern hair loss

More than 95% of hair loss problems in men are AGA [91]. Approximately 50% of men will have developed some degree of AGA by the age of 49, and around 80% of men will experience male pattern baldness by the age of 80 [92]. The incidence of pattern baldness varies from population to population and is based on genetic background. AGA shows a higher prevalence in Caucasian men compared to men of Asian or African descent [93–98].

AGA usually manifests at an early age and progresses slowly. Thinning of the hair can occur as early as the age of 12 or any time later in life. Most cases start between the ages of 15 and 25 [99]. The clinical course is gradual, consisting of acute episodic phases with increased loss of telogen hair alternating with periods when there is little shedding. The shedding may be seasonal in a small number of individuals [99]. For many individuals, the condition may seem stable for years [99]. Many men reach their maximum pattern by their forties, although hair density does decrease as they age further. Usually, there is a positive family history. However, in one study 12% showed a completely negative family history [100].

Clinical features

Hair loss is patterned and nonscarring, with preservation of follicular ostia. The gradual replacement of strong, thick, and pigmented terminal hair by fine vellus-like hair on the scalp of adult men with AGA occurs in certain patterns. In men, there is a frontal hairline recession associated with thinning or balding on the crown or vertex. There are exceptions, with certain individuals showing no recession and only vertex thinning.

In 1951, Hamilton produced the first grading scale after examining 312 Caucasian men and 214 Caucasian women. The Hamilton scale ranges from type I to type VIII (Figure 2.2). Type I represents the prepubertal scalp with terminal hair growth on the forehead and all over the scalp; types II and III show gradual

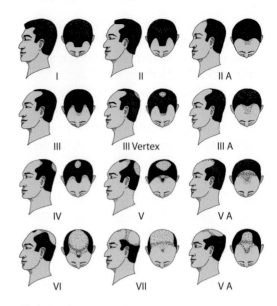

Figure 2.2
Norwood–Hamilton classification of hair loss based on severity.

frontal, mostly M-shaped recession of the hairline; types IV, V, and VI show additional gradual thinning in the vertex area; and types VII and VIII show a confluence of the balding areas and leave hair only around the back and the sides of the head [17].

In 1975, Norwood modified the classification based on a study of the degree of alopecia in 1000 Caucasian males of different ages. He included variations on the middle grades IIIa, IVa, and Va that show a more prominent gradual recession of the middle portion of the frontal hairline and type III vertex, which is characterized by a loss of hair mainly in the tonsure area and a frontotemporal recession that never exceeds that of type III [101] (Figures 2.3 and 2.4). These patterns are not restrictive, and some men can present with a female pattern (Figures 2.5, 2.6, and 2.7).

Norwood and Lehr [102] report that 10% of their male AGA patients present with a female AGA pattern. Ebling and Rook [103] used a scale of five grades of alopecia. They also described different variants of balding in different ethnic groups and both genders. Class A represents the Caucasian variant with the eventual persistence of a central lock; class B describes the Asian variant of AGA, characterized by a denuding of the frontal hairline and diffuse thinning in the frontoparietal area; C describes a Mediterranean or Latin variant, which corresponds to the Hamilton scale; and D represents the female pattern with diffuse thinning and for the most part persistence of the frontal hairline [103,104].

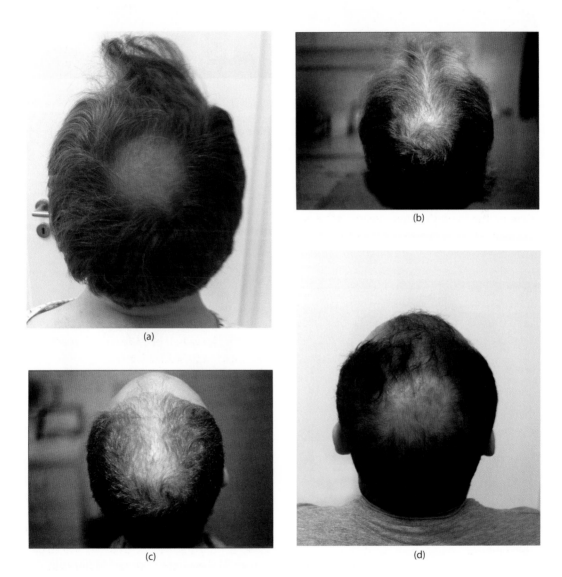

Figure 2.3
(a) Norwood–Hamilton stage III vertex, the patient showed bitemporal recession and slight thinning in the frontoparietal area. (b) Early Norwood–Hamilton stage IV, with the emergence of a bridge connecting lateral portions of the scalp. (c) Late Norwood–Hamilton stage IV, with the bridge less intact. (d) Norwood–Hamilton stage V, with the bridge gone but still with a significant number of miniaturized hairs on the top of the scalp.

(Continued)

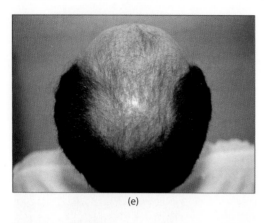
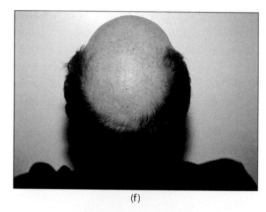

(e) (f)

Figure 2.3 (*Continued*)
(e) Norwood–Hamilton stavge VI, with very little hair on the top of the scalp. (f) Norwood–Hamilton stage VII, with preservation of the horseshoe of hair at the sides and back of the scalp.

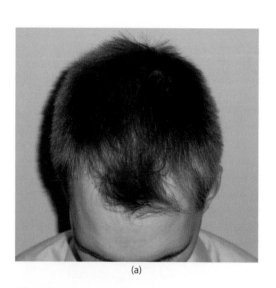
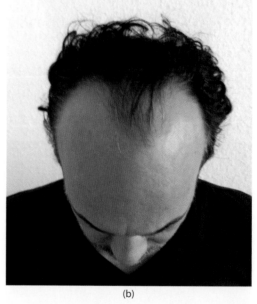

(a) (b)

Figure 2.4
(a) A 23-year-old patient with Norwood–Hamilton stage III showing the classic M hairline with frontotemporal recession; (b) a 42-year-old patient with advanced Norwood–Hamilton stage III.

(*Continued*)

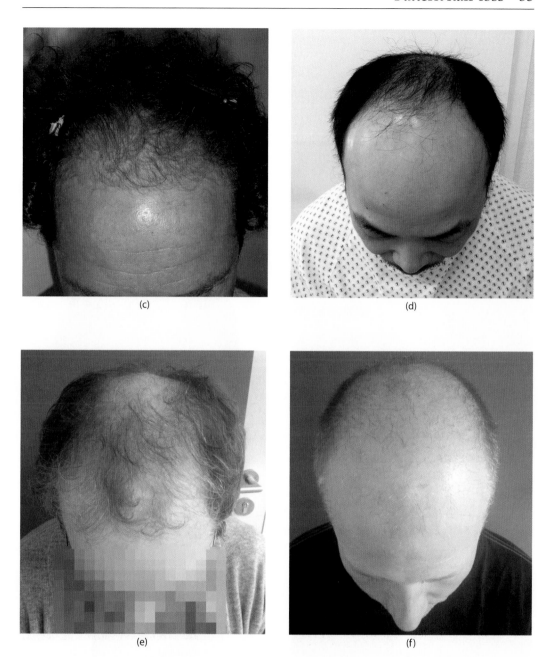

Figure 2.4 (*Continued*)
(c) A 41-year-old patient with Norwood–Hamilton Stage IIIa with frontal recession; (d) a
45-year-old patient with Norwood–Hamilton stage IVa showing marked frontal recession
and parietal thinning; (e) a 51-year-old patient with Norwood–Hamilton stage V;
(f) a 49-year-old patient with Norwood–Hamilton stage VI.

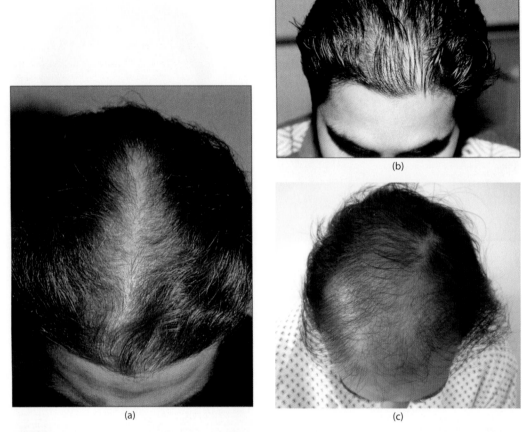

Figure 2.5
(a) A 14-year-old male with the Ludwig stage I pattern; (b) a 17-year-old male with Ludwig stage I; (c) a 36-year-old patient with Ludwig stage III.

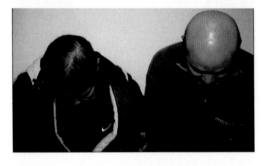

Figure 2.6
Patterns of hair loss can intermix within the same family and within the same sex. Norwood–Hamilton stage VII in a 48-year-old father (right) and Ludwig stage I occurring in his 20-year-old son (left).

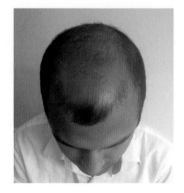

Figure 2.7
A 31-year-old patient with Norwood–Hamilton stage VI but with remaining frontal hairline.

Diagnosis

The diagnosis of androgenic alopecia in men can be usually established based on clinical presentation. A thorough inspection of the entire scalp is essential in every patient. Miniaturized hairs can usually be seen clinically or with a 10- to 100-fold magnifying device (dermatoscope or trichoscope) or with the help of contrast paper placed over a part. A pull test should be performed on different areas of the entire scalp to rule out diffuse shedding. Global photography is helpful to track disease progression and document therapy success.

Laboratory tests

Laboratory workup is usually not necessary in men with AGA unless there is concomitant diffuse hair loss. Although the complete genetic picture is not clear, there is a genetic test (HairDX™) that tests for a gene polymorphism and may predict the chances of future AGA development [20,21]. For young patients concerned about hair loss, this test may help to define the value of early treatment initiation. Moreover, a test that predicts responsiveness to treatment with finasteride is available [105].

Management of androgenetic alopecia in men

Finasteride

In 1997, the Food and Drug Administration (FDA) approved finasteride for use in the United States at a dose of 1 mg/day in men with AGA. Finasteride is the most common treatment approach for male AGA. It is a synthetic 4-azasteroid compound that is a specific inhibitor of type II 5α-reductase. 5α-Reductase type II is an intracellular enzyme that converts testosterone into dihydrotestosterone (DHT), resulting in significant decreases in serum and tissue DHT concentrations [106–112]. Finasteride does not have any hormonal properties in itself [106,107] and has no estrogenic, antiestrogenic, or progestational effects. A study by Roberts et al. [111] confirmed that finasteride 1 mg daily was the optimal dose, with 1 mg and 5 mg superior to lower doses such as 0.2 mg daily. The daily 5 mg dose was not more efficacious than the 1 mg dose.

Finasteride 1 mg is to be taken every day, on a regular schedule, with or without food. The bioavailability after oral intake is 65% [113]. Ninety percent of circulating finasteride is bound to plasma proteins and can cross the blood–brain barrier. Finasteride is metabolized in the liver, and therefore caution should be exercised in patients with liver function abnormalities [113]. Dosage does not need to be adjusted in case of renal insufficiency [113]. Finasteride does not affect the cytochrome P450–metabolizing enzyme system, and no drug interactions have been reported [113].

Finasteride is well tolerated, and side effects occur in less than 2% of patients [107,113]. Side effects include 1.8% decreased libido (1.3% placebo), 1.3% erectile dysfunction (0.7% placebo), and 0.8% decreased ejaculate volume (0.4% placebo) [107,114]. There was no significant difference in the placebo group for each of these side effects taken alone, but there is a statistical difference when all side effects are considered together (3.8% vs. 2.1%) [106,107,115,116]. Side effects will subside spontaneously in 58% of those who decide to continue the treatment and are reversible on cessation of treatment [117].

A study by Overstreet et al. [118] confirmed that finasteride 1 mg daily for 48 weeks did not affect spermatogenesis or semen production in men aged 19–41 years. However, some isolated case reports have also been published on the effect of low-dose finasteride on DNA changes in sperm [119], motility, and sperm counts [120,121]. These patients were under investigation for oligospermia and infertility when these findings were discovered. Significantly, these parameters improved after stopping the drug [122].

The effect on prostate volume and serum prostate-specific antigen (PSA) in this young population without benign prostate hypertrophy was small and reversible on discontinuation of the drug [118]. Finasteride can decrease PSA levels by 50% in older men [123]. The University of British Columbia Hair Research and Treatment Centre recommends that older men take a baseline PSA prior to initiation of therapy with finasteride. We also advise the patient's family doctor to double the PSA value while patients are taking finasteride.

Recently, there was a discussion on a possible "post-finasteride syndrome" triggered by some publications that are based on standardized interviews and surveys [124–126]. The studies revealed that the subjects reported new-onset persistent sexual dysfunction (low libido, erectile dysfunction, and problems with orgasm) associated with the temporal use of finasteride. These findings have been widely discussed on the Internet and in lay press. These rare side effects are now included in Merck's patient product information in the United States, and in public assessment reports of the Medicines and Health Regulatory Agency of the United Kingdom and the Medical Products Agency of Sweden [122]. However, so far there are no evidence-based data supporting a causal link between finasteride and persistent sexual dysfunction in the numerous double-blinded, placebo-controlled studies using finasteride 1 mg for hair loss.

In view of the conflicting and continuing data and importance of the subject, the International Society of Hair Restoration Surgery has established the Task Force on Finasteride Adverse Event Controversies to evaluate published data and make recommendations (http://www.ishrs.org/article/update-international-society-hair-restoration-surgery-task-force-finasteride-adverse-event) [122] (Figure 2.8).

Minoxidil

Minoxidil is a piperidinopyrimidine derivative originally used as an oral antihypertensive as a smooth muscle vasodilator. The mechanism of action is not fully understood. It has been shown to have a mitogenic, nonhormonal effect on epidermal cells leading to prolonged survival time [127,128] as well the capacity to induce increased proliferation on hair follicles in vitro [128]. Studies of follicles in vitro from the stump-tailed macaque show a significantly increased DNA synthesis in follicular keratinocytes and perifollicular epithelium but not in epidermal keratinocytes [129]. Plucked anagen hair bulbs from men applying minoxidil show a significant increase in proliferation index measured by DNA flow cytometry [130].

A change in intracellular calcium homeostasis has been suggested, because minoxidil is converted to minoxidil sulfate, a potassium channel agonist that increases potassium channel permeability, leading to the entry of calcium into the cells. This active metabolite is believed to be responsible for hair growth stimulation. The sulfotransferase enzyme (SULT1A1) activity in the hair follicle correlates with minoxidil response. There is a test that can measure this active metabolite and may predict how one might respond to therapy [131].

Minoxidil 5% solution or foam twice daily is approved for the treatment of AGA in men. The effectiveness of minoxidil has been shown in multiple clinical studies. Outcome parameters included hair counts, macrophotographs, and hair weight. The improvement in hair counts reflects a reversal from miniaturized vellus-like hairs to thicker visible terminal hairs. Initial clinical studies measured efficacy of minoxidil on vertex thinning, and subsequent studies confirmed that minoxidil works equally well on frontal scalp thinning [132].

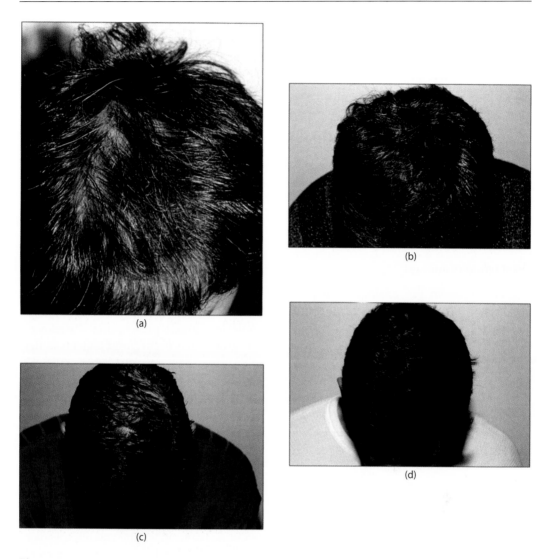

Figure 2.8
A 24-year-old male with androgenetic alopecia (AGA) (a) before the use of finasteride 1 mg/day and (b) 1 year later, showing improvement. A 33-year-old male with AGA (c) before the use of finasteride 1 mg/day and (d) after 11 months of therapy, showing improvement.

Side effects include contact dermatitis and a transient shedding during the first approximately 2 months of use. Use of 5% minoxidil in a commercially available foam vehicle that does not contain propylene glycol (potential irritant) reduces the incidence of pruritus [132]. Several products that include minoxidil, sometimes combined with other active ingredients such as tretinoin, are available from different manufacturers in the United States.

Dutasteride

Dutasteride is a dual inhibitor of both types I and II 5α-reductase that inhibits the conversion of testosterone to DHT. It is currently approved for treatment of benign prostatic hyperplasia. It is not approved by the FDA for the treatment of AGA. Only in Korea has dutasteride at a dose of 0.5 mg daily been recently approved for the treatment of MPHL. In several studies, it was shown that dutasteride improves hair growth in MPHL more rapidly and to a greater degree than finasteride at a dose of 2.5 mg/day [115,133]. However, its safety profile remains unclear. Side effects of dutasteride, which have been reported in the treatment of prostatic enlargement, include breast tenderness and enlargement and a prolonged reduced sperm count in addition to decreased libido, erectile dysfunction, and decreased ejaculate volume [134,135]. No statistically significant associations were observed between 5α-reductase inhibitors and breast cancer [136].

Prostaglandin analogs

The prostaglandin F2α analogs latanoprost and bimatoprost are used in treating ocular hypertension and glaucoma. A noted side effect is increased eyelash hair growth, a feature that has been investigated in several studies. Bimatoprost is now available as a treatment for eyelash growth [137]. More recently, latanoprost has been investigated for its potential to promote scalp hair growth. Latanoprost significantly increased hair density compared with baseline and placebo and may also encourage pigmentation [138]. Another recent study showed that topical bimatoprost 0.3% applied once daily significantly increased scalp hair growth compared to vehicle in subjects with mild to moderate AGA. However, the same study showed that topical minoxidil 5% applied twice daily in an open-label manner showed higher efficacy than any of the bimatoprost doses tested [139].

Ketoconazole

Ketoconazole is an imidazole antifungal agent; it is effective for the treatment of dermatitis and dandruff, and its action on scalp microflora may benefit those with AGA-associated follicular inflammation [140,141]. However, ketoconazole is also an antiandrogen and has been suggested to improve hair growth in AGA through androgen-dependent pathways [141,142]. Studies using ketoconazole shampoo 2% on MPHL showed increased hair density in addition to increased size and proportion of anagen follicles compared to those using a nonmedicated shampoo [141]. Ketoconazole shampoo can be utilized in conjunction with other AGA treatments [143]. Shampoos containing 2% ketoconazole are available over the counter in some countries; but in the United States, 1% is available over the counter, whereas 2% is a prescription.

Light therapy

Laser sources have become very popular in medical and nonmedical areas. Manufacturers and suppliers oftentimes guarantee hair regrowth, and various devices are available without prescription. Paradoxical hair growth has occurred in patients undergoing laser hair removal when relatively low-energy fluences were used [41]. The mechanism of action of this phenomenon is unknown [144]. One theory suggests an increase in blood flow in the dermal papilla.

Treatment protocols include 15- to 30-minute treatments on alternating days for 2–4 weeks tapering to one to two treatments per week for 6–12 months, followed by biweekly and once per month maintenance treatments. A change in texture and improvement in hair quality has been reported in patients using laser devices [145,146]. Low-level laser light sources appear to be safe to use in the treatment of hair loss. However, these authors feel that more double-blinded, placebo-controlled studies for the assessment of hair growth and density are necessary to evaluate the efficacy and safety of low-level laser therapy. More studies are also necessary to understand the mechanism of action.

Hair restoration surgery

Hair restoration surgery is an excellent treatment option for men with AGA Norwood–Hamilton stages III–V. The occipital area is

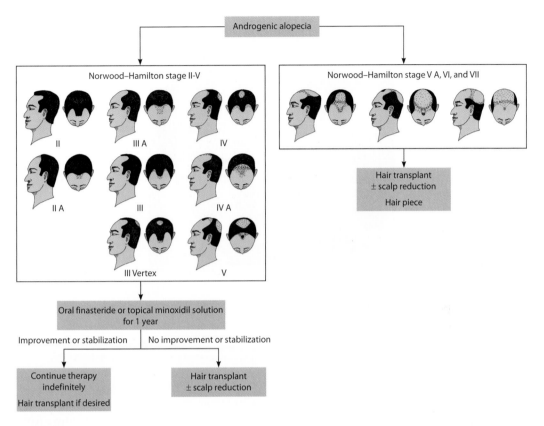

Figure 2.9

An algorithmic approach to the treatment of male androgenetic alopecia: the UCSF–UBC treatment protocol for androgenetic alopecia in men. (Courtesy of Jerry Shapiro, Vera H. Price, and Harvey Lui.)

usually not affected by the miniaturization process of AGA; therefore, hair from this "safe" zone can be taken and redistributed to the front, parietal area and vertex. The patient needs to understand that hair restoration surgery cannot create the density that the patient had before the hair loss started. But even with a lower density, scalp coverage and satisfying cosmetic results can be achieved (see Chapter 7).

Wigs and hair pieces

If hair loss exceeds Norwood–Hamilton stage V and progresses to stages VI and VII, full scalp coverage cannot be achieved with hair restoration surgery as the donor supply does not equal the demand. If full hair is

desired, hair pieces are an excellent option. Modern, well-designed hair pieces are nowadays almost undetectable and comfortable to wear (see Chapter 8) (Figures 2.9 and 2.10).

Female pattern hair loss

AGA together with telogen effluvium is the most common complaint of women in the everyday hair clinic. FPHL has a postpubescent onset [147]. However, a few cases of MPHL and FPHL have been reported in children [148]. It is noted that 25%–38% of women are affected with FPHL [149]. The expression pattern, age of onset, and final degree of hair loss show great interindividual differences.

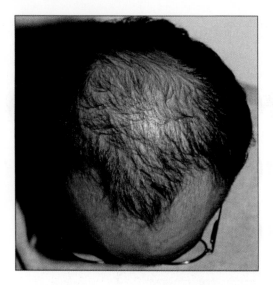

Figure 2.10
A good candidate for medical treatment of male androgenetic alopecia (note the presence of miniaturized hair).

Clinical features

The clinical presentation of AGA in women is classically divided into three stages of severity. In 1977, Ludwig described the presentation of the female type of AGA as grades I–III (Figure 2.11a). He described grade I as follows: perceptible thinning of the hair on the crown, limited in the front by a line situated 1–3 cm behind the frontal hairline. Grade II was described as follows: pronounced rarefaction of the hair on the crown within the area seen in grade I. Grade III was described by Ludwig as follows: full baldness within the area seen in grades I and II [150] (Figure 2.11). Figure 2.12 shows women with AGA presenting according to Ludwig's classification of grades I–III. Ludwig emphasized the preservation of the frontal fringe despite a diffuse thinning in the frontoparietal area and the progression of hair loss with age. However, FPHL can present with frontotemporal recession [151]; the temporal area is usually not completely devoid of terminal hair follicles, but the hair is markedly thinner and shorter. Olsen et al. [152] described the "Christmas tree pattern" as the most common presentation of FPHL, displaying a frontal accentuation of hair loss with or without thinning of the frontal fringe (Figure 2.13).

The severity of FPHL is not necessarily age related, as severe FPHL can occur in young adults. Other clinical variations of FPHL include diffuse thinning or thinning on the lateral scalp (Figure 2.14). Moreover, hair loss in women can present in male patterns involving complete frontotemporal recession and vertex thinning (Figure 2.15) [153].

Venning and Dawber [151] examined 564 women aged over 20 years. They found that 80% of premenopausal women had thinning in the Ludwig pattern and 13% had Norwood–Hamilton types II–IV patterns. After menopause, the proportion exhibiting the male pattern increased to 37% and, although they did not progress beyond Hamilton stage IV, some had marked M-shaped recession at both temples [151] (Figure 2.12b).

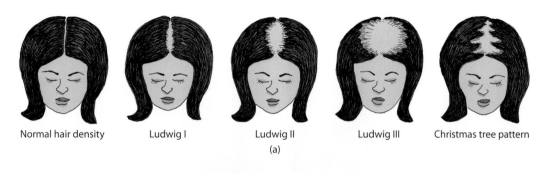

Normal hair density   Ludwig I   Ludwig II   Ludwig III   Christmas tree pattern

(a)

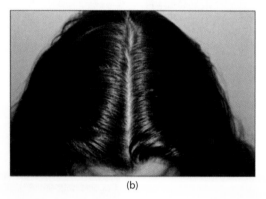

(b)

Figure 2.11
(a) Ludwig classification and Christmas tree pattern of female androgenetic alopecia (AGA), showing the three different stages of severity; (b) the characteristically narrow division of bare scalp between areas of combed hair ("part," "parting") found in a woman without AGA.

Diagnosis

The identification of FPHL is usually not difficult if the alopecia occurs in a classical clinical pattern. The diagnosis can be more difficult if the hair loss is more diffuse over the entire scalp or if it occurs together with other hair loss conditions such as telogen effluvium, diffuse alopecia areata, or mild forms of cicatricial alopecias. FPHL is a non-scarring alopecia with the preservation of follicular ostia. It is characterized by its special pattern; a variation in hair shaft diameter; and the occurrence of miniaturized, vellus-like hairs that sometimes can only be seen with a magnifier or trichoscopy. A clinical examination of the entire scalp should be performed. To rule out diffuse shedding, a pull test can easily be performed during the consultation. In FPHL, the hair pull test is only positive in an active stage. Usually, the pull test is negative in the occipital area.

Dermoscopy or videodermoscopy examination of the scalp skin helps to identify the presence of follicular ostia and the occurrence of miniaturized hair. Standardized scalp photography, especially of the part area, is very helpful as a qualitative assessment of the progression of hair loss and as therapy control. Quantitative diagnostic methods include trichogram, phototrichogram, and scalp biopsy.

Laboratory tests

In women, a laboratory test for thyroid-stimulating hormone (TSH) is recommended, because of the frequency of thyroid abnormalities and the difficulty of distinguishing AGA from telogen effluvium. Ferritin levels

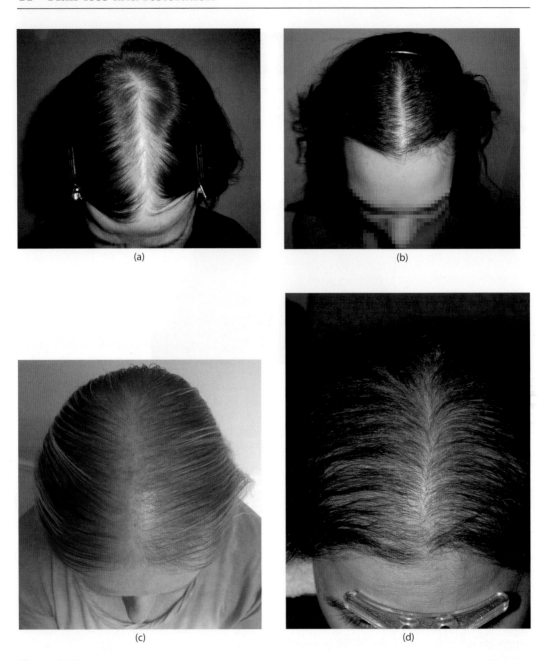

(a)   (b)

(c)   (d)

Figure 2.12

(a, b) Ludwig stage I: a widening of the division of bare scalp between areas of combed hair ("part," "parting") may be the first complaint of the female patient. She will also notice her ponytail diameter may be reduced one-third to one-half of what it used to be. The elastic band that she usually uses to tie up her ponytail can now be wound several times around her hair in contrast to only once or twice, as before; (c, d) Ludwig stage II: the width of the division of bare scalp (part, parting) is now considerably more evident than in Ludwig stage I.

(Continued)

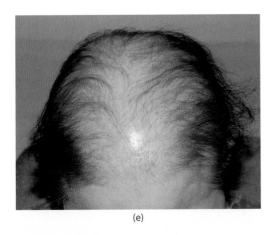

(e)

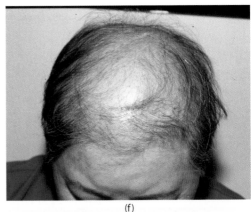

(f)

Figure 2.12 (*Continued*)
(e, f) Ludwig stage III: considerable loss of hair.

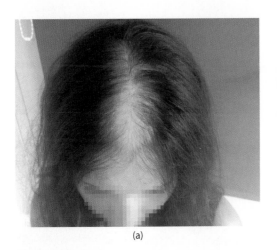

(a)

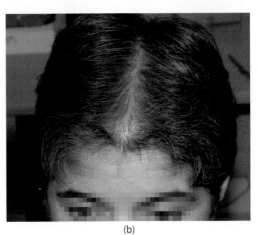

(b)

Figure 2.13
(a, b) Female pattern hair loss with frontal accentuation (Christmas tree pattern).

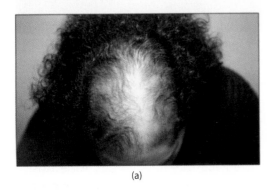

(a)

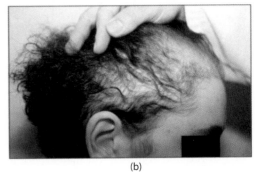

(b)

Figure 2.14
Female androgenetic alopecia may be totally diffuse, involving not only (a) the centroparietal area, but also (b) the sides and the back of the scalp.

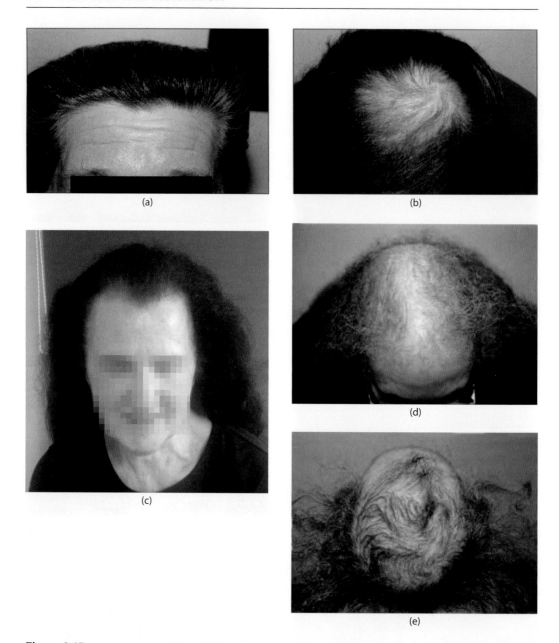

Figure 2.15

(a, b) A rare case of a 55-year-old male with absolutely no recession and simply vertex thinning. (c) A 69-year-old female patient with Norwood–Hamilton stage III; (d) a female with androgenetic alopecia (AGA) with a Norwood–Hamilton stage V pattern; (e) a female with AGA with a Norwood–Hamilton stage VI pattern.

are also ordered routinely on menstruating females, as low iron levels can trigger a telogen effluvium that may mimic AGA. Tests for vitamin D, vitamin B12, selenium, and zinc are also recommended to rule out sources for an underlying telogen effluvium. An extensive laboratory workup for androgens is not recommended for a routine visit. Women with irregular periods and/or other signs of androgen excess should be at least checked for free and total testosterone as well as DHEA-S. If elevated androgen levels are found, patients should be sent to an endocrinologist and/or gynecologist for further workup.

Management

Minoxidil

Only two pharmaceutical treatments have been approved by the FDA for the therapy of FPHL: 2% minoxidil solution [154,155] and, only recently, 5% minoxidil foam. Its use is indicated in women older than 18 years with mild to moderate hair loss, Ludwig stage I or II. Twice daily application of 1 mL minoxidil is recommended. In a double-blinded, placebo-controlled trial, 2% minoxidil used twice daily resulted in minimal hair regrowth in 50% of women and moderate hair regrowth in 13% of women after 32 weeks of treatment, compared with rates of 33% and 6%, respectively, in the placebo group ($P <$ .001) [154]. In a randomized, placebo-controlled trial of 5% and 2% topical minoxidil solutions in the treatment of FPHL after 48 weeks of therapy, both 2% and 5% minoxidil doses were superior to placebo for hair count, scalp coverage, and hair growth [156]. Efficacy can be assessed after 6–12 months of treatment [157]. Minoxidil is applied directly onto the dry scalp, 25 drops (or 1 mL) twice a day, on the frontoparietal and vertex area. Studies have shown 75% of absorption in the first 4 hours after application; therefore, the scalp and hair should not be washed for at least 4–6 hours after application [158].

Side effects of topical minoxidil therapy include contact dermatitis attributed to propylene glycol with dryness, itching, and erythema in approximately 7% of patients using the 2% minoxidil solution and a higher incidence with the 5% solution because of the increased content of propylene glycol. Symmetrical facial hypertrichosis on the malar areas and forehead affect up to 7% of patients [159,160]. This is possibly due to a

local transfer of the drug or a systemic effect. Hypertrichosis disappears within 4 months after discontinuation of therapy and frequently decreases even with continuous use after 1 year. Less than 1 in 1000 patients experience tachycardia and decreased blood pressure. Patients with heart problems should be cautious and use the medication with approval from their family physician or cardiologist.

In the first 6 weeks of treatment, one-third of patients will experience increased shedding, especially if the patient had active shedding before the treatment began. The use of 5% minoxidil may be considered in women who do not have a response to 2% minoxidil or who want more aggressive management. Minoxidil is a lifelong therapy and should not be used in pregnant or nursing women (Figures 2.16 through 2.18).

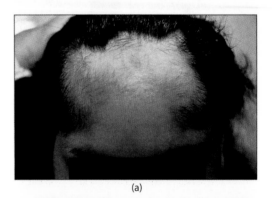

(a)

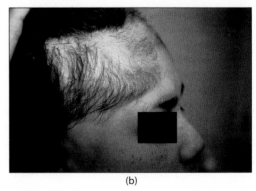

(b)

Figure 2.16
Hypertrichosis of the face can occur in women using topical minoxidil solution. (a) Frontal view; (b) lateral view.

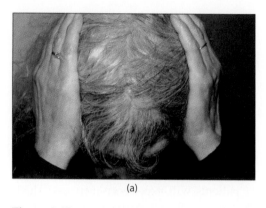
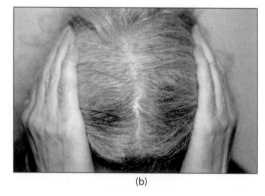

(a)   (b)

Figure 2.17
A 53-year-old female with androgenetic alopecia (a) before topical minoxidil solution and (b) after 8 months of topical minoxidil solution, showing marked improvement.

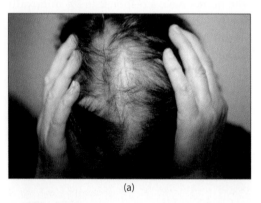
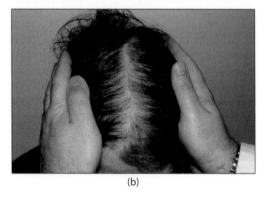

(a)   (b)

Figure 2.18
A 40-year-old female with androgenetic alopecia (a) before topical minoxidil solution and (b) after 6 months of use of topical minoxidil, showing marked improvement, with narrowing of her part/parting.

Finasteride

Finasteride is not approved for women. Its efficacy in FPHL is still controversial. Finasteride has no affinity for the androgen receptor and has no androgenic, estrogenic, antiestrogenic, or progestational effects. A multicenter double-blind, placebo-controlled randomized study of finasteride, 1 mg/day, in postmenopausal women with FPHL showed negative results. Scalp biopsies revealed no differences in the anagen to telogen ratio and the terminal hair to miniaturized hair ratio [161]. However, Camacho [162] reported hair regrowth using finasteride 2.5 mg/day in 41 women with FPHL and seborrhea, acne, hirsutism, and alopecia. Thai and Sinclair [163] administered finasteride 5 mg/week to a 67-year-old postmenopausal woman with FPHL without signs of hyperandrogenism. After 12 months of therapy, the woman showed a marked increase in hair density [163].

Trüeb et al. [164] reported effectiveness of finasteride at a dosage of 2.5 mg/day in four postmenopausal women and 5 mg/day in one postmenopausal woman after 6 months of treatment. Iorizzo et al. [165] were able to show an improvement in hair density in 62% out of 37 premenopausal women after 1 year of treatment with finasteride 2.5 mg/day and oral contraceptive (containing 3-mg drospi-renone, a synthetic progestin analog of spironolactone, and 30-μg ethinyl estradiol). Finasteride was generally well tolerated [166].

Women who are or potentially may be pregnant should not take finasteride or handle crushed or broken tablets [167]. Finasteride tablets are coated to prevent contact with the active ingredients during manipulation. The risk of teratogenicity in humans has not been directly evaluated, but there is a risk that finasteride exposure during pregnancy may cause hypospadias in the developing male fetus [168]. Exposure to semen of men who are taking finasteride does not pose a risk to a pregnant woman's male fetus.

Dutasteride

Dutasteride is an inhibitor of types I and II 5α-reductase [169]. It is approved at a dose of 0.5 mg daily for the treatment of symptomatic benign prostatic hyperplasia [169]. Little knowledge on efficacy and side effects is available for the treatment of FPHL with dutasteride. Dutasteride was administered orally to a 46-year-old woman who had shown nonresponsiveness to 5% minoxidil and limited improvement with finasteride 1 mg/day; after 6 months of therapy, significant improvement was observed and after 9 months the clinical diagnosis of androgenic alopecia could no longer be made in this patient. No side effects were observed [170]. Moftah et al. used a dutasteride-containing preparation as mesotherapy in 86 women. They found a photographic improvement in 62.8% of patients and an increase in mean hair diameter. Patient self-assessment showed statistically significant improvement compared to placebo ($P < .05$) [171].

5α-Reductase inhibitors are used off-label for the treatments for FPHL. Neither finasteride nor dutasteride is approved by the FDA for use in women. Women of childbearing age have to be advised to use effective means of contraception while taking any of these drugs, as these agents are known teratogens and may cause hypospadias in the development of the male fetus. More studies are necessary for the evaluation of the safety profile of these drugs for the treatment of men and women with AGA.

Cyproterone acetate

Cyproterone acetate (CPA) is a synthetic derivative of 17-hydroxyprogesterone. It acts as an androgen receptor antagonist with weak progestational and glucocorticoid activity [172]. It also inhibits the steroidogenic enzyme 21-hydroxylase, reducing the production of aldosterone and to a lesser extent 3β-hydroxysteroid dehydrogenase, both of which are needed to synthesize cortisol [172]. CPA is available in Europe, Canada, and South America. It is usually combined with ethinyl estradiol as a birth control pill [173].

For the treatment of FPHL, a regimen with 100 mg CPA daily on days 5–15 of the menstrual cycle and 50 μg of ethinyl estradiol on days 5–25 or 50 mg of CPA daily on days 1–10 of the cycle and 35 μg of ethinyl estradiol on days 1–21 has been suggested [174]. In a randomized 12-month clinical trial in 66 women, 33 women with FPHL used topical minoxidil 2% plus combined oral contraceptive, whereas 33 women received CPA 52 mg daily plus ethinyl estradiol 35 μg for 20 days of the cycle. The latter combination resulted in greater hair density in women with hyperandrogenism [175]. Side effects from CPA are irregular menstrual cycles, weight gain, breast tenderness, loss of libido, depression, and nausea.

Spironolactone

Spironolactone is a synthetic 17-lactone drug, which is a renal competitive aldosterone antagonist with a mild antiandrogenic effect by blocking the androgen receptor and preventing its interaction with dihydrotes-terosterone [176]. In the adrenal gland, the essential androgen synthesis is decreased by depleting cytochrome P450. Spironolactone is 98% protein bound and the primary metabo-lite, canrenone, is at least 90% protein bound, which contributes to the diuretic activities of spironolactone. Drug absorption is increased by food; spironolactone is metabolized in the liver and excreted in urine and bile [176]. The maximum androgen suppression is reached after 4–12 months; dosages of 200 mg daily are required.

Spironolactone may have a preventative effect in FPHL and may reduce shedding in individuals without hyperandrogenism, but it has failed to show significant hair regrowth [177]. The main side effect is men-strual irregularities (decreasing the dose to 50–75 mg/day and adding oral contracep-tives or continuing 2 to 3 months of therapy may correct this side effect). Spironolactone is contraindicated in patients with renal insufficiency, hyperkalemia, pregnancy, and abnormal uterine bleeding and women with genetic predisposition for breast cancer [177].

17α- and 17β-estradiol

In Europe, topical 17α- and 17β-estradiol are commercially available for the treat-ment of FPHL. Studies showed increased anagen and decreased telogen rates after topical treatment compared with pla-cebo treatment [178,179]. The underlying pathways of 17α-estradiol-induced hair regrowth are unknown. Niiyama et al. [180] showed that 17α-estradiol is able to dimin-ish the amount of DHT formed by human hair follicles after incubation with testos-terone while increasing the concentration of weaker steroids.

Recently, it has been shown that hair fol-licles in women with FPHL express more aromatase activity compared to male hair follicles [179]. Under the influence of

17α-estradiol, an increased conversion of testosterone to 17β-estradiol and andro-stenedione to estrone takes place in hair follicles derived from the occiput, which might explain the beneficial effects of estro-gen treatment in FPHL [179,181]. Women who were taking aromatase inhibitors were shown to develop FPHL more rapidly [182]. Another theory about the effectiveness of estradiol is the systemic induction of SHBG and therefore the reduction of free, bioavail-able testosterone [77].

Prostaglandin analogs

Recently, latanoprost was investigated for its potential to promote scalp hair growth. Latanoprost significantly increased hair density compared with baseline and placebo and may also encourage pigmentation [138]. Scalp injections of bimatoprost 0.03% weekly for 12 weeks and then biweekly for 4 weeks were attempted as a novel treatment for FPHL in a 59-year-old female without success [183]. This novel treatment reinforces that further pilot studies with prostaglandin analogs are necessary to determine efficacy [139].

Low-level light therapy

Like in MPHL, low-level laser light sources can be considered as a treatment option. The treatment appears to be safe, and its efficacy has been shown in one study [145]. However, more studies are necessary to understand the mechanism of action and to evaluate the effi-cacy of these devices.

Hair restoration surgery

Hair transplantation is another treatment option for women with FPHL. Hair fol-licles are taken from the occipital scalp and implanted into the area of thinning. Optimal candidates for hair transplantation are those with high donor hair density and frontal accentuation of hair loss. Prior to hair

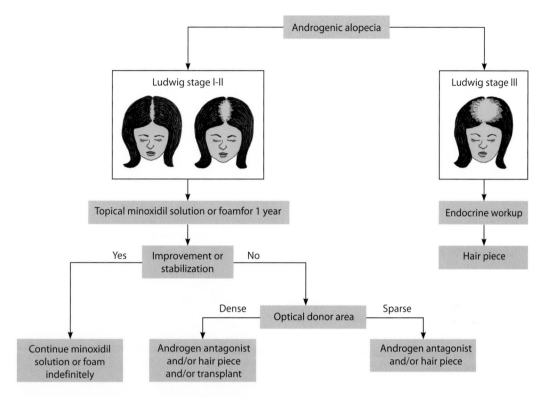

Figure 2.19
An algorithmic approach on the treatment of female androgenetic alopecia: the UCSF–UBC Treatment Protocol for androgenetic alopecia in women. (Courtesy of Jerry Shapiro, Vera H. Price, and Harvey Lui.)

restoration procedures in women, underlying causes for telogen effluvium should be ruled out. It is important that the patient understands the risks, benefits, and limitations of the procedure. An additional treatment with medical therapy is recommended to stop further hair loss of preexisting hair. Final results are usually seen 6–8 months after the surgery (see Chapter 7).

Wigs and hair pieces

Scalp prostheses are practical for patients who are not candidates for hair restoration surgery, women with extensive hair loss, and/or patients without satisfying improvement after using medical therapy. Wigs and hair pieces can provide excellent cosmetic results, especially when they are custom

made. It is usually easier to overcome the reluctance to wear a scalp prosthesis if the hair piece blends in nicely with the preexisting hair, if it is comfortable to wear, and if the patient is exposing her natural hairline (see Chapter 8) (Figure 2.19).

Pathology

The histologic features of AGA are similar in males and females [184]. Vertical sections show terminal hairs and follicular stelae in the subcutaneous tissue and reticular dermis and terminal and vellus hairs and stelae in the papillary dermis [184–186]. Stelae are the residual fibrous tracts that mark the upward migration of the catagen, telogen, or

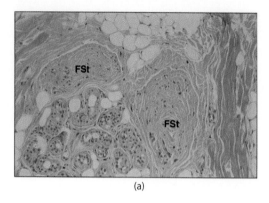

(a)

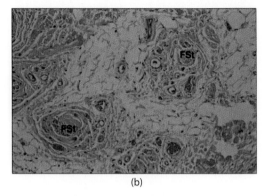

(b)

Figure 2.20
(a, b) Stelae or fibrous streamers (FSt) commonly seen in androgenetic alopecia. (Courtesy of Dr. Magdalena Martinka.)

miniaturizing hair shaft and bulb (Figure 2.20). Horizontal sections show distinctive changes in papillary and reticular dermis and in the deeper subcutaneous sections. In papillary dermis, terminal, vellus, and vellus-like hairs are identified. Vellus and vellus-like hairs are less than 0.03 mm in diameter. Primary vellus hairs are small hairs, have a thin outer root sheath, and originate in the upper half of the dermis (Figure 2.21). Vellus-like hairs are miniaturized hairs that have a thick outer root sheath and originate from a terminal hair rooted in reticular dermis or subcutaneous fat with underlying stelae (Figure 2.22).

Usually, hairs on the horizontal section are arranged in follicular bundles of two to four hairs with sebaceous glands and arrector pili muscle [185] (Figures 2.23 and 2.24). This patterning is typical of scalp hair. In reticular dermis, there are no vellus or vellus-like hairs. Terminal hair bulbs predominate in the anagen phase. Catagen and telogen terminal hairs are noted as well. In subcutaneous fat, only the deeper anagen terminal hairs are present (Figure 2.25).

Follicular counts vary from level to level. Normally, upper papillary dermis counts are around 40–50. In the reticular dermis the number is usually reduced to 35, and in

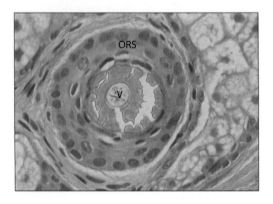

Figure 2.21
Primary vellus hair (V) with a small hair shaft and small outer root sheath (ORS). (Courtesy of Dr. Magdalena Martinka.)

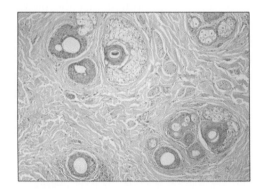

Figure 2.22
Secondary vellus hair (V) with small hair shaft and large outer root sheath (ORS), indicating true miniaturization. (Courtesy of Dr. Magdalena Martinka.)

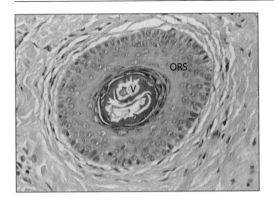

Figure 2.23
Follicular bundles with miniaturized hairs.
(Courtesy of Dr. Magdalena Martinka.)

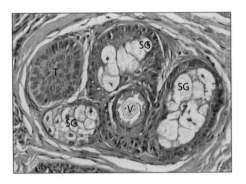

Figure 2.24
A close-up of a follicular bundle in androgenetic alopecia, showing a vellus hair (V)
and a telogen hair (T). Note the prominence
of sebaceous glands (SGs) when hairs are
miniaturized. (Courtesy of Dr. Magdalena
Martinka.)

the fat it is usually around 30. The different
follicular counts in papillary dermis and
reticular dermis are due to the number of
vellus hairs present in the papillary dermis.
The difference in follicular counts between
reticular dermis and fat is due to the number
of terminal telogen hairs. In AGA, the total
number of follicular counts is usually normal
in the papillary dermis. However, Whiting
[185] has seen a reduction in 10% of cases of
AGA, indicating a decreased capacity for follicular regrowth in a small number of AGA
patients.

Ratios of anagen to telogen and terminal to
vellus change in AGA. Normally, 90%–94%
of hairs are in anagen and 6%–10% are in
telogen. In AGA, as few as 80% of hairs are
found to be in anagen and up to 20% are in
telogen. In AGA, because miniaturization is
due to the shortening of the anagen phase,
with no decrease in telogen, there is clearly
an increase in telogen hairs. The terminal to
vellus ratio is normally 7:1. In AGA, the ratio
is 2:1, indicating a marked shift to miniaturization in AGA. A characteristic microscopic
finding in AGA is volumetric reduction of
terminal follicles. Initially, the follicles are
only minimally decreased in diameter, but
eventually a mixture of follicular sizes is
apparent. Sebaceous glands seem enlarged

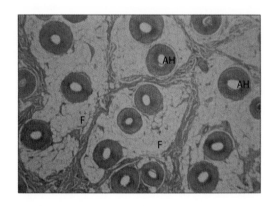

Figure 2.25
In androgenetic alopecia, subcutaneous fat
(F) contains anagen hairs (AHs). (Courtesy
of Dr. Magdalena Martinka.)

in relation to these miniaturized follicles.
Arao–Perkins bodies may be seen. These are
small clusters of elastic fibers in the neck of
dermal papillae. They are clumped in catagen and located at the lowest point of origin
of follicular stelae. Stacks of these Arao–
Perkins bodies may be seen, like rungs of
ladders, in these stelae of miniaturized anagen hairs.

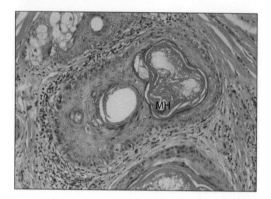

Figure 2.26
Inflammatory infiltrate in androgenetic alopecia is not uncommon. Note the perifollicular lymphocytic infiltrate around this follicular bundle, which contains a miniaturized hair (MH). (Courtesy of Dr. Magdalena Martinka.)

One-third of patients with AGA show mild inflammation, just as one-third of normal controls do. Forty percent of patients with AGA show moderate lymphohistiocytic inflammation, compared to only 10% of normal controls [184] (Figure 2.26). The role of inflammation is controversial. Possible causes for inflammation include seborrheic dermatitis; actinic damage; and the application of comedogenic, irritant, sensitizing, or otherwise toxic cosmetics and grooming agents to the scalp. Even porphyrins elaborated by follicular bacteria and activated by ultraviolet light could cause some inflammation. These causes may be more pronounced in the less-protected scalp [184].

Differential diagnosis

Usually, the diagnosis of AGA is not a difficult one in men. However, in women the diagnosis may be more difficult. The diagnosis of AGA is usually supported by the following cardinal features:

- Focal balding pattern with miniaturized hairs
- Gradual onset with progression
- Thinning with or without gradually developing bare patches
- Onset after puberty
- Negative pull test

The other two diagnoses that may be difficult to distinguish are telogen effluvium and alopecia areata, which are discussed at length in Chapters 3 and 5. Telogen effluvium is usually generalized, with an abrupt onset, and frequently has an identifiable trigger. There is thinning, with no bare patches (Figure 2.27). Shedding is prominent. Onset is at any age, but usually not childhood. The pull test is positive with telogen hairs. Alopecia areata is usually randomly patchy, but can be generalized. Onset is usually abrupt, with remissions and relapses. Onset is at any age, with over 60% presenting under the age of 20. Shedding is prominent, with a positive pull test for both dystrophic anagen and telogen hairs. Overlapping of AGA and alopecia areata can occur. It is expected that 1.7% of patients with AGA have had, or will have, alopecia areata. This may have great significance if one is contemplating hair transplantation surgery for AGA. If an AGA patient has a previous recent or remote history of alopecia areata, he or she must be warned that that it could recur after surgery.

The 4.0-mm scalp biopsy with transverse sectioning is the best laboratory test to distinguish AGA from alopecia areata or telogen effluvium.

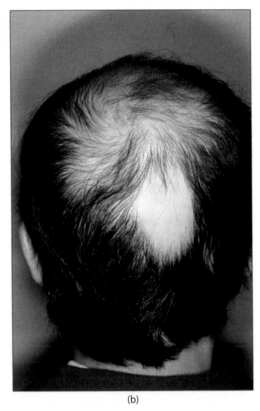

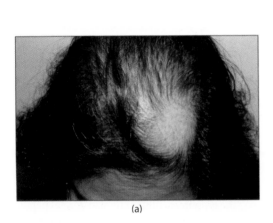

(a)

(b)

Figure 2.27

Overlapping of androgenetic alopecia (AGA) and alopecia areata (AA) can occur. It is expected that almost 2% of patients with AGA have had, have, or will have AA. This may have great significance if one is contemplating hair transplantation surgery for AGA. If an AGA patient has a previous, recent, or remote history of AA, he or she must be warned that that it could recur after surgery. (a) A 25-year-old female with female AGA with a 6-month history of a patch of AA; (b) a 35-year-old male with AGA with a 3-month history of a patch of AA.

References

1. Hanneken S et al., Androgenetic alopecia. Current aspects of a common phenotype. *Der Hautarzt*, 2003. **54**(8): 703–12.
2. Terry RL and Davis JS, Components of facial attractiveness. *Percept Motor Skills*, 1976. **42**: 918–23.
3. Franzoi SL, Anderson J, and Frommelt S, Individual differences in men's perceptions of and reactions to thinning hair. *J Soc Psychol*, 1990. **130**(2):209–18.
4. Cash TF, The psychological effect of androgenetic alopecia in men. *J Am Acad Dematol*, 1992. **26**: 926–31.
5. Cash TF, The psychosocial consequences of androgenetic alopecia: A review of the research literature. *Br J Dermatol*, 1999. **141**(3): 398–405.
6. Cash TF, Price VH, and Savin RC, Psychological effects of androgenetic alopecia on women: Comparisons with balding men and with female control subjects. *J Am Acad Dermatol*, 1993. **29**(4): 568–75.

7. Maffei C et al., Personality disorders and psychopathologic symptoms in patients with androgenetic alopecia. *Arch Dermatol*, 1994. **130**: 868–72.

8. Wells PA, Willmoth T, and Russel RJH, Does fortune favour the bald? Psychological correlates of hair loss in males. *Br J Psychol*, 1995. **86**: 337–44.

9. Girman CJ et al., Effects of self-perceived hair loss in a community sample of men. *Dermatology*, 1998. **197**: 223–9.

10. Budd D et al., The effects of hair loss in European men: A survey in four countries. *Eur J Dermatol*, 2000. **10**(2): 122–7.

11. Rushton DH, Androgenetic alopecia in men: The scale of the problem and prospects for treatment. *Int J Clin Pract*, 1999. **53**(1): 50–3.

12. Paschier J, Erdman J, and Hammiche F, Androgenetic alopecia: Stress of discovery. *Psychol Rep*, 2006. **98**(1): 226–8.

13. Trüeb RM, Von der hipokratischen Glatze zum "Gen-Shampoo." In *Haare—Praxis der Trichology*, Trüeb RM, Editor. 2003. Darmstadt: Steinkopff Verlag. p. 1–6.

14. Giacometti L, Facts, legends and myths about the scalp throughout history. *Arch Dermatol*, 1967. **95**: 629–31.

15. Montagna W, Phylogenetic significance of the skin of man. *Arch Dermatol*, 1963. **88**: 1–19.

16. Montagna W and Uno H, The phylogeny of baldness. In *Biopathology of Pattern Alopecia*, Baccareda-Boy A, Moretti G, and Fray JR, Editors. 1968. Basel: Karger. p. 9–24.

17. Hamilton JB, Patterned loss of hair in man; types and incidence. *Ann NY Acad Sci*, 1951. **53**: 708–28.

18. Randall VA, The use of dermal papilla cells in studies of normal and abnormal hair follicle biology. *Dermatol Clin*, 1996. **14**(4): 585–94.

19. Hibberts NA, Howell AE, and Randall VA, Balding hair follicle dermal papilla cells contain higher levels of androgen receptors than those from non-balding scalp. *J Endocrinol*, 1998. **156**(1): 59–65.

20. Randall VA, Hibberts NA, and Hamada K, A comparison of the culture and growth of dermal papilla cells from hair follicles from non-balding and balding (androgenetic alopecia) scalp. *Br J Dermatol*, 1996. **134**(3): 437–44.

21. Randall VA, Androgens and human hair growth. *Clin Endocrinol*, 1994. **40**(4): 439–57.

22. Randall VA et al., Androgen action in cultured dermal papilla cells from human hair follicles. *Skin Pharmacol Physiol*, 1994. **7**(1–2): 20–6.

23. Randall VA, Role of 5 alpha-reductase in health and disease. *Baillière's Clin Endocrinol Metab*, 1994. **8**(2): 405–31.

24. Randall VA, Thornton MJ, and Messenger AG, Cultured dermal papilla cells from androgen-dependent human hair follicles (e.g. beard) contain more androgen receptors than those from non-balding areas of scalp. *J Endocrinol*, 1992. **133**(1): 141–7.

25. Randall VA et al., Mechanism of androgen action in cultured dermal papilla cells derived from human hair follicles with varying responses to androgens in vivo. *J Invest Dermatol*, 1992. **98**(6 Suppl): 86S–91S.

26. Randall VA, Thornton MJ, and Hamada K, Androgens and the hair follicle. Cultured human dermal papilla cells as a model system. *Ann N Y Acad Sci*, 1991. **642**: 355–75.

27. Thornton MJ et al., Effect of androgens on the growth of cultured human dermal papilla cells derived from beard and scalp hair follicles. *J Invest Dermatol*, 1991. **97**(2): 345–8.

28. Randall VA, Androgens: The main regulator of human hair growth. In *Hair and Its Disorders*, Camacho FM, Randall VA, and Price VH, Editors. 2000. London: Martin Dunitz Ltd. p. 69–82.

29. Kligman AG, The human hair cycle. *J Invest Dermatol*, 1959. **33**: 307–16.

30. Randall VA and Ebling FJ, Seasonal changes in human hair growth. *Br J Dermatol*, 1991. **12**(2): 146–51.

31. Ellis JA, Sinclair R, and Harrap SB, Androgenetic alopecia: Pathogenesis and potential for therapy. *Expert Rev Mol Med*, 2002. **19**(2002): 1–11.

32. Braun-Falco O and Christophers E, Hair root patterns in male pattern alopecia. In *Biopathology of Pattern Alopecia*. 1 ed. Baccareda-Boy A, Moretti G, and Fray JR, Editors. 1968. Basel: Karger. p. 141–5.

33. Rushton DH, Ramsay ID, and Norris MJ, Natural progression of male pattern baldness in young men. *Clin Exper Dermatol*, 1991. **16**: 188–92.

34. Courtois M, Loussouarn G, and Hourseau S, Hair cycle and alopecia. *Skin Pharmacol Physiol*, 1994. **7**(1–2): 84–9.

35. Chumlea WC, Rhodes T, and Girman CJ, Family history and risk of hair loss. *Dermatology*, 2004. **209**(1): 33–9.

36. Bergfeld WF, Androgenetic alopecia: An autosomal dominant disorder. *Am J Med*, 1995. **98**(1A): 95S–8S.

37. Carey AH, Chan KL, and Short F, Evidence for a single gene effect causing polycystic ovaries and male pattern baldness. *Clin Endocrinol*, 1993. **38**(6): 653–8.

38. Kuster W and Happle R, The inheritance of common baldness: Two B or not two B? *J Am Acad Dermatol*, 1984. **11**(5 Pt 1): 921–6.

39. Carey AH, Waterworth D, and Patel K, Polycystic ovaries and premature male pattern baldness are associated with one allele of the steroid metabolism gene CYP17. *Hum Mol Genet*, 1994. **3**(10): 1873–6.

40. Panchaprateep R and Asawanonda P, Insulin-like growth factor-1: Roles in androgenetic alopecia. *Exp Dermatol*, 2014. **23**(3): 216–8.

41. Morton CC et al., Human genes for insulin-like growth factors I and II and epidermal growth factor are located on 12q22—q24.1, 11p15, and 4q25—q27, respectively. *Cytogenet Cell Genet*, 1986. **41**(4): 245–9.

42. Imperato-McGinley J, 5Alpha-reductase-2 deficiency and complete androgen insensitivity: Lessons from nature. *Adv Exp Med Biol*, 2002. **511**: 121–31.

43. Ellis JA, Stebbing M, and Harrap SB, Genetic analysis of male pattern baldness and the 5alpha-reductase genes. *J Invest Dermatol*, 1998. **110**(6): 849–53.

44. Axt-Gadermann M, Schlichting M, and Kuster W, Male-pattern baldness is common in men with X-linked recessive ichthyosis. *Dermatology*, 2003. **207**(3): 308–9.

45. Garton RA et al., Association of a polymorphism in the ornithine decarboxylase gene with male androgenetic alopecia. *J Am Acad Dermatol*, 2005. **52**(3 Pt 1): 535–6.

46. Konig A et al., An X-linked gene involved in androgenetic alopecia: A lesson to be learned from adrenoleukodystrophy. *Dermatology*, 2000. **200**(3): 213–8.

47. Hillmer AM et al., Susceptibility variants for male-pattern baldness on chromosome 20p11. *Nat Genet*, 2008. **40**(11): 1279–81.

48. Li R et al., Six novel susceptibility loci for early-onset androgenetic alopecia and their unexpected association with common diseases. *PLoS Genet*, 2012. **8**(5): e1002746.

49. Liang B et al., Genetic variants at 20p11 confer risk to androgenetic alopecia in the Chinese Han population. *PLoS One*, 2013. 26;**8**(8): e71771.

50. Ellis JA, Stebbing M, and Harrap SB, Polymorphism of the androgen receptor gene is associated with male pattern baldness. *J Invest Dermatol*, 2001. **116**(3): 452–5.

51. Hillmer AM et al., Genetic variation in the human androgen receptor gene is the major determinant of common early-onset androgenetic alopecia. *Am J Hum Genet*, 2005. **77**(1): 140–8.

52. Hamilton JB, Male hormone stimulation is a prerequisite and an incitant in common baldness. *Am J Anat*, 1942. **71**: 451.

53. Hamilton JB, The role of testosterone secretion as indicated by the effect of castration in man and by studies of pathological conditions and the short life-span associated with maleness. *Recent Prog Horm Res*, 1948. **3**: 257.

54. Simpson NB and Barth JH, Hair patterns: Hirsuties and androgenetic alopecia. In *Diseases of the Hair and Scalp*. 3 ed. Dawber R, Editor. 1997. Oxford: Blackwell Science Ltd. p. 101–21.

55. Severi G, Sinclair R, and Hopper JL, Androgenetic alopecia in men aged 40-69 years: Prevalence and risk factors. *Br J Dermatol*, 2003. **149**(6): 1207–13.

56. Sawaya ME, Androgen metabolism in androgenetic alopecia. In *Trichology. Diseases of the Pilosebaceous Follicle*. 1 ed. Camacho F and Montagna W, Editors. 1997. Madrid: Aula Medica Group. p. 317–23.

57. Zouboulis CC and Degitz K, Androgen action on human skin—From basic research to clinical significance. *Exp Dermatol*, 2004. **13**(Suppl 4): 5–10.

58. Fritsch M, Orfanos CE, and Zouboulis CC, Sebocytes are the key regulators of androgen homeostasis in human skin. *J Invest Dermatol*, 2001. **116**(5): 793–800.

59. Chen W, Thiboutot D, and Zouboulis CC, Cutaneous androgen metabolism: Basic research and clinical perspectives. *J Invest Dermatol*, 2002. **119**(5): 992–1007.

60. Courchay G, Boyera N, and Bernard BA, Messenger RNA expression of steroidogenesis enzyme subtypes in the human pilosebaceous unit. *Skin Pharmacol Physiol*, 1996. **9**(3): 169–76.

61. Itami S, Kurata S, and Takayasu S, 5Alpha-reductase activity in cultured human dermal papilla cells from beard compared with reticular dermal fibroblasts. *J Invest Dermatol*, 1990. **94**(1): 150–2.

62. Itami S, Kurata S, and Sonoda T, Mechanism of action of androgen in dermal papilla cells. *Ann N Y Acad Sci*, 1991. **642**: 385–95.

63. Harris G, Azzolina B, and Baginsky W, Identification and selective inhibition of an isozyme of steroid 5 alpha-reductase in human scalp. *Proc Natl Acad Sci U S A*, 1992. **89**(22): 1087–91.

64. Grino PB, Griffin JE, and Wilson JD, Testosterone at high concentrations interacts with the human androgen receptor similarly to dihydrotestosterone. *Endocrinology*, 1990. **126**(2): 1165–72.

65. Cunliffe WJ and Bottomley WW, Antiandrogens and acne. A topical approach? *Arch Dermatol*, 1992. **128**(9): 1261–4.

66. Cusan L, Dupont A, and Belanger A, Treatment of hirsutism with the pure antiandrogen flutamide. *J Am Acad Dermatol*, 1990. **23**(3 Pt 1): 462–9.

67. Vigersky RA, Mehlman I, and Glass AR, Treatment of hirsute women with cimetidine. *N Engl J Med*, 1980. **303**(18): 1042.

68. Kidwai BJ and George M, Hair loss with minoxidil withdrawal. *Lancet*, 1992. **340**(8819): 609–10.

69. Sawaya ME and Hordinsky MK, Advances in alopecia areata and androgenetic alopecia. *Adv Dermatol*, 1992. **7**: 211–26.

70. Cheung-Flynn J, Prapapanich V, and Cox MB, Physiological role for the cochaperone FKBP52 in androgen receptor signaling. *Mol Endocrinol*, 2005. **19**(6): 1654–66.

71. Hoffmann R, Male androgenetic alopecia. *Clin Exp Dermatol*, 2002. **27**(5): 373–82.

72. Hoffmann R, Androgenetische Alopezie. Der Hautarzt, 2004. **55**: 89–111.

73. Peleg S, Schrader WT, and O'Malley BW, Sulfhydryl group content of chicken progesterone receptor: Effect of oxidation on DNA binding activity. *Biochemistry*, 1988. **27**(1): 358–67.

74. Cumming DC, Yang JC, and Rebar RW, Treatment of hirsutism with spironolactone. *J Am Med Assoc*, 1982. **247**(9): 1295–8.

75. Frieden IJ and Price VH, Androgenetic alopecia. In *Pathogenesis of Skin Disease*. 1 ed. Thiers BH and Dobson RL, Editors. 1989. New York: Churchill Livingstone. p. 41–9.

76. Hatch R et al., Hirsutism: Implications, etiology, and management. *Am J Obstet Gynecol*, 1981. **140**(7): 815–30.

77. Vexiau P et al., Role of androgens in female-pattern androgenetic alopecia, either alone or associated with other symptoms of hyperandrogenism. *Arch Dermatol Res*, 2000. **292**(12): 598–604.

78. Kasick JM et al., Adrenal androgenic female-pattern alopecia: Sex hormones and the balding woman. *Cleve Clin Q*, 1983. **50**(2): 111–22.

79. Futterweit W et al., The prevalence of hyperandrogenism in 109 consecutive female patients with diffuse alopecia. *J Am Acad Dermatol*, 1988. **19**(5 Pt 1): 831–6.

80. Miller JA et al., Low sex-hormone binding globulin levels in young women with diffuse hair loss. *Br J Dermatol*, 1982. **106**(3): 331–6.

81. Montalto J et al., Plasma C19 steroid sulphate levels and indices of androgen bioavailability in female pattern androgenic alopecia. *Clin Endocrinol*, 1990. **32**(1): 1–12.

82. Giagulli VA et al., Precursors of plasma androstanediol- and androgen-glucuronides in women. *J Steroid Biochem*, 1989. **33**(5): 935–40.

83. Vermeulen A et al., Hormonal effects of an orally active 4-azasteroid inhibitor of 5 alpha-reductase in humans. *Prostate*, 1989. **14**(1): 45–53.

84. Gormley GJ et al., Effects of finasteride (MK-906), a 5 alpha-reductase inhibitor, on circulating androgens in male volunteers. *J Clin Endocrinol Metab*, 1990. **70**(4): 1136–41.

85. Herrera CRD et al., Baldness and coronary heart disease rates in men from the Framingham Study. *Am J Epidemiol*, 1995. **142**(8): 828–33.

86. Lotufo PA et al., Male pattern baldness and coronary heart disease: The Physicians' Health Study. *Arch Intern Med*, 2000. **160**(2): 165–71.

87. Matilainen VA, Makinen PK, and Keinanen-Kiukaanniemi SM, Early onset of androgenetic alopecia associated with early severe coronary heart disease: A population-based, case-control study. *J Cardiovasc Risk*, 2001. **8**(3): 147–51.

88. Matilainen V, Koskela P, and Keinanen-Kiukaanniemi SM, Early androgenetic alopecia as a marker of insulin resistance. *Lancet*, 2000. **356**(9236): 1165–6.

89. Hawk E, Breslow RA, and Graubard BI, Male pattern baldness and clinical prostate cancer in the epidemiologic follow-up of the First National Health and Nutrition Examination Survey. *Cancer Epidemiol Biomarkers Prev*, 2000. **9**: 523–7.

90. Giles GG et al., Androgenetic alopecia and prostate cancer: Findings from an Australian case-control study. *Cancer Epidemiol Biomarkers Prev*, 2002. **11**(6): 549–53.

91. Proctor PH, Hair-raising. The latest news on male-pattern baldness. *Adv Nurse Pract*, 1999. **7**(4): 39–42, 83.

92. Blumeyer A et al., Evidence-based (S3) guideline for the treatment of androgenetic alopecia in women and in men. *J Dtsch Dermatol Ges*, 2011. **9**(6 Suppl): S1–57.

93. Hamilton JB, Patterned loss of hair in man; types and incidence. *P Ann NY Acad Sci*, 1951. **53**: 708–28.

94. Takashima I, Iju M, and Sudo M, Alopecia androgenetica—Its incidence in Japanese and associated conditions. In *Hair Research Status and Future Aspects*, Orfanos CE, Montagna W, and Stuttgen G, Editors. 1981. New York: Springer Verlag. p. 287–93.

95. Tang PH et al., A community study of male androgenetic alopecia in Bishan, Singapore. *Singapore Med J*, 2000. **41**(5): 202–5.

96. Paik JH et al., The prevalence and types of androgenetic alopecia in Korean men and women. *Br J Dermatol*, 2001. **145**(1): 95–9.

97. Pathomvanich D, Thienthaworn P, and Manoshai S, A random study of Asian male androgenetic alopecia in Bangkok, Thailand. *Dermatol Surg*, 2002. **28**(9): 804–7.

98. Setty LR, Hair pattern of the scalp of white and Negro males. *Am J Phys Anthropol*, 1970. **33**: 49–55.

99. Orfanos CE, Androgenetic alopecia: Clinical aspects and treatment. In *Hair and Hair Diseases*, Orfanos CE, Editor. 1990. Berlin: Springer-Verlag. p. 485–527.

100. Salamon T, Genetic factors in male pattern alopecia. In *Biopathology of Pattern Alopecia*, Baccaredda-Boy GMA and Frey JR, Editors. 1968. New York: Karger. p. 39–49.

101. Norwood OTT, Male-pattern baldness. Classification and incidence. *South Med J*, 1975. **68**: 1359–70.

102. Norwood OT and Lehr B, Female androgenetic alopecia: A separate entity. *Dermatol Surg*, 2000. **26**(7): 679–82.

103. Ebling FJ and Rook A, Male-pattern alopecia. In *Textbook of Dermatology*. 2 ed. Rook A, Wilkinson FS, and Ebling FJ, Editors. 1972. Oxford: Blackwell Science. p. 49–66.

104. Camacho F and Montagna W, Current concept and classification. Male androgenetic alopecia. In *Trichology*, Camacho F and Montagna W, Editors. 1997. Madrid: Aula Medica Group. p. 328–9.

105. Keene S and Goren A, Therapeutic hotline. Genetic variations in the androgen receptor gene and finasteride response in women with androgenetic alopecia mediated by epigenetics. *Dermatol Ther*, 2011. **24**(2): 296–300.

106. Kaufman KD, Androgen metabolism as it affects hair growth in androgenetic alopecia. *Dermatol Clin*, 1996. **14**(4): 697–711.

107. Kaufman KD, Olsen EA, and Whiting D, Finasteride in the treatment of men with androgenetic alopecia. Finasteride Male Pattern Hair Loss Study Group. *J Am Acad Dermatol*, 1998. **39**(4 Pt 1): 578–89.

108. Gormley GJ, Stoner E, and Bruskewitz RC, The effect of finasteride in men with benign prostatic hyperplasia. The Finasteride Study Group [see comments]. *New Engl J Med*, 1992. **327**(17): 1185–91.

109. Stoner E, The clinical development of a 5 alpha-reductase inhibitor, finasteride. *J Steroid Biochem Mol Biol*, 1990. **37**(3): 375–8.

110. Drake L, Hordinsky M, and Fiedler V, The effects of finasteride on scalp skin and serum

androgen levels in men with androgenetic alopecia. *J Am Acad Dermatol*, 1999. **41**(4): 550–4.

111. Roberts J, Clinical dose ranging studies with finasteride, a type 2 5alpha reductase inhibitor in men with male pattern hair loss. *J Am Acad Dermatol*, 1999. **41**(4): 555–63.

112. Sawaya ME, Novel agents for the treatment of alopecia. *Semin Cutan Med Surg*, 1998. **17**(4): 276–83.

113. Monography CPA, Minoxidil and finasteride. In *Compendium of Pharmaceuticals and Specialties* (CPS). 34 ed. 1999. Ottawa.

114. Leyden J, Dunlap F, and Miller B, Finasteride in the treatment of men with frontal male pattern hair loss [see comments]. *J Am Acad Dermatol*, 1999. **40**(6 Pt 1): 930–7.

115. Gupta AK and Charrette A, The efficacy and safety of 5α-reductase inhibitors in androgenetic alopecia: A network meta-analysis and benefit-risk assessment of finasteride and dutasteride. *J Dermatolog Treat*, 2014. **25**(2): 156–61.

116. Mella JM et al., Efficacy and safety of finasteride therapy for androgenetic alopecia: A systematic review. *Arch Dermatol*, 2010. **146**: 1141–50.

117. Price VH, Treatment of hair loss. *New Engl J Med*, 1999. **341**(13): 964–73.

118. Overstreet JW, Fuh VL, and Gould J, Chronic treatment with finasteride daily does not affect spermatogenesis or semen production in young men. *J Urol*, 1999. **162**(4): 1295–300.

119. Tu HY and Zini A, Finasteride-induced secondary infertility associated with sperm DNA damage. *Fertil Steril*, 2011. **95**(2125): e13–4.

120. Chiba K et al., Finasteride-associated male infertility. *Fertil Steril*, 2011. **95**(1786): e9–11.

121. Collodel G, Scapigliati G, and Moretti E, Spermatozoa and chronic treatment with finasteride: A TEM and FISH study. *Arch Androl*, 2007. **53**: 229–33.

122. Mysore V, Finasteride and sexual side effects. *Indian Dermatol Online J*, 2012. **3**(1): 62–5.

123. Matzkin H, Barak M, and Braf Z, Effect of finasteride on free and total serum prostate-specific antigen in men with benign prostatic hyperplasia. *Br J Urol*, 1996. **78**(3): 405–8.

124. Irwig MS and Kolukula S, Persistent sexual side effects of finasteride for male pattern hair loss. *J Sex Med*, 2011. **8**: 1747–53.

125. Traish AM et al., Adverse side effects of 5α-reductase inhibitors therapy: Persistent diminished libido and erectile dysfunction and depression in a subset of patients. *J Sex Med*, 2011. **8**: 872–84.

126. Ganzer CA, Jacobs AR, and Iqbal F, Persistent sexual, emotional, and cognitive impairment post finasteride: A survey of men reporting symptoms. *Am J Mens Health*, 2014. Jun 13. pii: 1557988314538445. [Epub ahead of print].

127. Baden HP and Kubilus J, Effect of minoxidil on cultured keratinocytes. *J Invest Dermatol*, 1983. **81**(6): 558–60.

128. Cohen RL et al., Direct effects of minoxidil on epidermal cells in culture. *J Invest Dermatol*, 1984. **82**(1): 90–3.

129. Kurata S, Uno H, and Allen-Hoffmann BL, Effects of hypertrichotic agents on follicular and nonfollicular cells in vitro. *Skin Pharmacol Physiol*, 1996. **9**(1): 3–8.

130. Goren A et al., Clinical utility and validity of minoxidil response testing in androgenetic alopecia. *Dermatol Ther*, 2014. Aug 12. doi: 10.1111/dth.12164. [Epub ahead of print].

131. Goren A et al., Novel enzymatic assay predicts minoxidil response in the treatment of androgenetic alopecia. *Dermatol Ther*, 2014. **27**(3): 171–3.

132. Mirmirani P et al., Similar response patterns to 5% topical minoxidil foam in frontal and vertex scalp of men with androgenetic alopecia: A microarray analysis. *Br J Dermatol*, 2014. Sep 10. doi: 10.1111/bjd.13399. [Epub ahead of print].

133. Jung JY et al., Effect of dutasteride 0.5 mg/d in men with androgenetic alopecia recalcitrant to finasteride. *Int J Dermatol*, 2014. Jun 5. doi: 10.1111/ijd.12060. [Epub ahead of print].

134. Wu XJ et al., Dutasteride on benign prostatic hyperplasia: A meta-analysis on randomized clinical trials in 6460 patients. *Urology*, 2014. **83**(3): 539–43.

135. Amory JK et al., The effect of 5alpha-reductase inhibition with dutasteride and finasteride on semen parameters and serum hormones in healthy men. *J Clin Endocrinol Metab*, 2007. **92**(5): 1659–65.

136. Bird ST et al., Male breast cancer and 5α-reductase inhibitors finasteride and dutasteride. *J Urol*, 2013. **190**(5): 1811–4.

137. Beer KR et al., Treatment of eyebrow hypotrichosis using bimatoprost: A randomized, double-blind, vehicle-controlled pilot study. *Dermatol Surg*, 2013. **39**(7): 1079–87.

138. Blume-Peytavi U et al., A randomized double-blind placebo-controlled pilot study to assess the efficacy of a 24-week topical treatment by latanoprost 0.1% on hair growth and pigmentation in healthy volunteers with androgenetic alopecia. *J Am Acad Dermatol*, 2012. **66**(5): 794–800.

139. Levy LL and Emer JJ, Female pattern alopecia: Current perspectives. *Int J Womens Health*, 2013. **5**: 541–56.

140. Piérard-Franchimont C et al., Ketoconazole shampoo: Effect of long-term use in androgenic alopecia. *Dermatology*, 1998. **196**(4): 474–7.

141. Debruyne FM and Witjes FA, Ketoconazole high dose (HD) in the management of hormonally pretreated patients with progressive metastatic prostate cancer. *Prog Clin Biol Res*, 1987. **243A**: 301–13.

142. Khandpur S, Suman M, and Reddy BS, Comparative efficacy of various treatment regimens for androgenetic alopecia in men. *J Dermatol*, 2002. **29**(8): 489–98.

143. Bernstein EF, Hair growth induced by diode laser treatment. *Dermatol Surg*, 2005. **31**(5): 584–6.

144. Rangwala S and Rashid RM, Alopecia: A review of laser and light therapies. *Dermatol Online J*, 2012. **18**(2): 3.

145. Munck A, Gavazzoni MF, and Trüeb RM, Use of low-level laser therapy as monotherapy or concomitant therapy for male and female androgenetic alopecia. *Int J Trichology*, 2014. **6**(2): 45–9.

146. Olsen EA, Pattern hair loss in men and women. In *Disorders of Hair Growth. Diagnosis and Treatment*. 2 ed. Olsen EA, Editor. 2003. Barcelona: McGraw-Hill Companies, Inc. p. 321–62.

147. Tosti A, Iorizzo M, and Piraccini BM, Androgenetic alopecia in children: Report of 20 cases. *Br J Dermatol*, 2005. **152**(3): 556–9.

148. Birch MP, Lalla SC, and Messenger AG, Female pattern hair loss. *Clin Exp Dermatol*, 2002. **27**(5): 383–8.

149. Ludwig E, Classification of the types of androgenetic alopecia (common baldness) occurring in the female sex. *Br J Dermatol*, 1977. **97**(3): 247–54.

150. Venning VA and Dawber RP, Patterned androgenic alopecia in women. *J Am Acad Dermatol*, 1988. **18**(5 Pt 1): 1073–7.

151. Olsen EA, Female pattern hair loss. *J Am Acad Dermatol*, 2001. **45**(3 Suppl): S70–80.

152. Shapiro J, Clinical practice. Hair loss in women. *N Engl J Med*, 2007. **357**(16): 1620–30.

153. DeVillez RL et al., Androgenetic alopecia in the female. Treatment with 2% topical minoxidil solution. *Arch Dermatol*, 1994. **130**(3): 303–7.

154. Whiting DA and Jacobson C, Treatment of female androgenetic alopecia with minoxidil 2%. *Int J Dermatol*, 1992. **31**(11): 800–4.

155. Blume-Peytavi U et al., A randomized, single-blind trial of 5% minoxidil foam once daily versus 2% minoxidil solution twice daily in the treatment of androgenetic alopecia in women. *J Am Acad Dermatol*, 2011. **65**(6): 1126–34.

156. Lucky AW et al., A randomized, placebo-controlled trial of 5% and 2% topical minoxidil solutions in the treatment of female pattern hair loss. *J Am Acad Dermatol*, 2004. **50**(4): 541–53.

157. Clissold SP and Heel RC, Topical minoxidil. A preliminary review of its pharmacodynamic properties and therapeutic efficacy in alopecia areata and alopecia androgenetica. *Drugs*, 1987. **33**(2): 107–22.

158. Stern RS, Topical minoxidil. A survey of use and complications. *Arch Dermatol*, 1987. **123**(1): 62–5.

159. Rietschel RL and Duncan SH, Safety and efficacy of topical minoxidil in the management of androgenetic alopecia. *J Am Acad Dermatol*, 1987. **16**(3 Pt 2): 677–85.

160. Price VH et al., Lack of efficacy of finasteride in postmenopausal women with androgenetic alopecia. *J Am Acad Dermatol*, 2000. **43**(5 Pt 1): 768–76.

161. Camacho FM, SAHA syndrome: Female androgenetic alopecia and hirsutism. *Exp Dermatol*, 1999. **8**(4): 304–5.

162. Thai KE and Sinclair RD, Finasteride for female androgenetic alopecia. *Br J Dermatol*, 2002. **147**(4): 812–3.

163. Trüeb RM, Finasteride treatment of patterned hair loss in normoandrogenic postmeno-pausal women. Swiss Trichology Study Group. *Dermatology*, 2004. **209**(3): 202–7.

164. Iorizzo M et al., Finasteride treatment of female pattern hair loss. *Arch Dermatol*, 2006. **142**(3): 298–302.

165. Camacho-Martinez FM, Hair loss in women. *Semin Cutan Med Surg*, 2009. **28**(1): 19–32.

166. Stout SM and Stumpf JL, Finasteride treatment of hair loss in women. *Ann Pharmacother*, 2010. **44**(6): 1090–7.

167. Shapiro J and Price VH, Hair regrowth. Therapeutic agents. *Dermatol Clin*, 1998. **16**(2): 341–56.

168. Roehrborn CG et al., Efficacy and safety of a dual inhibitor of 5-alpha-reductase types 1 and 2 (dutasteride) in men with benign pros-tatic hyperplasia. *Urology*, 2002. **60**(3): 434–41.

169. Olszewska M and Rudnicka L, Effective treatment of female androgenic alopecia with dutasteride. *J Drugs Dermatol*, 2005. **4**(5): 637–40.

170. Moftah N et al., Mesotherapy using dutasteride-containing preparation in treatment of female pattern hair loss: Photographic, morphometric and ultrustruc-tural evaluation. *J Eur Acad Dermatol Venereol*, 2013. **27**(6): 686–93.

171. Carmina E and Lobo RA, Treatment of hyperandrogenic alopecia in women. *Fertil Steril*, 2003. **79**(1): 91–5.

172. Karrer-Voegeli S et al., Androgen depen-dence of hirsutism, acne, and alopecia in women: Retrospective analysis of 228 patients investigated for hyperandrogen-ism. *Medicine (Baltimore)*, 2009. **88**(1): 32–45.

173. Sinclair R, Wewerinke M, and Jolley D, Treatment of female pattern hair loss with oral antiandrogens. *Br J Dermatol*, 2005. **152**(3): 466–73.

174. Vexiau P et al., Effects of minoxidil 2% vs. cyproterone acetate treatment on female androgenetic alopecia: A controlled, 12-month randomized trial. *Br J Dermatol*, 2002. **146**(6): 992–9.

175. Rathnayake D and Sinclair R, Use of spirono-lactone in dermatology. *Skinmed*, 2010. **8**(6): 328–32.

176. Shapiro J and Price VH, Hair regrowth. Therapeutic agents. *Dermatol Clin*, 1998. **16**(2): 341–56.

177. Orfanos CE and Vogels L, Local therapy of androgenetic alopecia with 17 alpha-estradiol. A controlled, randomized double-blind study (author's transl). *Dermatologica*, 1980. **161**(2): 124–32.

178. Hoffmann R et al., 17Alpha-estradiol induces aromatase activity in intact human anagen hair follicles ex vivo. *Exp Dermatol*, 2002. **11**(4): 376–80.

179. Niiyama S, Happle R, and Hoffmann R, Influence of estrogens on the androgen metabolism in different subunits of human hair follicles. *Eur J Dermatol*, 2001. **11**(3): 195–8.

180. Kim JH et al., The efficacy and safety of 17α-estradiol (Ell-Cranell® alpha 0.025%) solution on female pattern hair loss: Single center, open-label, non-comparative, phase IV study. *Ann Dermatol*, 2012. **24**(3): 295–305.

181. Rossi A et al., Aromatase inhibitors induce "male pattern hair loss" in women? *Ann Oncol*, 2013. **24**(6): 1710–1.

182. Emer JJ, Stevenson ML, and Markowitz O, Novel treatment of female-pattern andro-genetic alopecia with injected bimatoprost 0.03% solution. *J Drugs Dermatol*, 2011. **10**(7): 795–8.

183. Whiting DA, Scalp biopsy as a diagnostic tool in androgenetic alopecia. *Dermatol Ther*, 1998. **8**: 24–33.

184. Whiting DA, Diagnostic and predictive value of horizontal sections of scalp biopsy specimens in male pattern androgenetic alopecia. *J Am Acad Dermatol*, 1993. **28**(5 Pt 1): 755–63.

185. Headington JT, Transverse microscopic anat-omy of the human scalp. A basis for a mor-phometric approach to disorders of the hair follicle. *Arch Dermatol*, 1984. **120**(4): 449–56.

3 Telogen effluvium: Pathogenesis, clinical features, diagnosis, and management

Telogen effluvium (TE) together with female pattern hair loss is the most common diagnosis in women in the everyday hair clinic. TE is characterized by abrupt shedding of hair on the entire scalp as a result of an early, synchronous entry of hair follicles (>20%) into the telogen phase. Follicles that would normally complete a longer cycle by remaining in anagen phase prematurely enter telogen and are subsequently shed 2–3 months after the initiating event. TE is far more common in women compared to men. TE can be caused by numerous trigger factors and systemic disturbances such as fever, childbirth, crash diets, thyroid dysfunction, iron deficiency, prolonged anesthesia, chronic illness, and psychological stress/trauma.

Headington divided TE into five functional types [1]:

1. Immediate anagen release
2. Delayed anagen release
3. Short anagen
4. Immediate telogen release
5. Delayed telogen release

The most common cause of TE is an immediate anagen release (IAR). In this case, the initiating trigger factor prematurely switches off the anagen phase, which leads to the induction of catagen through terminal differentiation and apoptosis. Catagen and telogen follow its natural course. As a result, shedding becomes obvious 3–4 months after the initiating event, after the full completion of catagen and anagen. This type of TE is often caused by high fever, crash diets, thyroid dysfunction surgery, and drugs.

A delayed anagen release (DAR) occurs after a synchronous switch from a prolonged anagen phase to catagen and telogen. Prolonged anagen can be found in the second and third trimester of pregnancy or during the use of trichogenic substances such as minoxidil. Once the anagen-prolonging stimulus is detracted (after child birth or after discontinuation of the trichogenic drug) a high percentage of hair follicles enter the catagen phase, followed by telogen. Like in IAR, catagen and telogen follow their natural course and shedding starts 3–4 months after the withdrawal of the anagen-prolonging stimulus.

Short anagen (SA) is characterized by a persistent mild shedding in combination with a relatively short length of hair. The existence of SA syndrome has been postulated. SA phases have been found in patients with trichodental dysplasia and forms of hereditary hypotrichosis [2–5].

An immediate telogen release (ITR) can be regarded as an early induction of exogen and shortening of the telogen phase. This phenomenon occurs, for example, after starting topical minoxidil [6].

Delayed telogen release (DTR) is a phenomenon that is observed in mammals when they shed their winter coat in spring after a prolonged telogen phase during the cold season. Even though humans have an asynchronous hair cycle, climatic and seasonal changes may cause a prolonged telogen phase with a subsequent shedding as soon as the climatic conditions change [1].

Anagen effluvium

Anagen effluvium is a result of a disturbance of hair follicle matrix cells. The anagen phase is interrupted and the hair falls out 7–14 days after the initiating event without entering catagen or telogen. Two different types of anagen effluvium can be distinguished: (1) Dystrophic anagen effluvium, which can be caused by chemotherapy, radiation, toxins, or alopecia areata, and (2) IAR. Microscopic investigation of the hair bulbs, obtained from a hair pull test or trichogram, usually shows a tapered tip where the weakened hair shaft is broken shortly above the bulb (dystrophic hair) [7].

Immediate anagen hair release is characterized by an easy release of anagen hairs after gentle pulling. The anagen hair has a broom-shaped, pigmented bulb. In loose anagen hair syndrome, a condition that occurs in childhood as well as in AIDS-related trichopathy, the pulled anagen hairs are devoid of the inner and outer root sheath [8]. In the European literature, this presentation has been referred to as dysplastic anagen hair. Normal-appearing anagen hair with inner and outer root sheath can be found to some extent in every anagen effluvium, but especially in bullous dermatosis of the scalp with sub- or intraepidermal blisters.

Once the initiating trigger is removed, the hair usually regrows after around 120 days. Cases of incomplete recovery following multiagent chemotherapy have been reported [7].

Patients should be advised about scalp prostheses and other forms of headdresses.

Acute telogen effluvium

Pathogenesis

There are multiple possible pathogenetic factors leading to acute TE.

Thyroid influences

There is no consistent correlation between the degree and duration of hypothyroidism and the severity of hair loss [9]. Diffuse alopecia may sometimes be the first or only cutaneous sign of hypothyroidism [10]. A thorough history regarding weight gain, cold tolerance, and energy level is important. Patients usually respond to thyroxine replacement [11] unless the problem has been of very long duration and some follicles have atrophied. Severe thyrotoxicosis can also cause diffuse alopecia of the scalp [12].

Iron deficiency

Iron deficiency with or without anemia has been reported to be present in as many as 72% of women with diffuse alopecia [13]. Iron deficiency even in the absence of anemia (low hemoglobin) has also been reported by Hard [14]. Because androgenetic alopecia (AGA) and iron deficiency are both common conditions in women, the two occur together frequently. It is possible that TE from iron deficiency may unmask underlying AGA [15]. Table 3.1 shows possible etiological factors of iron deficiency.

Fever

Fever can cause an immediate anagen arrest followed by massive shedding 8–16 weeks after the bout. Hair loss can be quite severe, but is never total; usually not more than 30% of hair follicles are affected by IAR. TE after a fever episode is usually completely reversible.

Fever, which augments metabolic demands, would probably impair the ability of the rapidly multiplying follicular matrix cells to proliferate normally [16]. Endogenous pyrogens, such as interferons α and γ, may slow down matrix proliferation [16]. Interferons α and γ have been shown to decrease epithelial proliferation and to affect follicular matrix cells directly [17,18].

Postpartum

During pregnancy, anagen is prolonged, and, as a result, percentages of anagen hairs increase during pregnancy from 84% in the first trimester to 94% in the final trimester [19,20]. After parturition, there is a DAR, as described by Headington [1]; not every follicle is involved, therefore, the alopecia is never complete. Increased hair loss may occur 1–4 months after childbirth, and may continue for several months [21,22]. There may be aggravating factors, such as psychophysical trauma, blood loss, and low plasma protein. Postpartum TE usually fully recovers in 4–12 months unless there is an underlying AGA that can be treated after breast-feeding [9,22] (Figure 3.1).

Major interventions and prolonged anesthesia

Blood loss and surgery with prolonged anesthesia may cause TE [23,24] (Figure 3.2). Desai

Table 3.1

Decreased Iron Intake	Decreased Iron Absorption	Increased Iron Needs

Lack of iron sources in the diet
 	
 • Crash diets
 • Unbalanced vegetarian or vegan diets
	• Stomach and intestinal conditions
	 • Overdose of antacids
	 • Genetically slow iron resorbtion
		• Pregnancy
		 • Blood loss
		   • Heavy menstrual periods
		   • Frequent blood donation
		 • Stomach and intestinal conditions
		 • Parasites (hookworm)
		 • Rapid growth

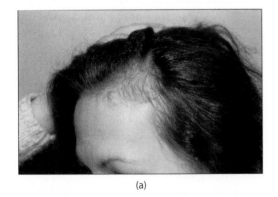

(a)

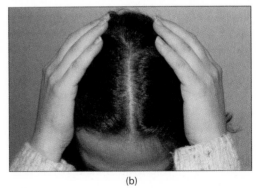

(b)

Figure 3.1

30-year-old female patient presenting with a 1-month history of abrupt diffuse hair shedding commencing 6 weeks after the birth of her last child. (a) Side view, showing frontotemporal thinning; (b) top view, showing a widening of the central part.

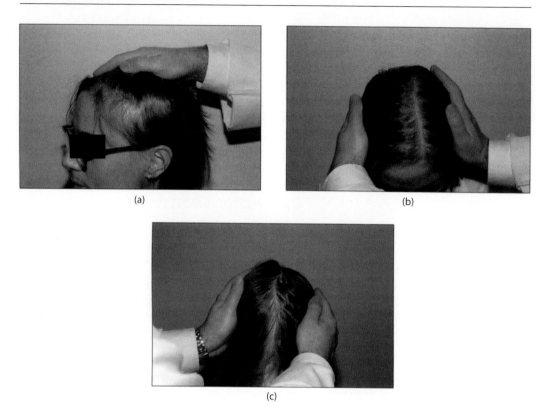

Figure 3.2
35-year-old female with a 6-week history of abrupt diffuse hair shedding commencing
8 weeks after bowel surgery. (a) Side view, showing marked thinning; (b) top view, showing
thinning of the central part; (c) occipital view, displaying a significant widening of the
parting.

and Roaf reported TE in a patient after prolonged surgery, with regrowth after 4 months [25]. This is clearly different from the patchy alopecia occurring after localized pressure from surgery [26].

Malignant disease, renal failure, hepatic disease, and malabsorption

TE may be caused by a number of systemic diseases. Hodgkin's disease may present with TE as its first sign [27]. This kind of hair loss is also referred to as "toxic telogen effluvium" [23]. In patients with chronic renal disease, scalp hair can become dry, brittle, and sparse. There may be shedding of scalp hair and in some cases thinning of body hair, including pubic or axillary hair [28,29].

Hepatic disease has been reported to be associated with diffuse alopecia. Zaun studied 53 patients who had either hepatitis, cirrhosis, or fatty liver [30]. He found increased telogen counts in 34 patients and evident hair loss in 11. The liver is the major site of amino acid interconversion. It has been suggested that disturbed liver metabolism of cystine and methionine may be related to alopecia [30].

When sparse hair and growth retardation are associated with chronic frequent loose, pale, and bulky stools, malabsorption should be investigated [9]. Inflammatory bowel disease has been reported to be associated with hair loss, particularly with Crohn's disease [31].

Crash dieting/hypoproteinemia

The primary form of protein malnutrition is most common in developing countries. In 2012, an estimated 17%, or 97 million children under 5 years of age in developing countries were underweight (Global Health Observatory, WHO 2012). In children, two different types due to protein malnutrition can be distinguished. Kwashiorkor is a severe form of protein–energy malnutrition. It is characterized by edema, irritability, anorexia, ulcerating dermatoses, sparse and depigmented hair and an enlarged liver with fatty infiltrates. Marasmus is defined as extreme weight loss and thinness due to a loss of subcutaneous fat and muscle throughout the body. Typical skin and hair changes due to protein malnutrition include scaly and dry skin, pigment changes in hair, decrease in hair thickness, and hair loss [8].

Malnutrition caused by unhealthy diets and rapid weight loss due to very low calorie diets (<1000 calories daily) can often cause immediate anagen arrest followed by TE. Eating disorders such as anorexia and bulimia are not uncommon. Obese adolescents sometimes inflict on themselves a diet of salads and fruits lacking in protein. This also can lead to hair loss. Rooth and Carlstrom noted hair loss, edemas, and weakness in 20 obese patients on a 200 calorie diet or on a total fast; these changes could be prevented by the addition of a small amount of protein [32].

Vitamin D

1,25-dihydroxyvitamin D3 and the vitamin D receptor (VDR) are involved in regulating skin biology. Studies using cultured keratinocytes, artificial human skin, and transgenic mouse models, as well as observations in patients with rickets, provide evidence of this pathway's importance in epidermal proliferation and differentiation and the hair growth cycle [15,33–35]. There is currently no evidence-based data to recommend vitamin D supplementation for various types of alopecia, but as vitamin D deficiency may contribute to the development of TE, serum levels should be checked in every patient with diffuse thinning and supplementation should be submitted if the levels are below normal.

Vitamin A

Vitamin A hypervitaminosis at a dose of over 50,000 IE daily can cause diffuse TE. An analogue effect can be noted as side effects of the retinoids Isotretinoin and Acitretin [8].

Zinc

Zinc is an essential factor of numerous enzyme systems including DNA- and RNA-polymerases [8,36]. Acquired zinc deficiency can cause TE and skin changes similar to seborrheic dermatitis. In severe cases, the patient may develop acrodermatitis enteropathica acquisita, which is characterized by periorificial and acral erosive dermatitis, alopecia, and diarrhea [37].

Copper

Inherited abnormalities in copper uptake lead to Menkes syndrome (kinky hair disease, trichopoliodystrophy). Acquired copper deficiency is rare but has been described in patients who received parenteral nutrition. Copper deficiency may lead to anemia, leucopenia, and hypopigmentation of hair shafts [8,38].

Selenium

Selenoproteins, proteins containing selenium in the form of the amino acid selenocysteine, seem to act as essential antioxidants in skin and play a significant role in keratinocyte growth and viability. Selenoprotein deficiency may lead to disturbance of the hair cycle. However, hair loss is described in a patient with excessive levels of selenium (selenosis/selenium intoxication) [39].

Essential fatty acids (vitamin F)

Deficiency of essential fatty acids is found in children with biliary atresia. Vitamin F deficiency may cause eczematous dermatitis on the scalp and eyebrows as well as TE [8,40].

Psychological stress, acute anxiety, and depression

Psychological stress is widely thought to be a cause of alopecia [16]. Acute anxiety, traumatic life events, or depression may cause TE [23]. There is literature that does support the notion of psychogenic TE [16,41,42].

Medications

These are discussed extensively in Chapter 4.

Clinical features

TE predominantly occurs in female patients. Patients report an abrupt onset of shedding, a reduction in hair density and their pony tail diameter, and hair thinning, especially on the temples (Figure 3.3). Women oftentimes present with a "bag sign," bringing in bags with hair that they have collected every day or over a couple of days (Figure 3.4). Women with TE can lose more than 300 hairs per day.

Diagnosis

The diagnosis is made by the patient's history. The determination of possible causes of TE can be tedious and time consuming. Multiple causes may be responsible for the development of TE. A thorough history of the evolution of the effluvium, review of systems and exposure to drugs, supplements, and chemicals, dietary history, history of recent illnesses, family history of pattern hair loss, menstrual and reproductive history, hair care practices, history of contact sensitivity, and evaluation of psychological

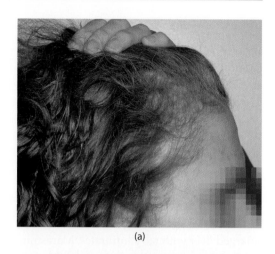

(a)

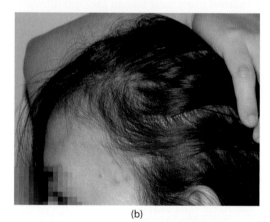

(b)

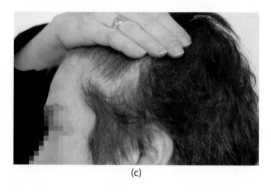

(c)

Figure 3.3
(a) 31-year-old female patient with acute TE 2 months after crash diet; (b) 23-year-old female patient with iron deficiency; and (c) 57-year-old female patient with TE 3 months after surgery. Note the marked thinning of the temples in all three cases.

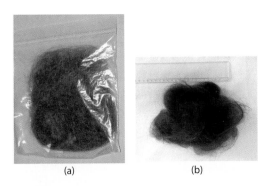

Figure 3.4
(a) "Bag sign" hair was collected over 14 days; (b) hair collected over 20 days by a patient with massive intoxication secondary to chemical cleaning agents.

stress are essential in the search for the etiology for TE [16].

A clinical examination of the entire scalp and a hair pull test are essential in the diagnosis of TE. The scalp examination may show a normal hair density, diffuse thinning, or pronounced thinning in the temporal area. The hair pull test is usually positive on the entire scalp or sometimes only in the occipital area. If hair regrowth of tapered coarse terminal hairs is already visible and the pull test appears to be negative, the TE is likely resolving. A scalp biopsy can help to confirm the diagnosis and to identify other concomitant hair disorders. Laboratory testing for ferritin and thyroid-stimulating hormone (TSH) is recommended, as iron deficiency and hypothyroidism are the most common metabolic causes of TE in women. Tests for vitamin D, vitamin B12, selenium, and zinc may also be considered.

Management

The removal of the cause is the major goal in the treatment of TE. Iron supplementation is recommended if the ferritin level is less than 70 ng/mL [43]. Borderline hypothyroidism can be difficult to identify. Women who complain of hair loss, depression, lack of energy, mental fatigue, cold intolerance, weight gain, and/or constipation may have hypothyroidism. TSH levels may fluctuate but are usually elevated, with normal or reduced thyroid hormone levels. If a thyroid dysfunction is suspected, the patient should be closely followed by an endocrinologist.

Women with TE are often most concerned about complete baldness. The patient has to be reassured that the condition does not lead to complete baldness, that the prognosis of hair regrowth is generally very good, and that the hair likely grows back around 6 months after removal of the initiating trigger.

Topical 2% or 5% minoxidil solution 1 ml twice daily can be helpful, especially in women with prolonged hair loss with unknown triggers or in patients with drug-related hair loss who are unable to discontinue the initiating medication.

Chronic telogen effluvium

Frequently encountered in dermatological practice is the woman who presents with chronic diffuse hair loss of unknown cause. Diffuse cyclic hair loss in women was first described by Guy et al. in 1959 [44]. They described a "not uncommon condition" presenting with transitory episodes of shedding lasting several weeks with no apparent cause. The typical patient is a "vigorous, otherwise healthy woman" who presents with diffuse hair loss that is cyclic and reversible. They considered this to be a physiological phenomenon. A modern term for this condition, coined by Whiting, is chronic telogen effluvium (CTE) [45]. CTE is defined as increased shedding of scalp hair on the entire scalp for longer than 6 months. Women who present with this type of hair loss frequently are upset and want a satisfactory explanation for their problem.

Pathogenesis

CTE is a form of diffuse hair loss affecting the entire scalp with no obvious cause [45,46]. Trigger factors include a persistent exposure to different stressors (drugs, endocrine or nutritive misbalance, chronic infections, collagenosis, or malignant diseases) [8]. It usually affects women 30 to 60 years of age who generally have a full head of hair before the onset of shedding. No underlying cause can be found in 30% of all cases of CTE [8].

Clinical features

Patients with CTE report persistent and massive shedding. The onset is usually abrupt, with or without a recognizable initiating factor. The degree of shedding is usually moderate to severe in the early stages. CTE tends to run a fluctuating course for several years. Females present with increased telogen shedding, generalized, but usually discrete thinning on the entire scalp, reduction in pony tail diameter, and moderately increased parting widths. A marked bitemporal recession may be present. The discrete hair thinning contrasts the intense emotional overtones brought about by this situation. This may initially lead to the differential diagnosis of psychogenic pseudoeffluvium.

Owing to the synchronization of the hair cycle, the amount of shed hair in CTE is greater than that in AGA, while miniaturized hairs are not a feature of the disorder. Overlap with AGA and/or psychogenic pseudoeffluvium is not uncommon. Scalp dysesthesia or a sensation of pain in the hair (trichodynia) is an accompanying symptom in a significant proportion of cases, and may correlate more with emotional upset than with actual hair loss.

Diagnosis

Like in acute TE, the diagnosis is based on the patient's history, examination of the

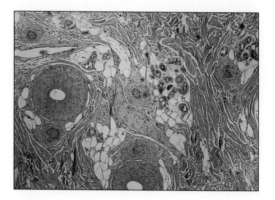

Figure 3.5
A histological transverse section of chronic telogen effluvium, showing a disproportionate number of telogen hairs on transverse section. (Courtesy of Dr. Magdalena Martinka.)

entire scalp, and pull test. Hair density and thickness are usually normal when measured with videodermoscopy. Scalp biopsies show an increased percentage of telogen hairs (Figure 3.5). In certain cases of CTE, laboratory testing may often show ferritin levels below the normal male reference range of 25–30 µg/L [47]. The normal ferritin levels for men and women differ in most laboratories. Usually, normal reference levels for women are considerably lower, as a large number of the "normal control" group are menstruating women. Van Neste and Rushton feel that topping ferritin levels to at least the lower limit for men may correct this problem to a certain degree [47]. These authors also feel that hemoglobin levels should be above the lower male range (greater than 13 g/dL) to maintain the normal anagen to telogen ratio of 9:1.

Management

Patients are particularly troubled by continuing hair loss, and fear total baldness. Repeated reassurance that the condition does not cause complete baldness is necessary. CTE does appear to be self-limiting in the long run. CTE is usually reversible. However, in those women who have a genetic predisposition to AGA, CTE may unmask their AGA, and hair will not necessarily grow back to the same density as before.

Nutritional supplements (except for iron when indicated) are not generally recommended. There is some evidence that taking excessive and unnecessary supplements could actually induce TE [47]. For example, large amounts of zinc in supplements (>25 mg/day) may affect iron absorption adversely [47].

Our approach to CTE is as follows: (1) confirm the diagnosis with a 4-mm scalp biopsy with transverse sectioning (see Figure 3.5); (2) make sure you have ruled out any underlying cause of TE; (3) top up ferritin levels to greater than 30 µg/L; the patient should be monitored every 4–6 months with repeat ferritin levels until they have reached this threshold level; and (4) prescribe topical minoxidil 5% solution or foam twice daily. We have found that topical minoxidil solution or foam is beneficial in maintaining hairs in anagen and increasing conversion of hairs from telogen to anagen.

Patients must be warned that initially there may be increased shedding with topical minoxidil solution or foam, as one must temporarily shed more telogen hairs to increase the eventual percentage of anagen hairs. We feel that it is likely that topping up ferritin levels will maximize the hair growth potential of topical minoxidil in menstruating women with low ferritin. However, further studies with double-blinded placebo controls analyzing the single and combinational benefits of supplemental iron and topical minoxidil solution/foam for CTE are needed.

References

1. Headington JT, Telogen effluvium. New concepts and review. *Arch Dermatol*, 1993. **129**(3): 356–63.
2. Giannotti A et al., Sporadic trichodental dysplasia with microcephaly and mental retardation. *Clin Dysmorphol*, 1995. **4**(4): 334–7.
3. Montalvan E et al., Trichodental dysplasia: A rare syndrome with distinct dental findings. *Pediatr Dent*, 2006. **28**(4): 345–9.
4. Barraud-Klenovsek MM and Trüeb RM, Congenital hypotrichosis due to short anagen. *Br J Dermatol*, 2000. **143**(3): 612–7.
5. Trüeb RM, Idiopathic chronic telogen effluvium in the woman. *Hautarzt*, 2000. **51**(12): 899–905.
6. Bamford JT, A falling out following minoxidil: Telogen effluvium. *J Am Acad Dermatol*, 1987. **16**(1 Pt 1): 144–6.
7. Sinclair R, Grossman KL, and Kvedar JC, Anagen hair loss. In *Disorders of Hair Growth – Diagnosis and Treatment*, Olsen EA, Editor. 2003. Madrid: McGraw Companies. p. 275–302.
8. Trüeb RM, Krankheitsbilder – Haarausfall als störung des haarzyklus. In *Haare – Praxis der Trichologie*, Trüeb RM, Editor. 2003. Darmstadt: Steinkopff Verlag. p. 184–208.
9. Rook A, Diffuse alopecia: Endocrine, metabolic and chemical influences on the follicular cycle. In *Diseases of the Hair and Scalp*, Dawber R, Editor. 1991. Oxford: Blackwell Scientific Publications. p. 136–66.
10. Jain VK, Kataria U, and Dayal S, Study of diffuse alopecia in females. *Indian J Dermatol Venereol Leprol*, 2000. **66**(2): 65–8.
11. Freinkel RK and Freinkel N, Hair growth and alopecia in hypothyroidism. *Arch Dermatol*, 1972. **106**(3): 349–52.
12. Williams R, Thyroid and adrenal interrelations with special reference to hypotrichosis and axillairis in thyrotoxicosis. *J Clin Endocrinol Metab*, 1947. **7**: 52.
13. Rushton DH et al., Biochemical and trichological characterization of diffuse alopecia in women. *Br J Dermatol*, 1990. **123**(2): 187–97.
14. Hard S, Non-anemic iron deficiency as an etiologic factor in diffuse loss of hair of the scalp in women. *Acta Derm Venereol*, 1963. **43**: 562–9.
15. Rasheed H et al., Serum ferritin and vitamin D in female hair loss: Do they play a role? *Skin Pharmacol Physiol*, 2013. **26**(2): 101–7.
16. Fiedler VC and Gray AC, Diffuse alopecia: Telogen effluvium. In *Disorders of Hair Growth – Diagnosis and Treatment*, Olsen EA, Editor. 2003. Madrid: McGraw Companies. p. 303–21.

17. Tabibzadeh SS, Satyaswaroop PG, and Rao PN, Antiproliferative effect of interferon-gamma in human endometrial epithelial cells in vitro: Potential local growth modulatory role in endometrium. *J Clin Endocrinol Metab*, 1988. **67**(1): 131–8.

18. Yaar M et al., Effects of alpha and beta interferons on cultured human keratinocytes. *J Invest Dermatol*, 1985. **85**(1): 70–4.

19. Lynfield Y, Effect of pregnancy on the human hair cycle. *J Invest Dermatol*, 1960. **35**: 323–7.

20. Pecoraro V, The normal trichogram of pregnant women. In *Advances in Biology of the Skin*, Montagna W and Dobson RL, Editors. 1969. Oxford: Pergamon Press. p. 203.

21. Schiff B, Study of postpartum alopecia. *Arch Dermatol*, 1963. **87**: 609.

22. Skelton J, Postpartum alopecia. *J Obstet Gynecol*, 1966. **94**: 125.

23. Camacho F, Alopecias due to telogen effluvium. In *Trichology Diseases of the Pilosebaceous Follicle*, Camacho FM, Editor. 1997. Madrid: Aula Medica Group SA. p. 403–9.

24. Thompson JS, Alopecia after ileal pouch-anal anastomosis. *Dis Colon Rectum*, 1989. **32**(6): 457–65.

25. Desai SP and Roaf ER, Telogen effluvium after anesthesia and surgery. *Anesth Analg*, 1984. **63**(1): 83–4.

26. Abel R, Postoperative (pressure) alopecia. *Arch Dermatol*, 1960. **81**: 34.

27. Klein AW, Rudolph RI, and Leyden JJ, Telogen effluvium as a sign of Hodgkin disease. *Arch Dermatol*, 1973. **108**(5): 702–3.

28. Lubach D, Dermatological changes in patients receiving long-term hemodialysis. *Hautarzt*, 1980. **31**(2): 82–5.

29. Scoggins R, Cutaneous manifestations of hyperlipidemia and uraemia. *Postgrad Med*, 1967. **41**: 357.

30. Zaun H, Wachstumsstorungen der kopfhaare als folge von hepatopathien. *Arch Klin Exp Derm*, 1969. **235**: 386–93.

31. Schattner A and Shanon Y, Crohn's ileocolitis presenting as chronic diffuse hair loss. *J R Soc Med*, 1989. **82**(5): 303–4.

32. Rooth G and Carlstrom S, Therapeutic fasting. *Acta Med Scand*, 1970. **187**(6): 455–63.

33. Amor KT, Rashid RM, and Mirmirani P, Does D matter? The role of vitamin D in hair disorders and hair follicle cycling. *Dermatol Online J*, 2010. **16**(2): 3.

34. Bollag WB, Mediator1: An important intermediary of vitamin D receptor-regulated epidermal function and hair follicle biology. *J Invest Dermatol*, 2012. **132**(4): 1068–70.

35. Jackson AJ and Price VH, How to diagnose hair loss. *Dermatol Clin*, 2013. **31**(1): 21–8.

36. Prasad AS, Discovery of human zinc deficiency and studies in an experimental human model. *Am J Clin Nutr*, 1991. **53**(2): 403–12.

37. Weismann K and Høyer H, Zinc deficiency dermatoses. Etiology, clinical aspects and treatment. *Hautarzt*, 1982. **33**(8): 405–10.

38. Olivares M and Uauy R, Copper as an essential nutrient. *Am J Clin Nutr*, 1996. **63**(5): 791S–6S.

39. Sengupta A et al., Selenoproteins are essential for proper keratinocyte function and skin development. *PLoS One*, 2010. **5**(8): e12249. doi: 10.1371/journal.pone.0012249.

40. Skolnik P, Eaglstein WH, and Ziboh VA, Human essential fatty acid deficiency: Treatment by topical application of linoleic acid. *Arch Dermatol*, 1977. **113**(7): 939–41.

41. Kligman A, Pathologic dynamics of human hair loss. *Arch Dermatol*, 1961. **83**: 175–98.

42. Dahlin PA, George J, and Nerette JC, Telogen effluvium: Hair loss after spinal cord injury. *Arch Phys Med Rehabil*, 1984. **65**(8): 485–6.

43. Trost LB, Bergfeld WF, and Calogeras E, The diagnosis and treatment of iron deficiency and its potential relationship to hair loss. *J Am Acad Dermatol*, 2006. **54**(5): 824–44.

44. Guy WB and Edmundson WF, Diffuse cyclic hair loss in women. *Arch Dermatol*, 1960. **81**: 205–7.

45. Whiting DA, Chronic telogen effluvium: Increased scalp hair shedding in middle-aged women. *J Am Acad Dermatol*, 1996. **35**(6): 899–906.

46. Whiting DA, Update on chronic telogen effluvium. *Exp Dermatol*, 1999. **8**(4): 305–6.

47. Van Neste DJ and Rushton DH, Hair problems in women. *Clin Dermatol*, 1997. **15**(1): 113–25.

4   Hair loss from drugs and radiation

Drugs and radiation can affect cell cycling and may lead to alopecia. This chapter reviews which drugs have been implicated in hair loss and explores the mechanisms of how pharmaceutical agents and radiotherapy can alter hair cycling and structure.

Drugs that cause alopecia

The true incidence of drug-related alopecia is hard to determine accurately. Practicing dermatologists make the diagnosis infrequently, but it is also true that they rarely see the majority of such patients: those receiving chemotherapy. Drugs are capable of producing a wide spectrum of alopecia, from complete baldness to slight, barely noticeable shedding. Subtle cases can be difficult to detect, and it is possible that many patients may lose small amounts of hair and never realize it. Even if they do notice it, the loss of hair is considered to be trivial, and so may go unreported or may be reported without adequate documentation.

The workup for any patient with hair loss must include a thorough drug history. Repeated questioning may be necessary because of forgetfulness or ignorance.

Drug-induced alopecia is usually confined to the scalp, although the eyebrows, the axillary and pubic regions, and the body may also be involved. The pattern of hair loss is almost always diffuse. Female androgenetic alopecia (AGA) poses a real problem, because it is very prevalent and can coexist with diffuse alopecia. A drug-induced alopecia can certainly unmask a tendency for AGA and accelerate the miniaturization process of AGA. The scalp itself is usually unremarkable, except in rare instances. Some drugs can cause a severe drug-induced lichenoid eruption of the scalp.

Certain laboratory tests such as scalp biopsy and blood work can be helpful in ruling out other causes of alopecia. A scalp biopsy with obligatory transverse sectioning will give you the anagen to telogen ratio and the terminal to vellus ratio, and will detect any inflammatory process. This will help to rule out AGA and alopecia areata, as well as to confirm an anagen or telogen effluvium (TE).

One must understand the basic mechanisms of hair growth and cycling to understand drug-induced hair loss. This is all reviewed in detail in Chapter 1. Each human scalp follicle produces hair cyclically and behaves independently of neighboring follicles. The scalp follicle passes through a growing, metabolically active phase known as anagen, which lasts 4–8 years. Following anagen, a brief transitional catagen phase of 2 weeks leads to a metabolically inactive resting telogen phase. The telogen phase lasts for 3 months, after which the club hair is shed as the hair follicle initiates a new cycle.

There are two mechanisms of drug-induced alopecia: direct and indirect effects. Direct effects include anagen growth interruption, precipitation of catagen, and disturbed keratinization, resulting in hair shaft damage. Indirect effects include causing a systemic disease (hypothyroidism or zinc deficiency) or a severe skin disease (lichenoid eruption or toxic epidermal necrolysis) of which alopecia is a feature.

Scalp follicles are in differing phases of the hair cycle and are randomly scattered over the scalp. Almost 90% of scalp follicles are in anagen, 10% in telogen, and 1% in catagen. Follicles are susceptible to noxious agents, usually when they are actively growing. During the anagen phase, the mitotic activity of the hair matrix is so high that it can be compared with the most actively kinetic tissues of the body, namely bone marrow and mucous membranes. For this reason, anagen hair matrix is highly susceptible to noxious events, whereas catagen and telogen follicles are relatively safe. The duration of anagen and telogen phases, the percentage of hairs in anagen and telogen phases, and the density of the follicles will account for the varying severity of alopecia in different areas of hair growth. The regions of the body with highest percentage of anagen hairs, such as the scalp and beard, are more likely to be affected by drugs than the regions of the body with the lowest percentage of anagen follicles, such as the eyebrows and eyelashes.

Drug-induced alopecia usually involves pharmaceutical alteration of the cycling process. Hair loss occurring a few days after drug intake indicates an effect on hair matrix cells. Hair loss developing weeks to months after drug intake may be due to hair matrix effects, but may result from changes in keratin production or changes in the hair cycle. If one excludes antimitotics, the most common mechanism by far for drug-induced alopecia is the precipitation of catagen. Of course, in the clinical setting, there is confusion, because many diseases for which drugs are administered also produce a precipitation of catagen. An example of such a dilemma is highlighted by Reeves and Maibach [1]. Ahmad [2] reported a case of cimetidine-induced alopecia but failed to take into account the fact that the stress from a duodenal ulcer might have caused the alopecia.

Anagen effluvium

Cytostatic drugs

Hair loss following chemotherapy causes severe anxiety. Patients are sometimes more afraid of the hair loss and cosmetic disfiguration than of the underlying disease or therapy itself. Around 8% of cancer patients refuse chemotherapy because of the fear of losing their hair [3]. Therapeutic options to prevent or treat chemotherapy-induced alopecia are very limited. Scalp cooling devices have shown some success in therapy regimens with taxane monotherapy [4–6].

Any drug that affects cell division can alter hair growth. Cytostatic drugs suppress hair matrix cell mitosis, impede hair cortex formation, and cause anagen effluvium in almost 100% of patients [7,8]. Chemotherapy-induced alopecia most prominently affects the highly proliferative matrix keratinocytes of anagen hair follicles, located in the hair bulb. The resultant hair contains fewer cells per unit length, is thin, and breaks easily.

Only the actively dividing matrix cells of anagen hairs are affected by cytostatic drugs. The intensity of damage to the cortex of the hair shaft depends on the drug dosage and the duration of its administration. A small single dose will produce constriction of the hair shaft. A large single dose that strongly suppresses mitosis produces a sharp point constriction. The hair breaks at the point of constriction, with hair fall beginning in 7–14 days (see Figure 4.1). Continued treatment with a smaller constant dose produces a slow decrease in hair shaft diameter to a tapered point. Combined therapy with two or more antimitotic agents has a greater effect than a larger dose of only one agent. A spectrum of changes seems to occur, and the predominant effect may depend on the dose and timing of the administration. In some cases, especially in patients subjected to multiple cycles of chemotherapy, hair follicle stem

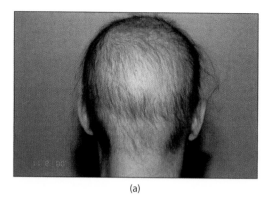
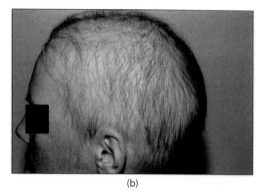

(a)   (b)

Figure 4.1

Anagen effluvium. A 33-year-old female patient with lymphoma on dacarbazine, bleomycin, doxorubicin, and vinblastine. Note the marked hair loss over the entire scalp. (a) Posterior view; (b) lateral view.

cells may also be damaged, which can lead to permanent hair loss.

Alopecia most commonly occurs with the use of doxorubicin (Adriamycin), cyclophosphamide, chlormethamine (mechlormethamine), methotrexate, fluorouracil, vincristine, daunorubicin, bleomycin, and hydroxycarbamide. Drugs that may aggravate alopecia when used in combination chemotherapy include chlorambucil, thiotepa, cytarabine, vinblastine, and dactinomycin.

Certain drugs affect specific phases of the mitotic process within the actively dividing hair matrix. Those drugs that are S-phase-specific include cytosine arabinoside, hydroxyurea, 6-mercaptopurine, and methotrexate. The M phase of mitosis is affected greatly by vincristine and vinblastine. Most of the cytotoxic agents are not phase specific; these include alkylating agents (cyclophosphamide, ifosfamide, melphalan, thiotepa, busulfan, carmustine, dacarbazine), nitrosoureas, antitumor antibiotics, procarbazine, and cisplatin.

Colchicine

Colchicine, used in the treatment of gout, has antimitotic activity operating through the failure of spindle formation. Cells with the highest rates of division are affected earliest [5]. Colchicine can produce diffuse hair loss in 1%–10% of cases. The mode of action is due to metaphase arrest [6]. Harms [7] reported a case of diffuse alopecia that occurred after 2 months of colchicine therapy. Hairs were dystrophic and broken off 1–2 cm above the scalp. Hair loss is dose dependent. It may persist for 1–3 months, and may be reversible even if the drug is continued [9].

Vasopressin

Vasopressin, a vasoconstrictor and antidiuretic pituitary hormone, has been reported to cause alopecia by causing anagen effluvium from cutaneous infarcts. All areas affected by anagen effluvium had normal hair growth after the medication was discontinued [10].

Table 4.1 lists the drugs that have been implicated as causing anagen effluvium [11].

Telogen effluvium

A large number of drugs have been reported to cause diffuse alopecia and TE. However, the cause–effect relationship between drugs and hair loss is very difficult to determine. The drug could cause a primary or secondary effect on the hair cycle. Many patients

Table 4.1
Drug-induced anagen effluvium

Asparaginase	Doxorubicin	Mitomycin
Bleomycin	Etoposide	Mitotane
Busulfan	Fluorouracil	Paclitaxel
Carboplatin	Gemcitabine	Pentostatin
Carmustine	Hydroxycarbamide	Procarbazine
Chlorambucil	Hydroxyurea	Thiotepa
Cisplatin	Idarubicin	Thioguanine
Colchicine	Ifosfamide	Topotecan
Cyclophosphamide	Lomustine	Vasopressin
Cytarabine	Mechlorethamine	Vinblastine
Dacarbazine	Medroxyprogesterone	Vincristine
Dactinomycin	Melphalan	Vinorelbine
Daunorubicin	Mercaptopurine	
Docetaxel	Methotrexate	

take more than one drug on a regular basis. A combination of drugs could aggravate the negative influence on hair growth. A thorough history should identify drugs that were started 3 months before the onset of hair loss. If the hair loss resolves after stopping the medication, the etiologic relationship between the drug and effluvium may be confirmed. The prognosis of hair regrowth after TE caused by medication is generally good unless the patient has an underlying AGA.

Tables 4.2 through 4.5 list the drugs that have been implicated as causing TE [11].

Anticoagulants

All forms of anticoagulants may induce hair loss. These include heparin and coumarins. TE occurs in more than 10% of patients, appears to be related to drug dosage, and tends to be more frequent in women (Figure 4.2).

Antithyroid drugs

Reversible alopecia is a constant finding in iatrogenic hypothyroidism, which occurs during the treatment of thyrotoxicosis. TE is frequently associated with hair dryness and brittleness. Antithyroid drugs that may produce TE include iodine, methylthiouracil, propylthiouracil, and carbimazole.

Psychopharmacologic medications

Lithium

Hair loss is a possible adverse effect of lithium carbonate, and may be noticed within weeks or years after commencing therapy [11]. Headington feels it is due to immediate anagen release. However, in those patients in whom the onset of the hair loss may take years, this mechanism is less likely. A correlation between hair loss and lithium blood level and/or dosage is suspected, but not established. In most reports, doses ranged from 0.4 to 1.5 g/day, with serum lithium assays between 0.5 and 1.4 Meq/L [12–17].

A review described 101 cases of lithium-related hair loss in over 25 years of use [18]. A 3-year survey of lithium-treated subjects

Table 4.2
Drug-induced telogen effluvium (incidence less than 1%)

Albendazole	Fluoxetine	Nisoldipine
Aldesleukin	Flurbiprofen	Nortriptyline
Altretamine	Fluroxamine	Octreotide
Amiloride	Foscarnet	Olanzapine
Amiodarone	Ganciclovir	Omeprazole
Amitriptyline	Grepafloxacin	Paroxetine
Amlodipine	Haloperidol	Prazosin
Amoxapine	Ibuprofen	Propafenone
Azathioprine	Imipramine	Propylthiouracil
Bromfenac	Indomethacin	Protriptyline
Bupropion	Ipratropium	Risperidone
Carvedilol	Ketoprofen	Ropinirole
Clofibrate	Lansoprazole	Sertraline
Clomiphene	Levothyroxine	Sparfloxacin
Clomipramine	Liothyronine	Sulindac
Desipramine	Lisinopril	Tacrine
Diethylstilbestrol	Losartan	Testosterone
Diflunisal	Meclofenamate	Tiagabine
Dopamine	Mefloquine	Tizanidine
Epinephrine	Mesalamine	Tocainide
Esmolol	Methimazole	Trimipramine
Estramustine	Mexiletine	Venlafaxine
Ethionamide	Nabumetone	Verapamil
Fenfluramine	Naproxen	Zaleplon
Fenoprofen	Naratriptan	
Flecainide	Nefazodone	

reported a 12% incidence of alopecia [16]. About 20% of patients on long-term lithium therapy, who had high lithium levels, reported hair thinning; 23% described their hair as also becoming straighter [19].

Patients on lithium who develop alopecia must undergo a thyroid function assessment because lithium is known for its ability to affect the thyroid gland. Hypothyroidism (commonly) and thyrotoxicosis (rarely) have been described in patients on lithium therapy, and both conditions may manifest with

hair changes [20,21]. There is a case report of alopecia areata occurring during lithium therapy [22]. This is probably coincidental.

Valproate

Valproic acid (VPA), once ingested, dissociates in the gastrointestinal tract into a salt or ionic form, valproate. VPA and divalproex (a stable combination of valproate sodium and valproic acid) may cause hair changes. A review of the literature mentions 643 cases of

Table 4.3
Drug-induced telogen effluvium (incidence of 1–5%)

Acyclovir	Cyclosporin	Lamotrigine
Allopurinol	Cytarabine	Letrozole
Amantadine	Dacarbazine	Leuprolide
Atorvastatin	Dactinomycin	Loratadine
Betaxolol	Delavirdine	Lovastatin
Bicalutamide	Dexfenfluramine	Nifedipine
Buspirone	Diclofenac	Pentosan
Captopril	Efavirenz	Riluzole
Carbamazepine	Fludarabine	Rofecoxib
Celecoxib	Gold	Tolcapone
Cetirizine	Granisetron	Topiramate

Table 4.4
Drug-induced telogen effluvium (incidence of more than 5%)

Acitretin	Interferon-α	Ramipril
Cidofovir	Isotretinoin	Terbinafine
Danazol	Leflunomide	Timolol
Granulocyte colony-stimulating factor	Levobunolol	Valproic acid
Heparin	Lithium	Warfarin
	Moexipril	

Table 4.5
Drug-induced telogen effluvium (exact incidence unreported) [46]

Acebutolol	Bisoprolol	Didanosine
Acetaminophen	Bromocriptine	Diethylstilbestrol
Acetohexamide	Chlorothiazide	Diflunisal
Aminophylline	Chlorotrianisene	Dopamine
Aminosalicylate sodium	Chloropropamide	Epinephrine
Amphotericin B	Chlorothalidone	Esmolol
Asparaginase	Cimetidine	Estrogen
Aspirin	Clonazepam	Ethambutol
Astemizole	Cyclophosphamide	Ethosuximide
Atenolol	Diazoxide	Etidronate
Bendroflumethiazide	Dicumarol	Etodolac

Table 4.5 (*Continued*)
Drug-induced telogen effluvium (exact incidence unreported) [46]

Famotidine	Methusuximide	Progestins
Felbamate	Methyldopa	Propranolol
Fenofibrate	Methylphenidate	Pyrimethamine
Fluconazole	Methyltestosterone	Quazepam
Fluoxymesterone	Methysergide	Quinidine
Fluvastatin	Metoprolol	Ranitidine
Gabapentin	Minoxidil	Ropinirole
Gemfibrozil	Misoprostol	Saquinavir
Gentamicin	Mitotane	Selegiline
Guanethidine	Mycophenolate	Simvastatin
Guanfacine	Nadolol	Sotalol
Halothane	Nalidixic acid	Spironolactone
Hydromorphone	Neomycin	Stanozolol
Hydroxychloroquine	Nimodipine	Sulfasalazine
Indinavir	Nitrofurantoin	Sulfisoxazole
Isoniazid	Ondansetron	Thalidomide
Itraconazole	Oral contraceptives	Thioguanine
Ketoconazole	Oxaprozin	Thioridazine
Labetolol	Paramethadione	Thiothixene
Lamivudine	Penbutolol	Tiopronin
Levodopa	Penicillamine	Trazodone
Loperamide	Penicillins	Triazolam
Lorazepam	Pergolide	Trimethadione
Loxapine	Phenytoin	Ursodiol
Maprotiline	Pindolol	Vitamin A
Mebendazole	Piroxicam	Zalcitabine
Mephenytoin	Pravastatin	Zidovudine
Mesoridazine	Prazepam	
Metformin	Probenecid	

valproate-induced alopecia [18], with a 0.5%–12.0% reported frequency [23,24]. Patients on VPA who develop hair loss tend to have a high valproate blood concentration [25]. It is not completely established whether alopecia is dose related, but usually dosage reduction leads to regrowth of hair in individuals with valproate-associated alopecia [26].

Carbamazepine

There are 177 documented cases of carbamazepine-induced alopecia [18], with a reported incidence of 1.6% and 6% [27,28]. A threefold dose reduction of 200 mg/day helped one female patient [29]. Carbamazepine and VPA possibly have different mechanisms of hair loss, despite a documented decrease in

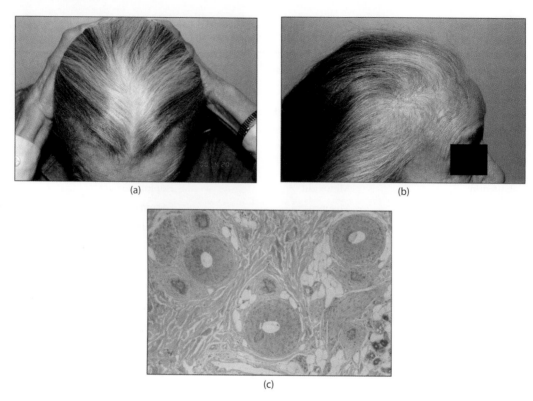

(a)   (b)

(c)

Figure 4.2
Telogen effluvium. A 63-year-old female patient on warfarin showing general shedding hair loss is not as marked as in anagen effluvium. (a) Top view with a slightly increased part width; (b) lateral view, illustrating marked thinning on the temples; (c) pathology of telogen effluvium, showing a disproportionate number of telogen hairs.

serum amounts of zinc and copper caused by both medications [30]. Some individuals may have an increased genetic predisposition to medicinal alopecia.

Tricyclic/tetracyclic antidepressants

A few instances of diffuse hair loss associated with tricyclic antidepressants (TCA) have been documented. All TCA versions have been implicated with alopecia: amitriptyline, amoxapine, despiramine, doxepin, imipramine, nortriptyline, and protriptyline. The tetracyclic antidepressant drugs maprotiline and trazodone may also result in hair loss. However, none of the monoamine oxide inhibitors are known to cause alopecia.

Serotonin reuptake inhibitors

Several serotonin reuptake inhibitors can also cause hair loss on rare occasions. Fluoxetine is the most frequently prescribed antidepressant, and with this there are 725 documented cases [18]. Sertraline has been reported in 46 instances [31,32] and paroxetine in 30 subjects [18]. The majority of these have a typical pattern of reversible diffuse alopecia, with a 2–6-month latency period. Sometimes alopecia may develop 1.5 years following fluoxetine introduction [33],[34]. In another case, a fluoxetine-induced alopecia was still evident 1.5 years after drug discontinuation [35].

Other antipsychotics/anxiolytics

Haloperidol, olanzapine, and respiridone have been documented as causing hair loss. Anxiolytic medicines of the barbiturate and benzodiazepine classes, as well as zolpidem, generally do not result in alopecia. Clonazepam is one exception. Buspirone is also associated with hair loss on rare occasions.

Oral contraceptives

Telogen hair is lost 2–3 months after discontinuation of treatment with oral contraceptives. Pathogenesis is probably similar to that in postpartum hair loss [36]. This is believed by Headington to be a delayed anagen release [37]. There is prolongation of the anagen phase, owing to the estrogens. The utilization of low-dose estrogen contraceptives is only occasionally associated with this effect.

Antihypertensive agents

Several antihypertensive agents are known to cause hair loss. Beta-blockers may have a direct toxic effect on the hair follicles. This side effect is reversible once medication is terminated.

Captopril can also cause hair loss. It may form a complex with zinc and thus decrease zinc levels, particularly in those patients with renal disease [38–41]. Low zinc levels can cause hair loss.

Topical ophthalmic beta-blockers

Topical ophthalmic beta-blockers can cause hair loss. Hair loss is not confined to the scalp alone, but also extends to eyelashes and eyebrows. Females are more commonly affected. It occurs 1–24 months after treatment. Significant recovery is seen after 4–8 months from the time the use of the solution is discontinued [39].

Interferons

TE occurs in 20%–30% of patients treated with interferons. There is no relationship between dosage and time of onset or severity of hair loss. In some cases, telogen loss subsides despite continuing treatment [42].

Keratin production interference

Thallium

Thallium is no longer used as a drug, but may be ingested accidentally in rodent poisons or contaminated foods. Thallium ingestion produces changes in the matrix cells, with subsequent disturbed keratinization. Intrafollicular thinning, accumulation of air bubbles in the hair shaft, breakage of the hair shaft, and the induction of telogen is seen in thallium alopecia. Available evidence indicates that thallium inhibits the utilization of cystine in the production of the keratin molecule. Acute poisoning produces hair loss in 10 days, along with ataxia, fatigue, joint pains, and weakness. Hair losses of several months' to years' duration, with muscle aches, have been reported in chronic thallium intoxication.

Retinoids

Soriatane and accutane can produce brittle, dry, unmanageable, loosely anchored hairs. Retinoid-induced alopecia has a later onset and is almost always reversible. It is due to a shortened anagen release, rather than an immediate anagen release, which is what is more commonly seen with other drugs. However, just like any TE, retinoids can certainly unmask a tendency for AGA. The package insert for accutane mentions hair loss. Diffuse hair loss is commonly observed during soriatane treatment, with evident alopecia occurring in about 20% of patients.

Cholesterol-lowering agents

Agents that block cholesterol synthesis through a variety of mechanisms can disrupt keratinization. Cholesterol is a component of cellular lipids, and its synthesis and metabolism are essential for the production of normal epidermal structures. Triparanol, which has been withdrawn from the market because of cataract induction, can cause significant alopecia, loss of hair color, and ichthyosis. Clofibrate may occasionally produce hair loss.

How to manage drug-induced alopecia

In cases where an effective therapeutic agent causes alopecia and no appropriate alternative can be found, an informed patient and physician should discuss the risks and benefits of continuing, stopping, or changing the dose or medication. The advantages and disadvantages of maintaining the drug must be reviewed. Such choices are especially difficult when the offending agent is otherwise effective. Similarly, the negative implications of stopping or changing the regimen also need to be considered. Decisions are based on alternative medications and hair loss severity and its emotional impact. More research may further clarify drug-induced hair loss issues, and offer new therapeutic recommendations.

The use of topical 5% minoxidil solution for drug-induced TE in those cases when the offending drug cannot be terminated or switched is certainly a therapeutic option we use at the University of British Columbia Hair Clinic. Minoxidil, which tends to maintain hairs in anagen and convert telogen hairs into anagen hairs more quickly, can be offered to the patient. During the early conversion of telogen to anagen hairs, there is surge of "telogen release." Patients may temporarily (for the first month of minoxidil application) experience more hair loss, shedding telogen hairs and subsequently replacing them with the more desired anagen hairs. Patients should be warned of this temporary setback.

For drug-induced anagen effluvium, topical minoxidil 5% solution has been reported to work [43]. We rarely need to use it, as the alopecia is usually reversible. The use of cooling scalp devices is still controversial [44, 45].

Alopecia after radiotherapy

The biologic effects of x-rays on hair follicles were first reported in the 1950s [46]. The development of effluvium after radiotherapy is dose dependent and evolves after a dose of 300–400 cGy (or rad) [47]. At this relatively low dose, anagen follicles usually recover quickly and completely. Single doses of >1200 cGy can cause a permanent inhibition of matrix cell proliferation that results in secondary cicatricial alopecia. Permanent hair loss after radiotherapy can be complete in the irradiated area or partial with a lower hair density and thickness and short hair cycles (Figures 4.3 and 4.4) [48]. Anagen hair turns into dystrophic anagen hair 72 hours after radiation.

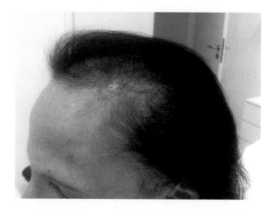

Figure 4.3
Permanent diffuse alopecia 5 years after radiotherapy.

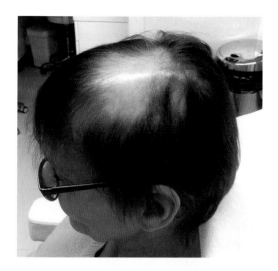

Figure 4.4
Patch of cicatricial alopecia 3 years after radiation of a skull metastasis from breast cancer.

The effluvium is usually abrupt and rapidly progressive. According to the anagen rate, approximately 80% of hair in the irradiated area will fall out [46,47]. If the damage to the hair matrix was not permanent, hair will usually completely grow back after 2–3 months.

Every patient who undergoes any form of radiotherapy should be informed about the total dose and the possibility of transient or permanent hair loss.

References

1. Reeves J and Maibach HI, *Drug- and Chemical-Induced Hair Loss*. 1983. Washington, DC: Horizon Books.
2. Ahmad S, Cimetidine and alopecia [letter]. *Ann Intern Med*, 1979. **91**(6): 930.
3. Hesketh PJ et al., Chemotherapy-induced alopecia: Psychosocial impact and therapeutic approaches. *Support Care Cancer*, 2004. **12**(8): 543–9.
4. Shin H et al., Efficacy of interventions for prevention of chemotherapy-induced alopecia: A systematic review and meta-analysis. *Int J Cancer*, 2014 Aug 1. doi: 10.1002/ ijc.29115.
5. van den Hurk CJ et al., Scalp cooling to prevent alopecia after chemotherapy can be considered safe in patients with breast cancer. *Breast*, 2013. **22**(5): 1001–4.
6. Betticher DC et al., Efficacy and tolerability of two scalp cooling systems for the prevention of alopecia associated with docetaxel treatment. *Support Care Cancer*, 2013. **21**(9): 2565–73.
7. Delaunay M, Cutaneous side effects of anti-tumor chemotherapy. *Ann Dermatol Venereol*, 1989. **116**(4): 347–61.
8. Dunagin WG, Clinical toxicity of chemotherapeutic agents: Dermatologic toxicity. *Semin Oncol*, 1982. **9**(1): 14–22.
9. Blankenship ML, Drugs and alopecia. *Australas J Dermatol*, 1983. **24**(3): 100–4.
10. Maceyko RF, Vidimos AT, and Steck WD, Vasopressin-associated cutaneous infarcts, alopecia, and neuropathy. *J Am Acad Dermatol*, 1994. **31**(1): 111–13.
11. Litt J, *Drug Eruption Reference Manual. Millennium Edition*. 2000. New York: The Parthenon Publishing Group.
12. Dawber R and Mortimer P, Hair loss during lithium treatment [letter]. *Br J Dermatol*, 1982. **107**(1): 124–5.
13. Eustace DP, Lithium-induced reaction [letter]. *Br J Psychiatr*, 1986. **148**: 752.
14. Jefferson J, Lithium and hair loss. *Int Drug Ther News*, 1979. **14**: 23.
15. Kusumi Y, A cutaneous side effect of lithium: Report of two cases. *Dis Nerv Syst*, 1971. **32**(12): 853–4.
16. Orwin A, Hair loss following lithium therapy [letter]. *Br J Dermatol*, 1983. **108**(4): 503–4.
17. Yassa R and Ananth J, Hair loss in the course of lithium treatment: A report of two cases. *Can J Psychiatr*, 1983. **28**(2): 132–3.
18. Pillans PI and Woods DJ, Drug-associated alopecia. *Int J Dermatol*, 1995. **34**(3): 149–58.
19. McCreadie RG and Morrison DP, The impact of lithium in South-west Scotland. I. Demographic and clinical findings. *Br J Psychiatr*, 1985. **146**: 70–4.
20. Freinkel RK and Freinkel N, Hair growth and alopecia in hypothyroidism. *Arch Dermatol*, 1972. **106**(3): 349–52.
21. Kirov G, Thyroid disorders in lithium-treated patients. *J Affect Disord*, 1998. **50**(1): 33–40.

22. Silvestri A, Santonastaso P, and Paggiarin D, Alopecia areata during lithium therapy. A case report. *Gen Hosp Psychiatr*, 1988. **10**(1): 46–8.

23. Davis R, Peters DH, and McTavish D, Valproic acid. A reappraisal of its pharmacological properties and clinical efficacy in epilepsy. *Drugs*, 1994. **47**(2): 332–72.

24. McKinney PA, Finkenbine RD, and DeVane CL, Alopecia and mood stabilizer therapy. *Ann Clin Psychiatr*, 1996. **8**(3): 183–5.

25. Klotz U and Schweizer C, Valproic acid in childhood epilepsy: Anticonvulsive efficacy in relation to its plasma levels. *Int J Clin Pharmacol Ther Toxicol*, 1980. **18**(10): 461–5.

26. Henriksen O and Johannessen SI, Clinical and pharmacokinetic observations on sodium valproate: A 5-year follow-up study in 100 children with epilepsy. *Acta Neurol Scand*, 1982. **65**(5): 504–23.

27. Mattson RH, Cramer JA, and Collins JF, A comparison of valproate with carbamazepine for the treatment of complex partial seizures and secondarily generalized tonic-clonic seizures in adults. The Department of Veterans Affairs Epilepsy Cooperative Study No. 264 Group. *New Engl J Med*, 1992. **327**(11): 765–71.

28. Verity CM, Hosking G, and Easter DJ, A multicentre comparative trial of sodium valproate and carbamazepine in paediatric epilepsy. The Paediatric EPITEG Collaborative Group. *Dev Med Child Neurol*, 1995. **37**(2): 97–108.

29. Ikeda T, Produced alopecia areata based on the focal infection theory and mental motive theory. *Dermatologica*, 1967. **134**(1): 1–11.

30. Suzuki T, Koizumi J, and Moroji T, Effects of long-term anticonvulsant therapy on copper, zinc, and magnesium in hair and serum of epileptics. *Biol Psychiatr*, 1992. **31**(6): 571–81.

31. Bourgeois J, Two cases of hair loss after sertraline use. *J Clin Psychopharmacol*, 1996. **16**(1): 91–2.

32. McDougle CJ, Brodkin ES, and Naylor ST, Sertraline in adults with pervasive developmental disorders: A prospective open-label investigation. *J Clin Psychopharmacol*, 1998. **18**(1): 62–6.

33. Jenike MA, Severe hair loss associated with fluoxetine use [letter]. *Am J Psychiatr*, 1991. **148**(3): 392.

34. Ogilvie AD, Hair loss during fluoxetine treatment [letter]. *Lancet*, 1993. **342**(8884): 1423.

35. Gupta S and Major LF, Hair loss associated with fluoxetine [letter]. *Br J Psychiatr*, 1991. **159**: 737–8.

36. Wong RC and Ellis CN, Physiologic skin changes in pregnancy. *J Am Acad Dermatol*, 1984. **10**(6): 929–40.

37. Headington JT, Telogen effluvium. New concepts and review [see comments]. *Arch Dermatol*, 1993. **129**(3): 356–63.

38. Brodin MB, Drug-related alopecia. *Dermatol Clin*, 1987. **5**(3): 571–9.

39. Fraunfelder FT, Meyer SM, and Menacker SJ, Alopecia possibly secondary to topical ophthalmic beta-blockers [letter]. *JAMA*, 1990. **263**(11): 1493–4.

40. Leaker B and Whitworth JA, Alopecia associated with captopril treatment [letter]. *Aust NZ J Med*, 1984. **14**(6): 866.

41. Smit AJ, Hoorntje SJ, and Donker AJ, Zinc deficiency during captopril treatment. *Nephron*, 1983. **34**(3): 196–7.

42. Tosti A, Misciali C, and Bardazzi F, Telogen effluvium due to recombinant interferon alpha-2b. *Dermatology*, 1992. **184**(2): 124–5.

43. Duvic M, Lemak NA, and Valero V, A randomized trial of minoxidil in chemotherapy-induced alopecia. *J Am Acad Dermatol*, 1996. **35**(1): 74–8.

44. Goldhirsch A, Kiser J, and Ross R, Prevention of cytostatic-related hair loss by hypothermia of a hairy scalp using a cooling cap. *Schweiz Med Wochenschr*, 1982. **112**(16): 568–71.

45. Katsimbri P, Bamias A, and Pavlidis N, Prevention of chemotherapy-induced alopecia using an effective scalp cooling system. *Eur J Cancer*, 2000. **36**(6): 766–71.

46. Ellinger F, Effects of ionizing radiation on growth and replacement of hair. *Ann N Y Acad Sci*, 1951. **53**(3): 682–7.

47. Lawenda BD et al., Permanent alopecia after cranial irradiation: Dose-response relationship. *Int J Radiat Oncol Biol Phys*, 2004. **60**(3): 879–87.

48. Severs GA, Griffin T, and Werner-Wasik M, Cicatricial alopecia secondary to radiation therapy: Case report and review of the literature. *Cutis*, 2008. **81**(2): 147–53.

5 Alopecia areata: Pathogenesis, clinical features, diagnosis, and management

Alopecia areata (AA) is a common, usually patchy, nonscarring hair loss condition affecting any hair-bearing surface. The lifetime risk in the United States has been estimated at 1.7% [1,2]. AA equally affects men and women. It is the most common hair loss complaint in children; approximately 20% of patients with AA are children and as many as 60% present with their first patch before the age of 20 [3,4] (Figure 5.1). Colombe et al. suggest a bimodal pattern for AA, with an early-onset form associated with greater severity, long duration, and family history of the disease and a late-onset form characterized by milder severity, shorter duration, and low family incidence [5] (Figure 5.2).

The exact cause of AA is unknown, but is likely to be an interaction between genetic and environmental factors. Many etiologic factors have been suggested to contribute to the development of AA, including stress, infectious agents, vaccinations, hormonal factors, and genetics [6–13]. Multiple factors may contribute to disease onset and severity. Most of the recent literature supports autoimmunity as the major pathogenic process in AA [6–16]. Several observations support this hypothesis. AA can be seen as an organ-specific autoimmune condition characterized by T cell–mediated attacks on the hair follicle [6,14–16]. The inciting antigenic stimulus is unknown. A dense peribulbar lymphocytic infiltrate and reproducible immunologic abnormalities are hallmark features of the condition.

Genetic factors

Genetic factors play an important role in the etiology of AA. There is a high frequency of a positive family history of AA in affected individuals, ranging from 10% to 42% of cases [17,18]. There is a significantly higher incidence of a positive family history in patients with early onset of AA [19]. Familial incidence of AA has been reported to be 37% in patients who had their first patch by 30 years of age and 7.1% with the first patch after 30 years of age [5,19–21]. Also, there have been reports of AA in identical twins [22–26], with up to 55% concordance rate in identical twins [25]. Scerri [26] presented a case of 11-year-old identical twin boys, with ophiasis occurring simultaneously.

Recently, a genomewide association study (GWAS) from the NIH-funded registry in AA has identified at least eight regions in the genome with evidence for association with AA [12] similar to rheumatoid arthritis and Crohn's disease and not to psoriasis. These genetic studies have identified several immune-related as well as end organ target-specific genes associated with AA, including CTLA4, ULBP3/6, IL2/21, and IL2RA. These genes may have some relevance to being targets for newer therapies. Preclinical studies using CTLA4-Ig have shown efficacy in preventing alopecia in the C3H/HeJ mouse model. This drug is already being used in studies involving rheumatoid arthritis [27].

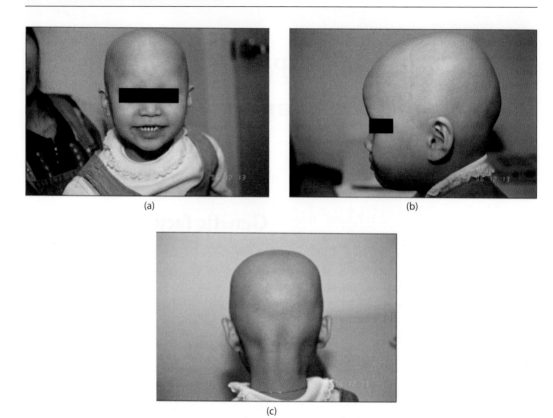

Figure 5.1
Alopecia universalis after 1 year in a 3-year-old girl. (a) Front view showing loss of hair on scalp, eyebrows, and eyelashes; (b) side view; (c) back view. This early onset form of alopecia areata (AA) is associated with greater severity, longer duration, and greater probability of a positive family history of AA. Human leukocyte antigens studies suggest this early onset group of severe AA patients is a genetically distinct group. They are prognostically and therapeutically distinguishable, too.

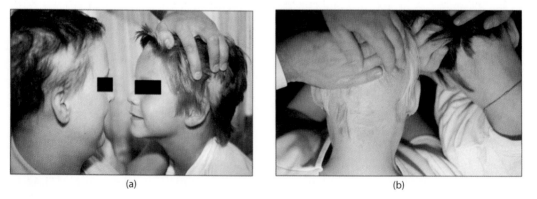

Figure 5.2
(a) Simultaneous circumscript alopecia in mother and son; (b) simultaneous ophiasis in mother and daughter.

Several closely linked genes, such as the human leukocyte antigens (HLA), are located on the short arm of chromosome 6, forming the major histocompatibility complex (MHC) [19,28]. The HLA complex has been investigated in AA patients because of the association of other autoimmune diseases with increased frequencies of HLA antigens [28,29]. Associations with both HLA class I (HLA-A, HLA-B, HLA-C) and class II (HLA-DR, HLA-DQ, HLA-DP) have been studied in AA. The earlier studies identified the association of AA with several class I antigens, such as HLA-A9, B7, and B8 [29], B12 [30], B18 [31], B13, and B27 [32]. However, some studies show no correlation with HLA class I antigens [33,34]. There has been an increased consistency in evidence-revealing associations between AA and HLA class II antigens.

Studies reveal a significant association of HLA-DR11 and DQ3 in patients with AA [5,20,21,33,35–40]. The HLA alleles DQB1*03 (DQ3) and HLA-DRB1*1104 (DR11) appear to be markers of general susceptibility for all forms of AA [5,20,21,33,35–40]. The HLA alleles DRB1*0401 (DR4) and DQB1*0301(DQ7) are markers for more severe long-standing alopecia totalis (AT)/ alopecia universalis (AU) [5,20,21]. The investigators [20] suggest that amino acid sequencing of the antigen-binding grooves of these HLA antigens may indicate the structure and identity of the elusive AA target antigens. Other investigators [35] also suggest that DRB3*52a may confer resistance to AA.

By identifying these HLA genetic correlations, we are a step closer to understanding the structure of the epitopes recognized by T cells, which are key to the follicular inflammatory immune response responsible for AA. Identification of the AA antigens will be a major step in understanding the mechanisms of AA and in the design of therapies for prevention and treatment. However, one must bear in mind that the presence of predisposing HLA is but one component in a cascade of factors leading to autoimmune disease.

AA is a complex trait expressed by a number of genes. Polygenic influences are clearly involved. There is up to an 8.8% increased frequency of AA in patients with Down syndrome, suggesting involvement of a gene located on chromosome 21 in determining susceptibility to AA (Figure 5.3) [41,42]. Thirty percent of patients with autoimmune-polyglandular syndrome have AA. The defective gene in this syndrome is mapped to chromosome 21, again implicating this chromosome [43]. Tarlow et al. reported an association between the severity of AA and inheritance of allele 2 of a five-allele polymorphism in intron 2 of the interleukin-1 receptor antagonist gene [44]. The IL-1 gene cluster on chromosome 2 includes genes for the proinflammatory IL-1 proteins, their cell membrane receptors, and the anti-inflammatory IL-1 receptor antagonist. Polymorphism within the IL-1 cluster may modulate IL-1 responses. IL-1 has a direct effect on hair growth. In hair follicle organ cultures, IL-1 inhibits growth of the hair fiber [45] and induces morphological changes that resemble those seen in AA [46].

In conclusion, many studies indicate that AA is a polygenic disease with certain genes correlated with susceptibility and others with severity. Most probably, there is an interaction between genetic and environmental factors that triggers the disease. At this point, the exact causative genes have not been discovered. With the discovery of animal models for AA, and with the final data on the Human Genome Project completed in 2003, it is expected that our understanding of this complex trait will be further clarified. Genetic research may ultimately explain why, how, and who develops AA.

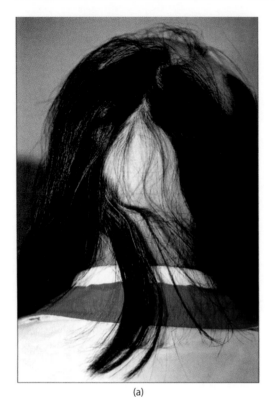
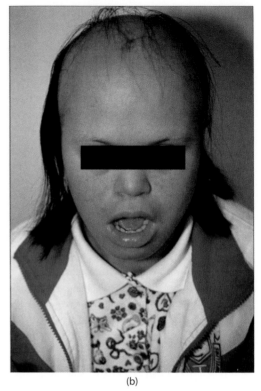

(a)   (b)

Figure 5.3
(a, b) Alopecia areata and Down syndrome. There is up to an 8.8% increased frequency of alopecia areata (AA) in patients with Down syndrome, suggesting involvement of a gene located on chromosome 21 in determining susceptibility to AA.

Immunological factors

Indirect clues for autoimmunity

There are reported associations between AA and classic autoimmune disorders. The main associations are with thyroid diseases and vitiligo. Several reports reveal an 8.0%–11.8% incidence of thyroid disease in patients with AA, compared to only 2% in the general population [47,48]. This evidence has been further confirmed by documentation of an increased prevalence of antithyroid antibodies [49] and thyroid microsomal antibodies [49]. However, Puavilai et al. showed no increase in microsomal antibodies compared to normal controls [50].

AA has been shown to have a significant association with vitiligo, with a fourfold greater incidence of vitiligo in AA patients [17,51,52]. Other studies have revealed an increased prevalence of gastric parietal cell antibodies and anti-smooth muscle antibodies in sera of patients with AA [53,54]. There are also reported associations of AA with pernicious anemia [53], diabetes mellitus [53], lupus erythematosus [55], myasthenia gravis [56–60], polymyalgia rheumatica [61], ulcerative colitis [60,62,63], celiac disease [64], lichen planus [65–69], and autoimmune polyendocrinopathy-candidiasis ectodermal dystrophy, also known as autoimmune polyglandular syndrome type 1 (APS-1) [43,70–72]. Thirty percent of patients with APS-1 have AA.

Successful treatment of AA with immunosuppressive agents such as oral cyclosporine [73,74] and systemic steroids [75] also supports the idea of immune-mediated pathogenesis in AA.

Direct clues for autoimmunity

Humoral immunity

Studies in the past with direct immunofluorescence have failed to show particular antibodies to epidermal cells or hair follicles in AA [76]. Studies of passive transfer of serum from AA patients to nude mice failed to inhibit hair growth in grafted transplants of human scalp skin [77]. However, Tobin et al. reported detection of antibodies to pigmented hair follicles by Western blotting in the sera of 100% of the AA patients examined, as compared to only 44% of normal controls [78]. In another study by Tobin et al. [79], much higher levels of autoantibodies to multiple structures of anagen hair follicles in AA patients have been reported, as compared to controls using indirect immunofluorescence. The antibody response to hair follicles in patients with AA has been found to be heterogeneous, because different patients develop different patterns of antibodies to different hair follicle structures. The most common target structures were the outer root sheath, followed by the matrix, inner root sheath, and hair shaft [79].

Cell-mediated immunity

AA can be seen as an autoimmune disease with a collapse of the hair follicles' immune privilege [80]. The immunopathogenesis of AA and the relevant autoantigens remains unclear.

Studies of cell-mediated immunity in AA have given conflicting results. Circulating total numbers of T lymphocytes have been reported as reduced [53,81] or normal [82]. Friedmann [53] suggested that the number of circulating T cells is reduced in AA, and that the level of this reduction is related to disease severity. In addition, he suggested

that the impairment of helper T cell function and the change in suppressor T cell numbers may also reflect changes in disease activity. A slight increase in helper T cells (CD4) and decrease in number of suppressor T cells (CD8), resulting in an increase in the ratio of helper to suppressor cells, may be correlated with the amount of hair loss [81].

The dense peribulbar lymphocytic infiltrate affecting anagen follicles is one of the most consistent and reproducible immunologic abnormalities in AA. The follicular infiltrate in AA is mainly composed of CD4+ and CD8+ T cells [14,16]. The cellular infiltrate first becomes evident around the bulbar blood vessels, particularly in the dermal papilla/capillary network, and consists mostly of T lymphocytes and, to a lesser extent, macrophages and Langerhans cells. The infiltrate is most prominent in active disease. The infiltrate subsides in inactive disease and disappears in the regrowth phase. Most of the T cells are activated, as can be seen by the expression of DR antigens and IL-2 receptors. The T cell helper to suppressor ratio is 2:1–4:1. The implication of these observations is that there may be an immune response to antigens in the lower half of hair follicles or in the peribulbar blood vessels in AA. The presence of cellular infiltrates around unaffected hair follicles suggests that the process precedes rather than results from injury to hair follicles.

CD8+ T cells especially seem to play a key role in the development of AA. It has been shown that the transfer of CD8+ cells alone induces localized AA-like hair loss in the C3H/HeJ mouse model [83,84], while the depletion of CD8+ T cells had some protective influence [85]. Gilhar [86] and Tsuboi [87] have shown that grafting affected scalp AA skin from humans onto severe combined immunodeficiency (SCID) mice results in regrowth of hair, with the disappearance of the T cell infiltrate. Tsuboi has shown that the CD8+ cells had disappeared completely from almost all portions of the hair follicle, while CD4+

cells still remained in the upper portions of the hair follicle. This may imply the greater importance of CD8+ in the expression of AA.

Furthermore, Gilhar et al. [86] reported that AA can be induced in human scalp explants from AA patients transplanted onto SCID mice by transfer of autologous T lymphocytes isolated from involved scalp. In this study, T lymphocytes that had been cultured with hair follicle homogenate along with antigen-presenting cells and melanocyte-derived protein were capable of inducing the changes of AA. These changes include hair loss, perifollicular T cell infiltration, and HLA-DR and intercellular adhesion molecule-1 (ICAM-1) expression of follicular epithelium. T cells that had not been cultured with follicular homogenate were not able to induce AA. The necessity of the follicular homogenate to inducing AA suggests that T cells recognize a follicular autoantigen. Furthermore, AA induction followed on injection with CD8+ cells cultured with follicular homogenate, but not on injection of the cultured CD4+ cells. This study also suggests that AA is mediated by T cells, particularly CD8+ cells [86].

Gilhar et al. recently showed that AA can be also induced by IL-2 stimulated NKG2D+/CD56+ immunocytes, which are mostly also CD8+ T cells [88]. Most recently, Bertolini et al. suggested that an abnormal interaction between mast cells and CD8+ T cells may play a functionally important role in the pathogenesis of AA [80].

For a medical condition to fit as an autoimmune disease, the following criteria should be met:

1. Unique antigens in the affected organ
2. An autoimmune response to that antigen
3. An autoimmune response specifically associated with the disease
4. The autoimmune response producing, not following, the condition
5. The disease being transferred passively by autoantibodies or T cells

For AA, many of the above criteria are indeed met. Increased frequency of hair-specific antibodies, antibodies to pigmented hair follicles, high levels of autoantibodies to multiple structures of anagen hair follicles, an increase in the ratio of helper to suppressor cells, and induction of AA on SCID mice by transfer of T lymphocytes cultured with follicular homogenates are evidence supporting the view that AA is an autoimmune disease targeting the hair follicle. Figure 5.4 illustrates some of the immunologic cascade events that take place in AA.

The hair follicle has a distinct immune system [89] that differs from that of its surrounding skin. The cellular components of the hair follicle immune system are composed of intrafollicular T lymphocytes and Langerhans cells, located exclusively in the distal outer root sheath, perifollicular mast cells, and macrophages [89]. There is also a unique expression

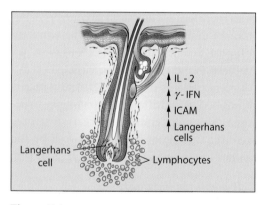

Figure 5.4

The pathogenesis of alopecia areata. Antigen-presenting cells, such as Langerhans cells, are increased in the bulb of the affected follicles. They present the responsible epitope to the peribulbar lymphocytes. This leads to a cascade of immunologic events with increased interleukin-2 (IL-2), gamma interferon (gIFN), and intercellular adhesion molecules (ICAM). This series of events helps to induce hair loss. This is considered to be a type 1 T helper cell response.

of follicular MHC class Ia/Ib and ICAM-1 [89]. Human hair follicles may even serve as a Langerhans cell reservoir. The epithelium of the proximal anagen hair follicle is immune privileged, since the inner root sheath and hair matrix do not express MHC class I molecules. This immune privilege may collapse in AA. A recent theory for AA proposed by Paus et al. [90] involves the upregulation of MHC antigens and/or downregulation of locally produced immunosuppressants (melanocyte-stimulating hormone, adrenocorticotropin, and transforming growth factor), allowing the immune system to recognize the immune-privileged hair follicle antigens, leading to onset of AA.

Cytokines

It appears that cytokines have a significant pathogenic role in AA. Cytokines are immunomodulators mediating inflammation and regulating cell proliferation. T helper cells produce cytokines divided into two subgroups depending on the pattern of cytokine production.

Type 1 T helper (Th1) cells produce interferon γ (IFN-γ) and IL-2. Type 2 helper (Th2) cells produce IL-4 and IL-5 [91]. Aberrant expression of cytokines of the Th1 type (see Figure 5.4) and IL-1β have been detected in affected areas of the scalp in patients with AA [92]. As hair regrows with topical immunotherapy, these cytokine profiles change.

IFN-γ is probably the main cytokine expressed in AA through a CD4+ Th1-mediated response. IFN-γ is produced by perifollicular or follicular antigen-presenting cells and is known to suppress anagen hair growth in dermal papilla cells [93]. Significantly increased serum levels of IFN-γ have been found in patients with AT and AU. This may reflect the state of disease activity and inflammation [94,95]. Monokine induced by IFN-γ (MIG) is a cytokine that is also found to be elevated in AA, and its level correlates with disease activity [96]. MIG mRNA

is mostly found in mononuclear cells in the peri- and intrabulbar infiltrate and also in the follicular papilla [97].

Cytokines derived from epidermal keratinocytes, interleukins IL-1 α, IL-1 β, and tumor necrosis factor-α (TNF-α) are potent inhibitors of hair follicle growth, and in vitro produce changes in hair follicle morphology similar to those in AA [46,92]. Interleukin 1 (IL-1) is an inducer of hair loss and a significant human hair growth inhibitor in vitro [98]. In transgenic mice an overexpression of IL-1α in the epidermis led to patchy hair loss resembling AA [99].

In human scalp areas affected by AA, an excessive expression of IL-1β is detected particularly at the early stages of the disease. Patients with an insufficient amount of IL-1 receptor antagonist, due to gene polymorphisms, show more progressive and severe forms of AA. Patients with more severe forms of AA have an increased frequency of the IL-1β 1,2 genotype [100], with allele 2 of the IL-1β + 3953 polymorphism exhibiting a strong association with increased production of IL-1β [101]. Philpott et al. showed that the effects of IL-1α and IL-1β in cultured hair follicles may be blocked by adding IL-1 receptor antagonist [46].

Although IL-2 and IFN-γ serum levels are mainly elevated in extensive disease states of AA, possibly implying that the progression to the extensive form may be mediated by Th1 cytokines, IL-1α and IL-4 are significantly elevated in patients with localized AA [97,102]. It is also considered that a disequilibrium in the production of cytokines, with a relative excess of proinflammatory and Th1 types, versus anti-inflammatory cytokines, such as IL-4 and IL-10, may be involved in the persistence of AA lesions [97,103]. Finally, it has been shown that steady-state levels of IL-10 mRNA increase after successful diphenylcyclopropenone treatment, making IL-10 an important inhibitor of Th1 cytokine production [97,98,104].

Along with IL-1α and IL-1β, TNF-α plays a major role in the pathogenesis of AA [105,106]. IL-1α, IL-1β, and TNF-α cause a decrease in the size of the matrix, disorganization of follicular melanocytes, and abnormal differentiation and keratinization of the precortical cells and the inner root sheath [46]. TNF-α levels in the skin correlate positively with plasma adrenocorticotropic hormone (ACTH) levels and cutaneous ACTH receptor expression levels under repeated stress in humans [107]. Elevated serum levels of B cell activating factor (BAFF), which belongs to the TNF family, were found in patients with AA [108,109]. BAFF may activate T cells and promote Th1 response, leading to the production of IFN-γ and perpetuation of disease activity [97,110].

Infection

There has been a report regarding the possibility of cytomegalovirus (CMV) infection found within the patches of scalp AA. This initial report showed a convincing positive association with CMV [111], but this has not been confirmed, as other investigators have reported negative findings [112–114]. The whole concept of molecular mimicry of the hair follicle with a virus is intriguing, but the evidence for a viral etiology of AA at this point in time is not conclusive.

Emotional stress

Several studies suggest that stress may be a precipitating factor in some cases of AA. Acute psychotrauma before the onset of AA [112–116], a higher number of stressful events in the 6 months preceding hair loss [116], higher prevalence of psychiatric disorders [117], and psychosomatic factors in patients with AA have been reported [118]. In contrast, there are reports revealing that emotional stress does not play any role in the pathogenesis of AA [119].

Intrinsically abnormal melanocytes or keratinocytes

Morphological analysis of follicles in active AA lesions has revealed regressive changes in the hair bulbs of anagen hair follicles [119–122]. Abnormal melanogenesis and melanocytes are common findings. This evidence, together with the presence of antibodies to pigmented hairs of AA, may explain some of the associated pigmentary anomalies seen clinically in acute AA and the preferential effect of AA on pigmented hairs. Also, degeneration of precortical keratinocytes has been shown in follicles of active AA lesions [120]. Abnormal melanosomes in clinically normal regions, together with degenerative changes, including vacuolation, in the outer root sheath of all hair follicles from non-balding lesions of AA [120] correspond well with the hypothesis of a subclinical condition of the disease in clinically normal areas of AA.

Neurological factors

It has been suggested that local changes in the peripheral nervous system at the level of the dermal papilla or bulge region may play a role in the evolution of AA because the peripheral nervous system can deliver neuropeptides that modulate a range of inflammatory and proliferative processes [123]. This theory has been supported by Hordinsky et al., who revealed a decrease in calcitonin gene-related peptide (CGRP) and substance P (SP) expression in the scalps of patients with AA [124]. The neuropeptide CGRP has a potent anti-inflammatory action [124,125], and neuropeptide SP is capable of inducing hair growth in the mouse [124,126]. In addition, application of capsaicin, which causes neurogenic inflammation and releases SP, to the entire scalp of two AA patients revealed an enhanced presence of SP in AA perifollicular nerves and induced vellus hair growth [127].

Alopecia areata animal models

Animal models have greatly helped understanding of the pathogenesis of AA. Animal models with spontaneous AA include the C3H/HeJ mouse [128], the Dundee experimental bald rat (DEBR) [129], and the Smyth chicken [130]. The Smyth chicken model also has vitiligo, and may suggest a link between vitiligo, melanogenesis, and the development of AA.

AA can be induced in normal C3H/HeJ mice using full-thickness skin grafts from affected C3H/HeJ mice [131]. AA developed 8–10 weeks after grafting. The ability to induce AA in a model suggests that, whereas individuals may be genetically predisposed toward AA, susceptibility genes are not enough to develop the condition. AA induction can also be used to produce large numbers of mice for testing pharmaceutical agents.

Animal models are used in research for new and improved treatments. Lui et al. have shown that leflunomide, an IL-2 inhibitor, has some efficacy in the DEBR rat [132]. Shapiro et al. [133] have shown efficacy of diphenylcyclopropenone (DPCP) in the C3H/HeJ mouse. Freyschmidt-Paul has shown the efficacy of squaric acid dibutyl ester (SADBE) in the C3H/HeJ AA mouse [134].

Animal models with AA-like hair loss are significantly useful in investigations regarding pathogenesis, disease behavior, efficacy, and side effects of available or future treatments.

Non-alopecia areata animal models

The hairless mouse has an autosomal recessive allelic mutation that maps to chromosome 14 [128,135]. These mice develop a normal pelage at about 14 days and then lose their hair over 1 week. Investigations have correlated this hairless gene in mice with congenital atrichia in humans.

Hox genes, particularly homeobox C13 (Hoxc13), play a significant role in follicular proliferation and differentiation [136]. Transgenic Hoxc13 deficient mice were unable to synthesize hair keratins and had sparse brittle hair [136]. More knowledge of Hoxc13 expression in epidermal appendages will in turn provide further insight into the functioning of the normal ordered follicle, which in turn will allow us to understand the disordered follicle more clearly [137].

Non-AA animal hair mutations may eventually help us to unravel the delicate mechanisms of the hair cycle and subsequently bring us closer to understanding the disordered hair follicle as it is found in AA.

Pathology

In early active AA, the hair cycle is abnormal, with hair follicles entering the telogen or late catagen stage prematurely in the involved areas [138]. There are distinct stages in the histopathology of AA: (a) acute alopecia, (b) persistent alopecia, and (c) recovery [139,140]. Figure 5.5 shows the transition from the acute stage to the chronic stage with a miniaturized anagen or telogen [139]. A peribulbar lymphocytic infiltrate ("swarm of bees") with no scarring is characteristic of the diagnosis of AA (Figure 5.4 and 5.6a through c). The inflammatory cellular infiltrate is composed chiefly of activated T lymphocytes together with macrophages and Langerhans cells [141,142]. Also, miniaturization of hairs, with numerous fibrous tracts along with pigment incontinence within these fibrous tracts, is appreciable (Figure 5.6d).

During the acute phase of hair loss, matrix cell and matrical melanocyte failure with a formation of dysplastic hair shafts is noted. Following complete matrix failure, the involved follicle enters the end-stage telogen.

Clinical course and hair cycle in alopecia areata

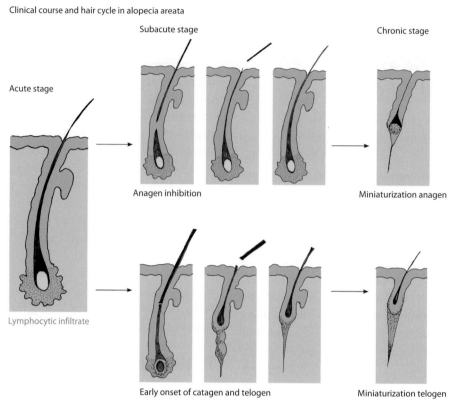

Figure 5.5
Acute, subacute, and chronic stages of alopecia areata. (From Whiting DA. *Arch Dermatol*, 2003. **139**(12): 1555–9.)

A decreased anagen to telogen ratio, resulting in marked increase in telogen and catagen hairs, can be observed in horizontal sections of scalp biopsies [142,143] (Figure 5.6e). The terminal to vellus ratio is decreased and even reversed by the increased numbers of miniaturized hairs. Inflammatory changes in the mid and upper dermis are generally not prominent unless many vellus hairs are affected by the disease.

In patients with long-standing persistent alopecia, the involved hair follicles arrest in the end-stage telogen phase. In these cases, peribulbar infiltration along with an increase in Langerhans cell numbers [144], a decrease in follicular density, and follicular miniaturization may be present. In patients with complete recovery, normal hair follicles with little or no peribulbar lymphocytic infiltration and no decrease in hair density are noted.

Eosinophils are also detectable in all stages of AA, within the peribulbar infiltrate and the fibrous tracts. Although clinical correlation is necessary, this feature is helpful in diagnosis of AA in some biopsy specimens without peribulbar lymphocytic infiltrate [145]. Mast cells were also noted in a small series of AA slides [146].

Electron-microscopic examination of microdissected hair follicles from AA scalps showed ultrastructural abnormalities in the dermal papillae of both lesional and clinically normal hair follicles [147]. This shows that, with patchy involvement, AA is not a localized process. Immunohistochemical evaluation of clinically normal AA specimens reveals a prominent expression of ICAM-1 in the dermal papilla and keratinocytes of the matrix and outer root sheath [148].

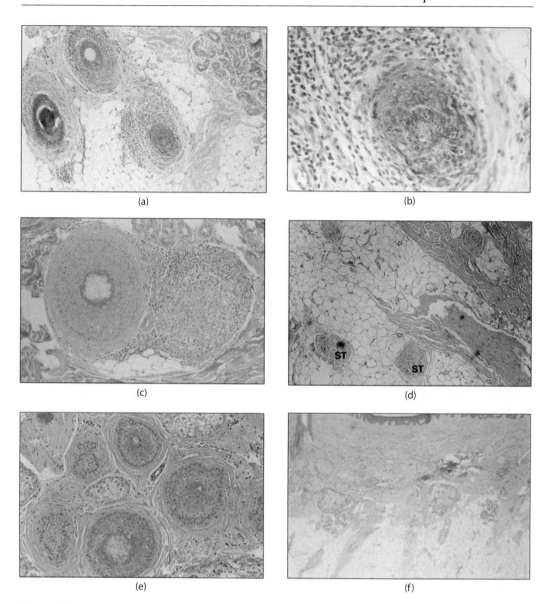

Figure 5.6

Histopathology of alopecia areata. (a) "Swarm of bees" noted in the deep subcutaneous peribulbar area of the follicle; (b) close-up of the lymphocytic infiltrate, with matrix destruction; (c) two follicles, with one showing marked lymphocytic infiltration, whereas the other does not. This highlights the fact that alopecia areata (AA) is a very heterogeneous condition, not only on the same scalp, but within the same follicular bundle; (d) follicular stellae (ST) remnants in AA; (e) the large number of telogen hairs in AA. Almost all follicles within this field are telogen; (f) reduction of follicular numbers in chronic AA. (Courtesy of Dr. Magda Martinka, Dr. David Shum, and Dr. Martin Trotter.)

Histopathologically, AA should be differentiated from androgenetic alopecia, telogen effluvium, trichotillomania, and syphilitic alopecia. In androgenetic alopecia, miniaturization of hairs is present with lack of lymphoid infiltration at the level of the bulb and a lack of pigment incontinence within fibrous tracts. In telogen effluvium, miniaturization of follicles is not present. Trichotillomania is characterized by empty anagen follicles, multiple catagen hairs, trichomalacia, and pigment casts in the follicular infundibulum. Syphilitic alopecia is very difficult to distinguish from AA. Presence of plasma cells along with no peribulbar eosinophils and abundant lymphocytes in the isthmus are features of syphilitic alopecia, whereas the presence of peribulbar eosinophils and lymphocytes strongly suggests AA [149].

Clinical features

AA can manifest with several different clinical features. Patients usually complain of abrupt hair loss and marked hair shedding. The characteristic lesion of AA is commonly a round or oval, totally bald, smooth patch involving the scalp or any hair-bearing area on the body (Figure 5.7a and d). The patch may have a mild peachy or pinkish-red color (Figure 5.7b, e and f). Hair loss is seen both as intact and as fractured hairs (Figure 5.7c and i). The intact hairs are dystrophic anagen or telogen hairs. The fractured hairs develop owing to damage involving both cortex and medulla, resulting in distal fractures [150]. These hairs are described as "exclamation mark" hairs, because the distal segment is broader than the proximal end (Figure 5.7g). The pull test may be positive at the margins of the patch, indicating very active disease. Although hair loss is usually asymptomatic in most cases, some patients describe paresthesias, with mild to moderate pruritus, tenderness, burning sensation or pain, before the appearance of the patches.

The clinical presentation of AA is subcategorized according to pattern or extent of the hair loss. If categorized according to pattern, the following forms are seen: patchy AA, round or oval patches of hair loss (most common); reticular AA, reticulated pattern of patchy hair loss; ophiasis band-like AA, hair loss in temporo-occipital scalp; ophiasis inversus (sisapho) [151], a rare band-like pattern of hair loss in the frontoparieto scalp (the exact opposite of ophiasis) [152]; and diffuse AA, a diffuse decrease in hair density over the entire scalp (Figure 5.8).

If categorized by extent of involvement, the following forms may be seen: AA, partial loss of scalp hair; AT, 100% loss of scalp hair; and AU, 100% loss of hair on scalp and body (Figure 5.9). Any hair-bearing surface can be affected. Where there is hair, there can be AA! Beard AA is very common, as well as body AA, affecting the limbs or the thorax area. (Figures 5.10 and 5.11).

Most patients present with the limited patchy type that is easily camouflaged. The initial regrowth in AA is often white, followed by repigmentation. Frequently, AA preferentially affects pigmented hair, and only the white hairs remain (Figure 5.12). Regrowth on one site and extension of the alopecia on another site may be seen at the same time in the same patient.

Nail dystrophy may be associated with AA. The reported incidence of onychodystrophy in AA ranges from 10% to 66% [153], depending on how diligently it is looked for. Changes may be seen in one, many, or all of the nails. The dystrophy may precede, coincide with, or follow resolution of the AA. Pitting with an irregular pattern or in organized transverse or

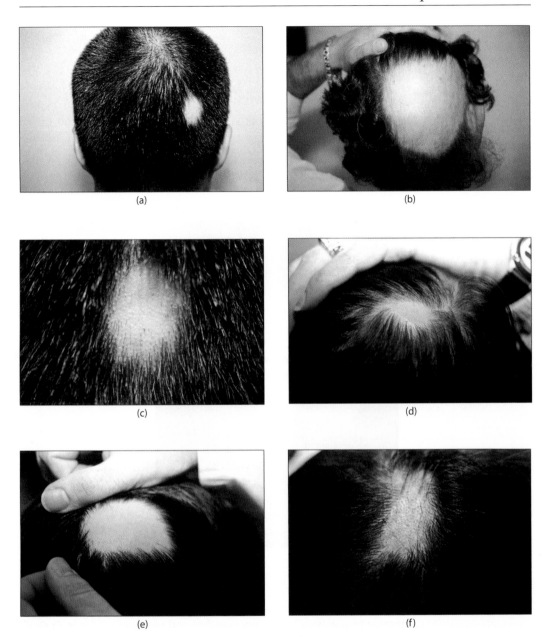

Figure 5.7

Alopecia areata circumscripta. Patients frequently present with just a patch. (a) A single small circular patch; (b) a single large circular patch totally devoid of hair, "bare as a baby's bottom"; (c) the patch may be skin-colored with broken-off hairs; (d) the color of an alopecia areata (AA) patch may be peach; (e) another peach-colored patch of AA; (f) the AA patch may be red. This patient complained of burning on the patch before the hair fell out.

(*Continued*)

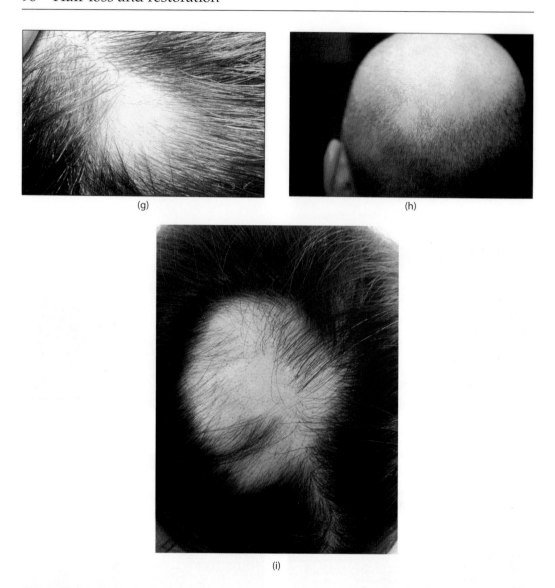

(g)

(h)

(i)

Figure 5.7 (*Continued*)
(g) Exclamation point hairs may be seen during an active phase of the condition. (Courtesy of Dr. Harvey Lui.) (h) Circumscript patches can be very constant and persistent. This is a patch on a 40-year-old male that has been present in the same place and has been the same size for 10 years. He has not had any other spots for over a decade. (i) Patch of AA with residual intact hairs.

longitudinal rows, trachyonychia (longitudinal striations resulting in sandpaper appearance), Beau's lines (grooves through the nail matching that of the lunula margin), onychorrhexis (superficial splitting of the nail extending to the free edge), thinning or thickening (pseudomycotic), onychomadesis (onycholysis with nail loss), koilonychia (concave dorsal nail plate), punctate or transverse leukonychia, and red spotted lunula may be associated with AA [154–158] (Figure 5.13).

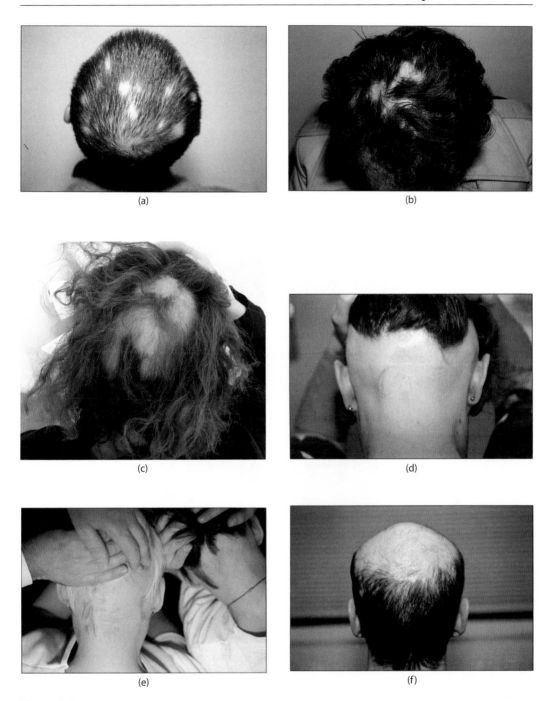

Figure 5.8
Clinical forms of alopecia areata (AA) based on pattern. (a) Patchy AA in multifocal areas;
(b) reticulated patches in AA; (c) reticulated and interconnected patches; (d) ophiasis
(e) simultaneous ophiasis in mother and daughter.

(*Continued*)

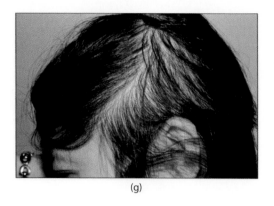

(g)

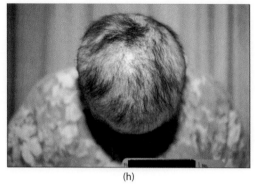

(h)

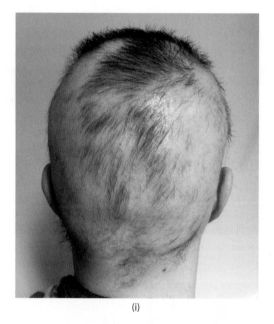

(i)

Figure 5.8 (*Continued*)
(g) Early diffuse AA with no distinct patches; (h, i) advanced diffuse AA.

Diagnosis

The diagnosis of AA can be usually established based on clinical presentation. A thorough inspection of the entire scalp and body is essential in every patient to identify all areas affected with AA. The presence of follicular ostia should be evaluated with a 10–100-fold magnifying device (dermatoscope or trichoscope) to rule out scarring alopecia. Exclamation point hairs as well as yellow and black dots can also be identified with trichoscopy [159–161]. A pull test should be performed to estimate disease activity in the margin of each lesion and on different areas of the scalp. Measurements of the single lesions with a ruler and photography of the patches can be helpful to track disease progression and to document therapy success. In diffuse AA, a trichogram can be useful and will display an increased number of dystrophic hairs. If the diagnosis is in doubt, a 4-mm punch biopsy is recommended from the margin of an active lesion [162].

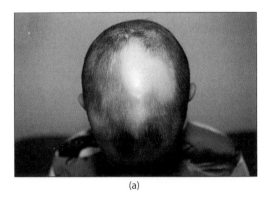
(a)

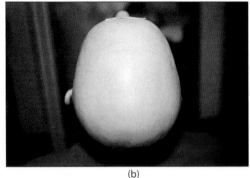
(b)

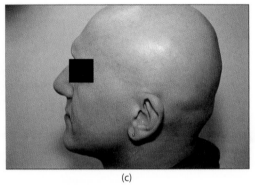
(c)

Figure 5.9
Clinical forms of alopecia areata (AA) based on extent. (a) AA with its characteristic circular patches; (b) alopecia totalis affecting 100% of the scalp; (c) alopecia universalis in an adult affecting all hairs on the body, including eyelashes and eyebrows.

Laboratory tests

Laboratory workup should involve a thyroid stimulating hormone (TSH) test as well as thyroid autoantibodies due to AA's frequent association with thyroid diseases including Hashimoto thyroiditis [50,163–167]. Tests for ferritin, vitamin D, vitamin B12, selenium, zinc, and copper may also be useful to rule out deficiencies that could possibly affect hair growth and regrowth [168].

Prognosis

The only predictable thing about the progress of AA is that it is unpredictable. Patients usually present with several episodes of hair loss and hair regrowth during their lifetime. The recovery from hair loss may be complete, partial, or nonexistent. The majority of patients will regrow their hair entirely within 1 year without treatment. However, 7%–10% can eventually end up with the severe chronic form of the condition. Poor prognostic indicators are atopy, the presence of other immune diseases, a positive family history of AA, a young age of onset, nail dystrophy, extensive hair loss, and ophiasis [118,162,169].

Differential diagnosis

Clinically, the differential diagnosis is usually between cicatricial alopecias, telogen effluvium, androgenetic alopecia (AGA), trichotillomania, traction alopecia, triangular

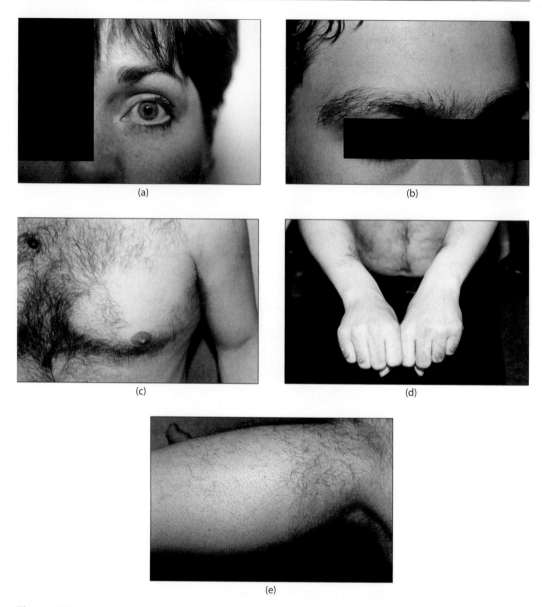

Figure 5.10
Extracranial alopecia areata (AA). (a) AA affecting just the eyelashes; (b) AA affecting one eyebrow; (c) AA affecting the chest; (d) AA affecting the dorsa of the arms; (e) AA affecting just the lateral portion of the leg.

temporal alopecia, pressure-induced alopecia, and tinea capitis (Figure 5.14). In telogen effluvium, hair loss is generalized over the whole scalp, whereas in AA it is usually patchy. Hairs that are shed are either telogen or dystrophic anagen in AA, and purely telogen in telogen effluvium. Patients with AGA usually show the typical predictable pattern of balding, and shedding is not prominent. The pull test is usually negative in AGA. In trichotillomania and traction alopecia, twisted and broken hairs are frequently

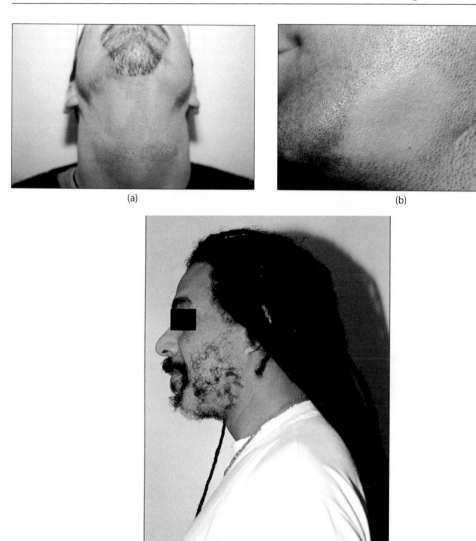

(a)

(b)

(c)

Figure 5.11
Alopecia areata (AA) of the beard is very common. (a) Random patches on the beard area;
(b) the characteristic peach color on AA of the beard; (c) extensive AA of the beard, but not
affecting the great head of dreadlocks.

evident. In tinea capitis, there is usually an inflammatory component. However, noninflammatory tinea capitis may be most difficult to distinguish from AA. Look for the characteristic scaling in tinea capitis. A potassium hydroxide preparation and fungal culture may be necessary to distinguish noninflammatory tinea capitis from AA. Wood's light examination may help if the patient is in or has been in an area where the fluorescent tineas predominate. In British Columbia as well as in Germany, the most common cause of tinea capitis is *Microsporum canis*, which does fluoresce.

Temporal triangular alopecia (TTA) may mimic AA. The lifetime incidence of TTA is

0.11% [170]. This is 10 times less frequent than AA. Lesions present as a triangular, oval, or lancet-shaped patch of non-scarring alopecia overlying the frontotemporal suture. There is controversy as to whether the lesions are present at birth or acquired later in life.

A biopsy may occasionally be necessary to distinguish TTA from AA. Histologically, peribulbar lymphocytic infiltrates are not present. Pressure-induced alopecia [170–174] (PIA) may also mimic AA. Usually a history of coma or surgery is present. Clinically,

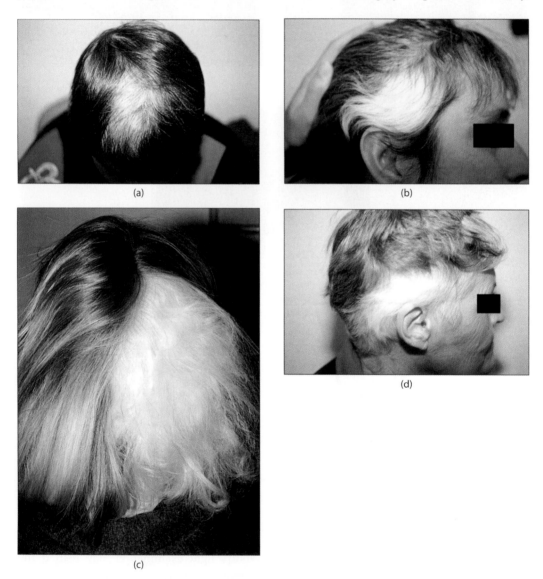

(a)

(b)

(c)

(d)

Figure 5.12
White hairs, vitiligo, and alopecia areata (AA). (a) Hair regrowth in a young child who had been diagnosed as a case of trichotillomania. The white hair regrowth proves the diagnosis had always been AA; (b and c) white regrowth on the side of the scalp; (d) white regrowth in an area of previous ophiasis.

(Continued)

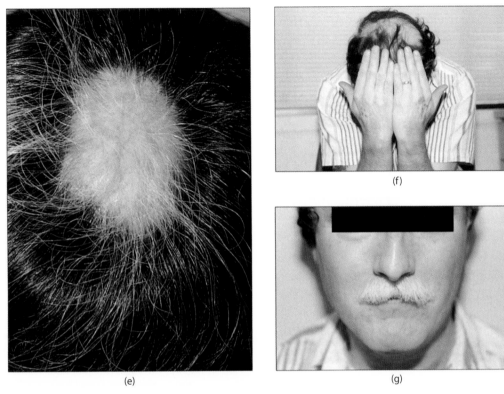

Figure 5.12 (*Continued*)
(e) Circumscript AA, sparing white hairs; (f) AA and vitiligo on the same person; (g) white moustache in a vitiliginous area in the patient.

there is usually some scarring with PIA. Occasionally in AA, the scalp may be so shiny and smooth that follicular ostia may be difficult to see, and patchy AA may be difficult to differentiate from pseudopelade.

Treatment

Modern therapy for AA is best appreciated within a historical framework. Bateman [175], in the 1800s, wrote about AA and concluded that the application of a caustic substance with the subsequent production of bullae was often successful in the treatment of AA. He advocated the use of ointments prepared with oil of mace, turpentine, mustard, and black pepper. Although this may seem crude, some current treatment regimens have similar objectives. They cause blisters and erythema, and an immunologic patient response to modify the perifollicular immunologic milieu. Despite the advance of medicine over the last 200 years, some of the fundamental principles in the treatment of AA remain unchanged.

There is great difficulty in evaluating the literature on treatment modalities for AA, because there is so much variability regarding baseline patient populations and the terms "successful regrowth" or "responders." Most studies have grouped patients with AT and AU with those with just patchy AA. There is no question that AT/AU is a distinct prognostic and therapeutic group, and results can be skewed by this more difficult and severely affected population. There is a

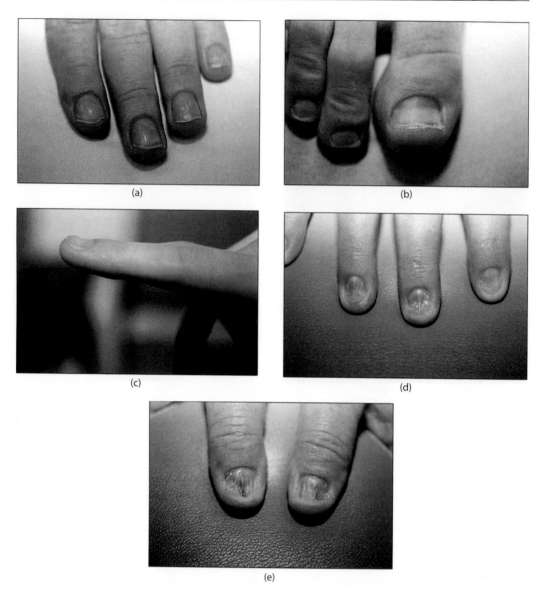

Figure 5.13
Nail changes and alopecia areata (AA). (a) Trachyonychia, and red-spotted lunula on the fingernails; (b) red-spotted lunula on the toenails; (c) koilonychia present in AA; (d, e) severe nail dystrophy in AA.

paucity of studies that distinguish AT/AU from patchy AA. This lack of stratification of the patient population can have a profound influence on evaluating therapeutic efficacy. Unfortunately, the treatment of AA is very difficult, and there are no consistently reliable treatments. Although the FDA has never approved any drug for AA, this does not mean that there are no effective treatments.

Evaluating efficacy is most difficult, especially for patchy AA, as it is so unpredictable and frequently improves on its own. To prove efficacy with sufficient power and statistical significance, large patient populations are necessary. Most published studies for AA have been small. Half-head studies are very powerful, but again, much of this published work has involved patient populations with a preponderance of AT/AU. In 1999,

Olsen et al. published *Alopecia Areata Investigational Assessment Guidelines.* These guidelines are very helpful in establishing criteria for selecting and assessing patients for clinical studies of AA, facilitating

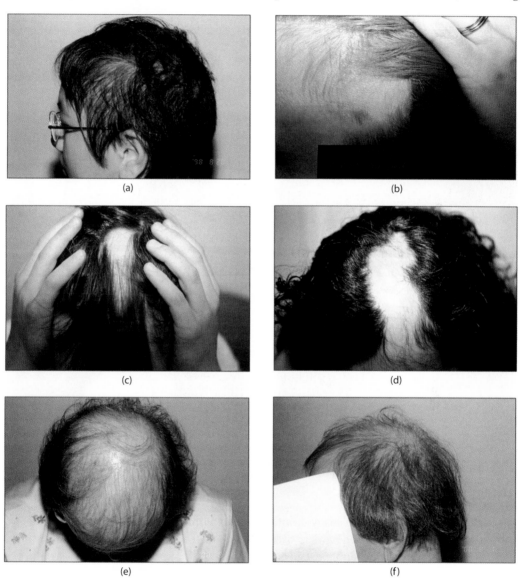

(a)   (b)

(c)   (d)

(e)   (f)

Figure 5.14
Differential diagnosis of alopecia areata (AA). (a) This is an early case of biopsy-proven diffuse AA, which can be difficult to differentiate from telogen effluvium; (b) temporal triangular alopecia can mimic AA; (c) AA may be linear and mimic morphea; (d) morphea mimicking AA. It is crucial to look for the presence of follicular ostia, which may be difficult to see on a shiny, smooth scalp; (e, f) AA mimicking AGA in a female patient.

(Continued)

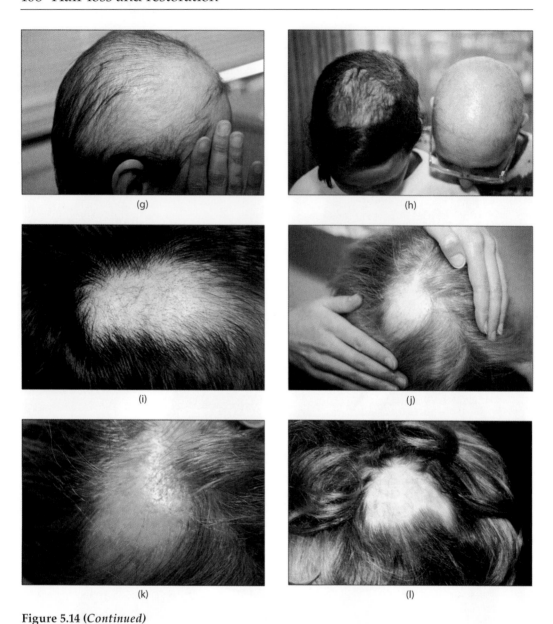

Figure 5.14 (*Continued*)
(g) Trichotillomania, which can easily mimic AA; (h) simultaneous trichotillomania in a mother and daughter; (i) broken hairs in trichotillomania; (j, k) pseudopelade mimicking AA. Note the loss of follicular ostia; (l) postsurgical pressure-induced alopecia can appear like AA, but usually has a significant scarred component to it.

collaboration, comparison of data, and measuring the extent of scalp involvement [176]. They highlight the fact that AT and AU are considered separate entities from AA, and must be separated out to determine the efficacy of any trichogenic agent. It is of paramount importance that dermatologists be knowledgeable and conscious of this important segregation when evaluating modalities in the treatment of AA. The terms "responder" and "successful regrowth" are not used in the same way from one study to another. The guidelines help us to evaluate successful regrowth. Most dermatologists consider successful regrowth to be cosmetically acceptable regrowth, meaning being able to abandon one's wig or cap. When comparing studies, it is important to ascertain clearly what the authors have defined as a "responder."

At present, all treatments are palliative, only controlling the problem and not curing the condition. All local treatments may help the treated areas, but do not prevent further spread of the condition. In addition, any mode of treatment may require long periods of usage, owing to the chronic nature of AA. At the present time, topical, intralesional, and systemic steroids, topical immunotherapy, anthralin, minoxidil, and photochemotherapy are available for the treatment of AA. Treatment guidelines for AA have been published by the American Academy of Dermatology [177]. All treatment plans for patients depend on three major factors: the extent of scalp involvement, the age of the patient, and the motivation level of the patient.

Corticosteroids

The main mechanism of action is immunosuppression. However, some biochemical abnormalities relating to steroid chemistry have been discovered in AA patients by Sawaya and Hordinsky [178]. They showed that patients with AA have abnormalities in glucocorticoid receptors (GCR) for type 2 binding. This receptor is found to influence long-term, slow-growth cellular processes. Scalp biopsies from 15 untreated AA patients showed a twofold increase in unoccupied GCR. This suggests suppressed cellular transcription. It was found that low concentrations of calmodulin stimulate a cytosol kinase, and thus hormone binding to GCR. This suggests that patients with AA have abnormalities in type 2 GCR activation because of abnormal calcium–calmodulin metabolism. These abnormalities may explain why patients with AA show a varied response in hair area growth when treated with glucocorticoids [178].

Intralesional corticosteroids

Intralesional corticosteroid injection is first line therapy for adult patients with less than 50% scalp involvement [179]. For circumscribed AA, intradermal corticosteroids remain the therapeutic standard [180]. Porter and Burton [181] demonstrated response rates of 64% using triamcinolone acetonide and 97% using the less soluble and more atrophogenic triamcinolone hexacetonide. Price [179], Shapiro [182], Mitchell and Krull [169,183], Whiting [183], Bergfeld [184], and Thiers [185] prefer triamcinolone acetonide. Concentrations of triamcinolone acetonide vary from 2.5 to 10.0 mg/mL diluted either in xylocaine or sterile saline. Price [179] prefers 10 mg/mL, Whiting [183] prefers 5–10 mg/mL, Shapiro [182] prefers 5 mg/mL, Bergfeld prefers 2.5–5.0 mg/mL [184], and Thiers [185] prefers 3.3 mg/mL.

In our hair clinic, for scalp AA, we inject a concentration of 5 mg/mL with a maximum total of 3 mL of triamcinolone acetonide. A weaker concentration of 2.5 mg/mL is used for the beard area and the eyebrows. Triamcinolone acetonide is administered with a 0.5-inch-long 30-gauge needle as multiple intradermal injections of 0.1 mL per site, approximately 1 cm apart. Initial regrowth is often seen in 4–8 weeks. Treatments are repeated every 4 to 6 weeks.

The main side effect is minimal transient atrophy. This can be prevented by avoiding injections that are too great in volume per injected site, too frequent, or too superficial (intraepidermal). Topical anesthesia cream (2.5% lidocaine and 2.5% prilocaine in a cream) in a thick layer with occlusion 1 hour before injection can be used. However, this cream can be difficult to use on the hairy scalp. Children under 10 years of age are not usually treated with intralesional steroids owing to the local pain at the injection sites. After 6 months of treatment, if there is no response, discontinue intralesional corticosteroids, because these patients may lack adequate corticosteroid receptors in the scalp [178] (Figure 5.15).

Topical Therapy

Topical corticosteroids

Topical corticosteroids are widely used in the treatment of AA. However, the evidence for their efficacy is limited. Clobetasol propionate [186,187], betamethasone valerate [188], fluocinolone acetonide [189,190], halcinonide

[191], and dexamethasone [192] have been reported to have some success [193].

Pascher et al. compared 0.2% fluocinolone acetonide cream twice a day to placebo in a half-head study. Unilateral regrowth was noted in 54% of patients in the treatment arm compared with 0% in the vehicle group [190]. A multicenter prospective, randomized, controlled, investigator-blinded trial in patients with less than 26% hair loss showed a greater than 75% hair regrowth rate in 61% of patients using 0.1% betamethasone valerate foam in comparison with 27% in the 0.05% betamethasone dipropionate lotion group [188]. Tosti et al. had success with unilateral application of 0.05% clobetasol propionate

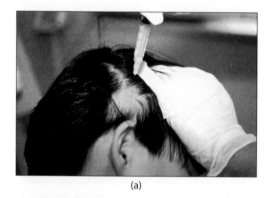
(a)

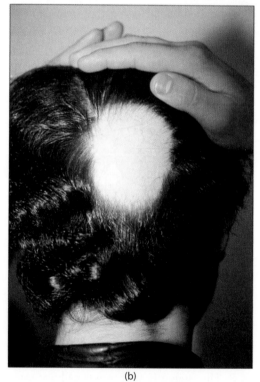
(b)

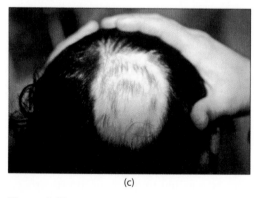
(c)

Figure 5.15
Intralesional corticosteroid injections for alopecia areata. (a) Injecting triamcinolone acetonide 5 mg/mL with a 3 mL syringe and a 30-gauge needle; (b) patch of alopecia before injection; (c) same patch after 2 months of injections.

(Continued)

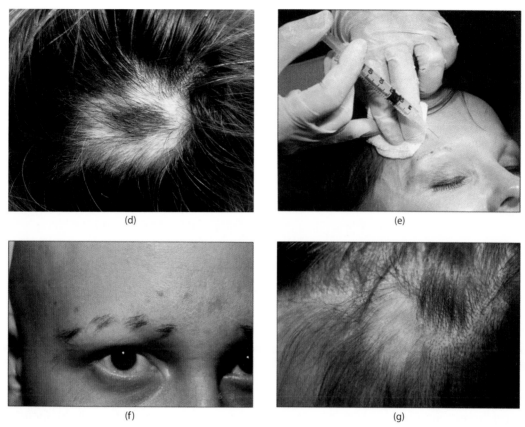

(d)   (e)

(f)   (g)

Figure 5.15 (*Continued*)
(d) Patch 2 months after injections with central regrowth and centrifugal expansion;
(e) injection of eyebrows with triamcinolone 2.5 mg/mL for a total of 0.5 mL per eyebrow;
(f) regrowth in eyebrow area after 4 weeks. Injections are performed every 4 weeks, with the
next set in between areas of regrowth; (g) atrophy secondary to injection with triamcinolone
acetonide 40 mg/mL, which is at least four to eight times what is recommended.

ointment under occlusion in patients with AT/AU; 17.8% of patients experienced a long-term benefit on the treated side [186]. Fiedler [194] believes that a combination of 0.05% betamethasone dipropionate cream and minoxidil may be more beneficial than either alone. She reports that quality of response in severe recalcitrant AA was fair to good after 16 weeks of treatment with placebo in 13%, with 0.05% betamethasone dipropionate in 22%, with 5% minoxidil in 27% and with 5% minoxidil, and 0.05% betamethasone dipropionate in 56%. This suggests a synergistic benefit of using both modalities.

Side effects of topical corticosteroids include folliculitis (more with ointment compared with foam formulations) and rarely skin atrophy and telangiectasia [186,190]. No significant modifications in cortisol and adrenocorticotropic hormone blood levels were observed [187].

Minoxidil

Minoxidil is a biologic response-modifier that enhances hair growth. Minoxidil stimulates follicular DNA synthesis, has a direct effect on the proliferation and differentiation

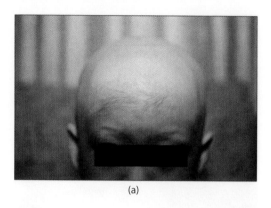
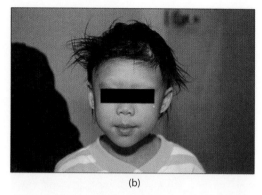

(a)   (b)

Figure 5.16

The use of minoxidil and topical betamethasone dipropionate. (a) A 4-year-old patient with a 2-year history of alopecia areata; (b) after 8 months of treatment, there was cosmetically acceptable regrowth. It is difficult to know if this was truly the effect of therapy or spontaneous regrowth.

of follicular keratinocytes in vitro, and regulates hair physiology independently of blood flow influences [195,196]. Minoxidil does not have an immunomodulatory effect [197].

Topical minoxidil 5% solution is the most effective concentration compared to other, lower concentrations [198–202]. There clearly is a dose–response effect [198–202]. Cosmetically acceptable hair regrowth using topical 5% minoxidil solution has been shown in approximately 40% of patients, with 20%–99% scalp involvement after 1 year [201]. More successful results are seen in less severe cases of the disease. This treatment should not be expected to be effective in patients with AT/AU [201]. In our clinic, we use topical minoxidil 5% solution for patchy AA. It must be applied twice daily. Initial hair regrowth is usually seen after 12 weeks. The response is usually maximized at 1 year. It must be continued until remission occurs. It can be used on the scalp and eyebrows. It can also be used on the beard area in men.

There are negative studies with topical minoxidil [203–205]. However, all these studies did not maximize on the 5% solution. More importantly, the majority of patients within these studies had AT/AU. One would not expect efficacy with topical 5% minoxidil solution in this difficult subpopulation.

The efficacy of minoxidil solution can be enhanced with anthralin or betamethasone dipropionate [194]. In combination with topical minoxidil, anthralin is applied 2 hours after the second minoxidil application. Betamethasone dipropionate cream is applied twice daily, 30 minutes after each use of minoxidil (Figure 5.16). Although combination therapy has been found to be more effective than monotherapy, this therapy is not effective in patients with AT/AU.

Side effects of minoxidil are rare. These include local irritation, allergic contact dermatitis, and facial hair growth (Figure 5.17), which tends to diminish with continued treatment. Systemic absorption is minimal [179].

Anthralin

Anthralin may have a nonspecific immunomodulating effect (anti-Langerhans cell), as it does in psoriasis [206]. Clinical irritation is not necessary for efficacy, just as clinical irritation is not necessary in psoriasis. There are citations in the literature that suggest that skin irritants are not effective in AA [207,208].

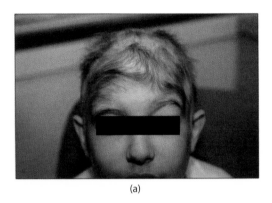
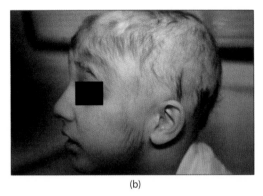

(a)   (b)

Figure 5.17
Hypertrichosis with topical minoxidil solution. (a, b) A 5-year-old boy who had used topical 5% minoxidil solution for over 6 months. There is marked symmetrical hypertrichosis on the forehead and cheeks.

Cosmetically acceptable regrowth has been reported to vary from 20% to 25% for patchy AA [209]. Schmoekel et al. [210] have shown with photographs that anthralin has benefit in a half-head study and is effective for patchy AA.

Anthralin 0.5%–1.0% cream is applied once daily [179,182,209,211]. Short-contact therapy is preferred. It is left on for 20–30 minutes daily for 2 weeks, and then 45 minutes daily for 2 weeks, up to a maximum of 1 hour daily. It is not to be used on the eyebrows or the beard area. Some patients may tolerate overnight therapy [179]. When therapy is effective, new hair growth is usually seen within 3 months. It may take 24 or more weeks for a cosmetically acceptable response. Because of its good safety profile, anthralin is a good choice for children. Combination therapy with minoxidil may have a synergistic effect, as was mentioned above [212].

Nelson and Speilvogel report a negative study with anthralin [213]. However, AT/AU patients were grouped in with patchy AA in this small study of 10 people, and it is not specified how many had AT/AU. It is unlikely that anthralin has as much efficacy, if any, in AT/AU as it does in patchy AA.

Side effects of anthralin are irritation, scaling, folliculitis, and regional lymphadenopathy. Patients are cautioned to avoid getting anthralin into the eyes, to protect treated skin against sun exposure, and to be aware of staining of the treated skin, clothes, and linens (Figure 5.18).

Topical immunotherapy

Topical immunotherapy is the most effective therapeutic modality with the best safety profile in the treatment of chronic severe AA. Systemic steroids may be the most effective modality, but their safety profile is unacceptable to most dermatologists. Three contact sensitizers have been used extensively in AA: DPCP, dinitrochlorobenzene (DNCB), and SADBE.

The mechanism of action of topical immunotherapy is unclear. The immuno-modulating effect of the topical sensitizers is supported by a decrease in the peribulbar CD4+/CD8+ lymphocyte ratio [214], and a shift in the position of the T lymphocytes away from perifollicular areas to the interfollicular area and dermis. It has been suggested that the immunogen may attract a new population of T cells into the treated

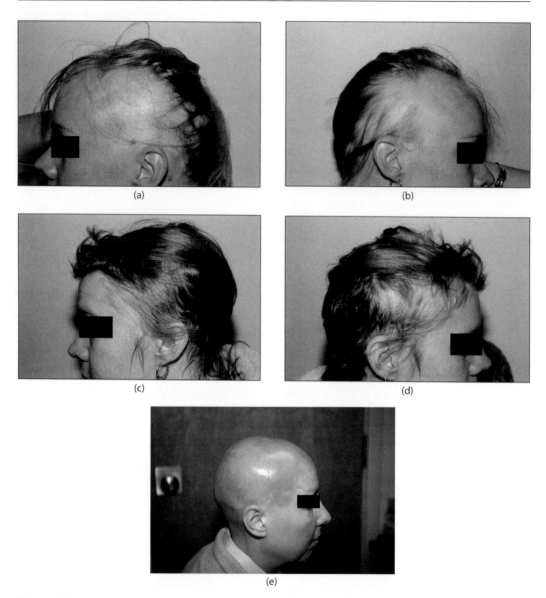

Figure 5.18
Anthralin for alopecia areata (AA). (a) A 27-year-old female with AA for 8 months. Baseline, left side; treated with anthralin 1% cream for 1 hour daily; (b) baseline, right side; untreated side; (c) 4 months of treatment: left (treated) side showing regrowth; (d) 4 months of treatment: right (untreated) side showing regrowth, but less than the treated side. There was clearly unilateral preference for the treated side; (e) marked redness can occur from anthralin.

area of the scalp that could eliminate the antigenic stimulus present in AA. Happle has proposed the concept of antigenic competition [214,215]. This theory presumes that the generation of T suppressor cells into the area may exert a nonspecific inhibitory effect on the autoimmune reaction to the hair-associated antigen, and thus allow hair to regrow. Immunogens may interfere with the initial or continued production of proinflammatory cytokines by the follicular keratinocytes. Careful dissection of the mechanism by which contact dermatitis is able to suppress AA is important, because it may be possible in the future to mimic the effect on the dermatitis by providing specific cytokines or specific inhibitors of cytokines.

Diphenylcyclopropenone

DPCP has been used not only in the treatment of AA, but also as an immunomodulator in the treatment of melanoma [216] and warts [217]. Efficacy in AA has varied from study to study. Van der Steen et al. [218] showed a response rate (in 139 patients) of 50.4%, with excellent or satisfactory results. Of 107 who showed a unilateral response, 30 relapsed and were resistant to further therapy. In 8 of those 107 a tolerance phenomenon was seen, defined as a required continuous increase in DPCP concentration until a concentration of 2.0% was reached without producing an adequate dermatitis, resulting in loss of all regrown hair. In 3 of 107 a paradoxical regrowth of hair on the untreated side of the scalp was seen. This phenomenon is known as castling.

MacDonald-Hull and Norris [219] reported 29% (8/28) of patients had a cosmetically acceptable result. MacDonald-Hull and Cunliffe [220] studied posttherapy relapse rates within 6 months after treatment. They found that 7 of 19 (37%) showed no hair loss after treatment had been stopped for 6 months. In 68%, the appearance of the scalp 6 months later was cosmetically acceptable, although 53% developed patchy alopecia and 10% lost all hair that had regrown. MacDonald and Hull et al. [220,221] reported further results with DPCP on a larger series of patients. Of 78 patients, 25 (32%) showed complete regrowth of hair. The authors felt that eliciting an allergic reaction was an integral part of successful treatment resulting in hair growth.

Wiseman et al. [222] utilized Kaplan–Meier survival analysis to determine cosmetically acceptable regrowth over time and a Cox regression model to determine factors predictive of regrowth in the largest series to date of 148 AA patients. Using the survival analysis model, the cumulative patient response at 32 months was 77.9%. A cosmetically acceptable endpoint was obtained in 17.4% of subjects with 100% hair loss, 60.3% of subjects with 75%–99% hair loss, 88.1% of subjects with 50%–74% hair loss, and 100% of subjects with 25%–49% hair loss. A lag period of 3 months was present between initiation of therapy and detection of the first clinical response. Factors affecting response were clearly extent of the condition and age of onset. Those patients with a younger age of onset are less likely to respond. It appears those with AT/AU and an early age of onset are prognostically a separate group. This fits well with the data of Colombe et al. [5] showing that this group is a distinct subpopulation of AA. Duration of condition, the presence of atopy, and nail changes were not correlated to response.

Gordon et al. [223] showed that 38% of 48 patients responded to DPCP with cosmetically acceptable regrowth. Pericin [116] showed that in 68 patients, 70.6% showed a response, with complete regrowth in 30.9%. The only prognostic indicator correlated with response was extent of the condition. Monk [224] showed cosmetically acceptable results in 33% (6/18). Hatzis et al. [225] showed satisfactory regrowth in 24% (11/45). Ashworth et al. showed efficacy in only 1/26 [226]. Orecchia and Rabiossi [227] also had a success rate of 1/26. Berth-Jones and Hutchinson [228] showed only an 18% response rate over 6 months, with no significant difference in response with inosine pranobex (inosiplex). Shapiro et al. [229] showed that topical 5% minoxidil solution combined with DPCP showed no benefit over DPCP alone.

Regarding children, MacDonald-Hull et al. [230] treated 12 children aged 5–15 years, with 33% showing complete regrowth. Six months after treatment was discontinued, three of the four children with complete regrowth maintained their hair.

DPCP is not mutagenic in the Ames test, and teratogenicity and organ toxicity could not be detected in the hen's egg test or in the mouse teratogenicity test [231]. Analysis on serum and urine samples following application of at least 0.5 mL of a 1% solution of diphency-prone to the scalp of 18 patients under treatment for AA revealed no detectable amounts of diphencyprone in any sample of serum or urine from these subjects. These data suggest that diphencyprone is not absorbed following application to the skin [232]. Commercial DPCP may contain a precursor, dibromoke-tone, that is positive in the Ames test [233,234]. It is therefore recommended that all DPCP samples be purified as described by van der Steen et al. [231] or that a pharmaceutical chemist perform high-pressure liquid chromatography on the DPCP sample to ensure that there are no detectable amounts of this dibromoketone compound. DPCP is degradable upon exposure to light, and must be stored in amber bottles. At our clinic, DPCP is dissolved in acetone and stored away from the staff in the refrigerator in a special container.

For adults with more than 50% scalp hair loss, topical immunotherapy with DPCP is our treatment of choice. We use DPCP on patients with less than 50% hair loss only if all other modalities have failed, such as intralesional corticosteroids, topical minoxidil 5% solution in combination with topical corticosteroids, or topical anthralin. As Peret et al. [235,236] suggest, patients should be thoroughly informed about the experimental character of the treatment, the lack of sufficient toxicologic data, the chance for regrowth, the possible side effects, and the possible failure to respond. Patients must be warned that the induction of an allergic contact dermatitis is a desired side effect, and one that

is necessary for a good result. A local ethics committee should be asked for consent.

We use DPCP as follows: Before commencing treatment, risks and benefits are carefully reviewed with all patients and an informed consent is signed. The patient is encouraged to meet with and observe other patients undergoing treatment.

Posttreatment guidelines for the patient include the following:

1. Scalp/hair should not be washed in the 48 hours following treatment.
2. The scalp must be protected from all sources of light. The wearing of a hair-piece or scarf is sufficient.
3. A commitment is made to return for weekly treatments for at least 24 weeks.
4. A low-potency topical corticosteroid is given to the patient for mild inflammatory reactions posttreatment. The physician must be notified of severe reactions.

DPCP is compounded in an acetone base and stored in opaque bottles to protect the solution from photodegradation. All bottles are dated on first use, because we have found that the shelf life after opening is approximately 6 months. We periodically check the DPCP for purity with high-pressure liquid chromatography. All the screw-top lid bottles of DPCP are stored in a large plastic bin with a lid to prevent both accidental spillage and inadvertent staff sensitization. The standard DPCP tray for AA includes the following concentrations: 0.0001%, 0.001%, 0.01%, 0.1%, 0.5%, 1.0%, and 2%. Intermediate concentrations may be necessary. The transition from 0.1% to 1.0% is best bridged with a 0.5% solution of DPCP (Figure 5.19). Although not routinely used, it has occasionally been necessary to use 0.05% and 0.25% strengths for sensitive patients.

Safety precautions must be implemented when handling DPCP, because of the risk of sensitization of staff administering the treatment. Gloves must be worn and caution used to prevent DPCP from coming in contact with the skin of the staff member. If the person administering the DPCP develops eczema, the use of a barrier cream and double gloving is helpful. A gown covering the arms should be worn and laundered after each treatment session. Spills should be wiped up immediately using a dry towel, followed by a moist towel, to eradicate all traces

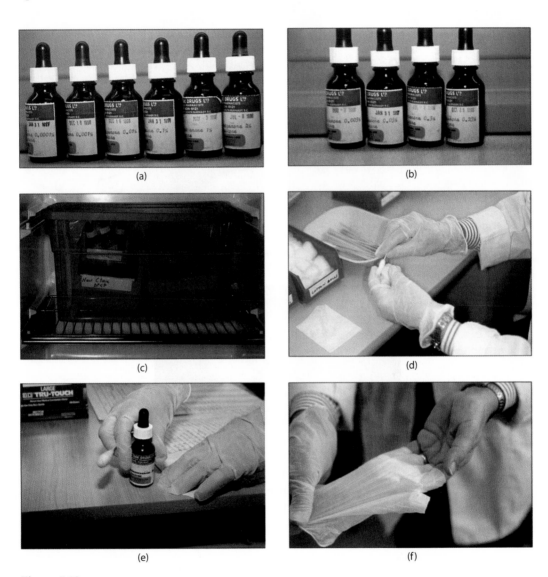

(a)

(b)

(c)

(d)

(e)

(f)

Figure 5.19
Topical immunotherapy for alopecia areata. (a) Standard diphenylcyclopropenone (DPCP) tray concentrations varying from 0.0001% to 2.0%; (b) intermediate concentrations may be necessary; (c) DPCP is stored away from the clinic in the refrigerator in a plastic container; (d) the cotton is wound around the stick to make a reinforced swab approximately three times the thickness of an average cotton-tipped applicator; (e) the physician or nurse must wear gloves when handling the bottles; (f) after the application, gloves must be removed carefully from the inside out.

(Continued)

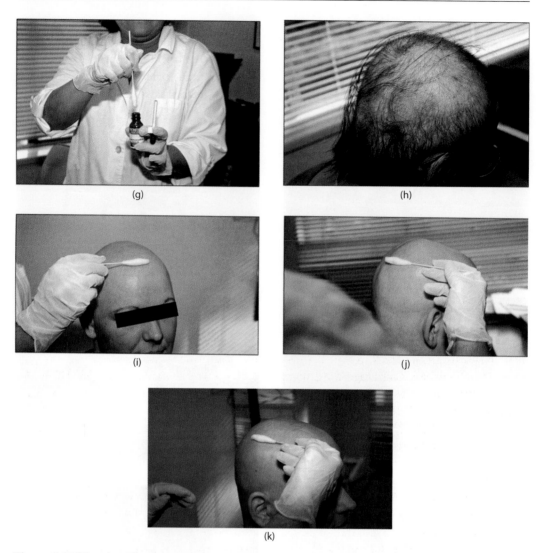

Figure 5.19 (*Continued*)
(g) Cotton swab is dipped directly into the bottle. If the swab needs to be remoistened, an eyedropper is used to saturate the swab; (h) an area that has been sensitized 1 week before with a 2% solution; (i, j) one coat is painted is the anteroposterior direction; (k) another coat is painted in the lateral direction. Only unilateral application is performed until hair regrowth is seen on one side.

of the DPCP. There is a report in the literature where DPCP treatment had to be abandoned in a clinic owing to the large number of staff becoming sensitized to DPCP [237].

The DPCP solution is applied to the scalp using a thick cotton swab that has been dipped into the bottle. If the swab needs to be remoistened, an eyedropper is used to saturate the swab and prevent contamination. These swabs are constructed with long wooden applicator sticks and cotton balls. The cotton is wound around the stick to make a firm swab approximately three times the thickness of an average cotton-tipped applicator (Figure 5.19). Cotton-tipped applicators do not retain enough moisture to paint the scalp adequately.

Once the patient commits to DPCP treatment, an initial sensitizing dose of 2% DPCP is administered to a 4 × 4 cm circular area on the occipital region of the scalp. Patients return for weekly visits until hair growth is established. After 1 week, if no reaction or only a mild to moderate reaction is observed, a 0.0001% solution is applied to half the scalp. Two coats are applied, the first coat in an anteroposterior direction and the second coat in a lateral direction. We avoid application to the nape of the neck, as well as the area where the tape for the hairpiece is applied. If this area becomes irritated, it is difficult for the patient to continue wearing a hairpiece. The nape of the neck is a very sensitive area that will react when other parts of the scalp do not. This can be confusing when attempting to titrate the patient to the correct dosage. Titration must be conducted carefully, because severe reactions can discourage the patient and precipitate discontinuation of treatment. If there is a marked reaction, we do not apply any solution until the following week.

DPCP is left on the scalp for 48 hours and then washed off. The patient must protect the scalp from light with a cap, wig, or scarf during this period, as DPCP is degraded when exposed to light. The following week, DPCP is reapplied to the same half of the scalp. The aim is to maintain erythema and pruritus, or a low tolerable eczema, on the treated side for 36–48 hours after application. The concentration is adjusted individually on the basis of the severity of the previous reaction. Concentrations vary (0.0001%, 0.001%, 0.01%, 0.05%, 0.1%, 0.5%, 1.0%, 2.0%). Once hair growth is established on one side, the other side is treated (see Figure 5.20). Each week when the patient returns, the severity of reaction and the presence of any hair growth are assessed. The tolerance to the discomfort from the eczema varies with patients. It is important to listen to your patients. It is better to be cautious than to be very aggressive and cause a severe reaction. If patients have discontinued treatment because of intolerable effects, it is difficult to get them to resume therapy. The strength can always be increased later when the patient becomes familiarized with the treatments.

Once full regrowth has occurred (Figures 5.20 and 5.21), the frequency of treatment is gradually reduced, using the rule of four: treatment is administered every other week for 4 weeks, then every third week for 4 weeks, and so on. This reduction of visits continues until the patient experiences some hair loss and establishes the maintenance requirement. Maintenance requirements vary with individuals and commonly range from biweekly to bimonthly treatments. One patient was able to discontinue treatments for 4 years before she experienced any hair loss. The requirement for maintenance therapy illustrates the palliative nature of the treatment.

Regrowth of hair will take at least 12 weeks. However, we have had patients that have taken 41 weeks to see unilateral regrowth. If the patient has not responded by 52 weeks, we consider the patient unlikely to respond, and we may abandon topical immunotherapy and proceed to another modality of therapy. In certain responders, most of the scalp regrows hair except for a few small areas refractory to DPCP. These resistant areas are treated with intralesional triamcinolone acetonide 5 mg/mL once monthly, and usually respond well (see Figure 5.22).

We have had a few patients that we identify as "slow growers." They consistently grow new hair in more areas and do not seem to lose hair. The process of complete regrowth is lengthy, with gradual new growth in multiple areas. Another phenomenon we have seen is the "initial nonresponder." These patients initially do not respond, and discontinue treatment. Within 2 years of stopping treatment, a small number of individuals have returned with hair growth only on the originally treated side. On recommencing treatment, growth was obtained (Figure 5.23).

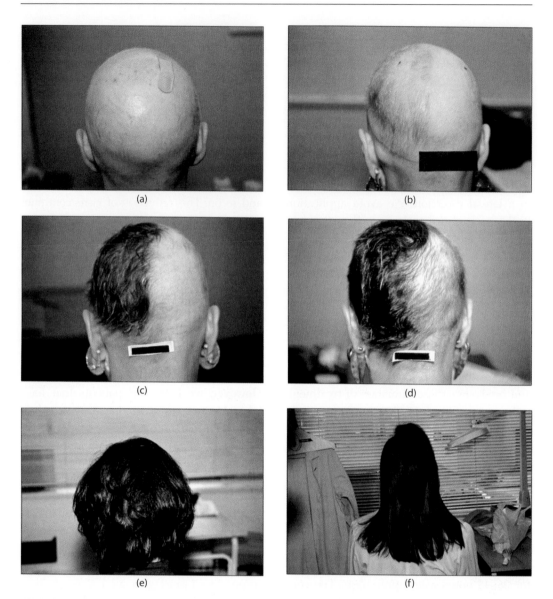

Figure 5.20
A 40-year-old female with an 18-year history of alopecia involving 99% of the scalp; (a) base-line; (b) 12 weeks of unilateral diphenylcyclopropenone treatment; (c) 24 weeks of unilateral treatment; (d) 30 weeks of treatment of the left side and 6 weeks on the contralateral side; (e) 1 year of treatment; (f) 5 years of intermittent treatment.

DPCP has been used with success to treat eyebrows. Extreme caution must be used. The patient should be lying flat, the eyes shielded with gauze, and the swab should be minimally moist. This is best done at the end of the treatment, after the scalp has been treated (see Figure 5.24).

Side effects include eczema (Figure 5.25), autoeczematization [238], severe blistering, and lymphadenopathy (Figure 5.26) in the

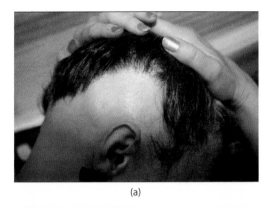

(a)

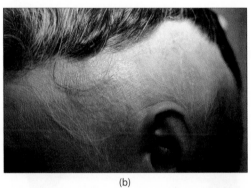

(b)

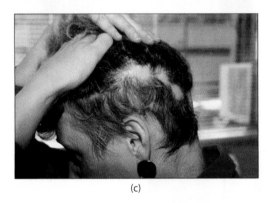

(c)

Figure 5.21
Ophiasis in a 43-year-old female of 2 years' duration; (a) baseline; (b) 12 weeks of diphenylcyclopropenone (DPCP) treatment, showing some white regrowth; (c) 24 weeks of DPCP treatment.

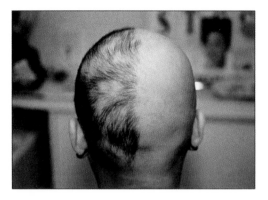

Figure 5.22
Unilateral treatment with diphenylcyclopropenone (DPCP), showing circular areas refractory to treatment. These refractory areas can be injected once monthly. DPCP is applied weekly for 3 weeks out of every month. Intralesional corticosteroid is injected once monthly.

neck behind the ears. Consort dermatitis to spouse/partner has also been reported [238]. Shah et al. [237] report the risk to medical and nursing staff. Pigment changes (Figure 5.27), such as hyperpigmentation, hypopigmentation [239], a combination of both referred to as "dyschromia in confetti" [240], and vitiligo [241–244] have been reported. Vitiligo is more common in AA patients, and because vitiligo has a tendency to Koebnerize onto inflamed skin, one must be very cautious about rapid extension of vitiligo in an AA patient who already has the condition. Vitiligo is a relative contraindication for treatment with topical immunogens. Extreme caution should be exercised when treating patients of dark pigmentation. Contact urticaria [245,246], severe dermographism [247], and erythema multiforme [248] have also been reported. Because of the possible side effects, we do not ever give DPCP to the patient for self-application.

DPCP is contraindicated in pregnancy, although teratogenicity has not been demonstrated. All female patients are counseled to use reliable birth control while on DPCP. At our clinic, six women have become pregnant while on DPCP therapy, despite all the warnings on the informed consent form. DPCP therapy was immediately halted once

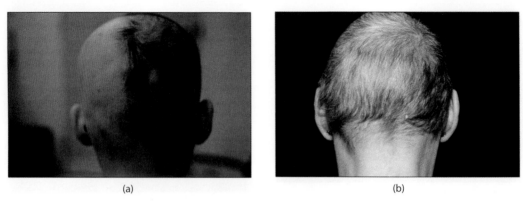

(a) (b)

Figure 5.23
Delayed diphenylcyclopropenone response. The patient had been treated unilaterally for
6 months without a response. (a) She returned to the clinic after treatment had been discontinued for 6 months with a unilateral response on the treated side; (b) both sides were then
subsequently treated with full regrowth.

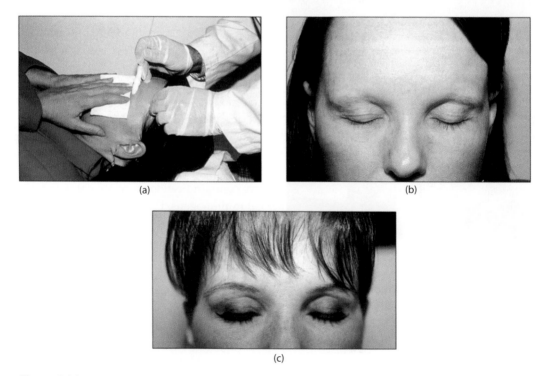

(a) (b)

(c)

Figure 5.24
Treatment of eyebrows with diphenylcyclopropenone (DPCP). (a) Position used to apply
DPCP to eyebrows. Eyes are well shielded; (b) baseline before treatment in a 40-year-old
female with no eyebrows for 18 years; (c) complete regrowth with treatment.

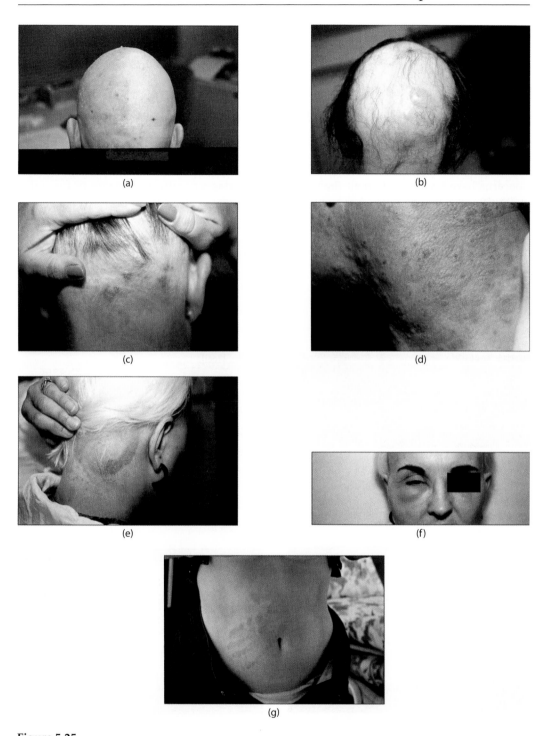

Figure 5.25
Eczematous eruptions from diphenylcyclopropenone. (a) Unilateral eczematous response 1 week after application. This reaction is too strong. No application for 1 full week with a lower concentration applied the following week. (b) Marked bulla formation is possible; (c–e) the neck area is a common area for a bad reaction; (f) frontal unilateral edema and eczema; (g) contact dermatitis to remote areas.

our clinic was informed. All six pregnancies have produced normal children.

Dinitrochlorobenzene

Daman et al. [249] first reported regrowth of hair in two patients following application of DNCB. The overall efficacy of DNCB treatment for AA has been investigated and has varied from 25% to 89% [250,251]. Concerns have been raised about the safety of DNCB. DNCB is rapidly absorbed after topical application, with 53% recoverable in the urine. Excretion is primarily renal, and

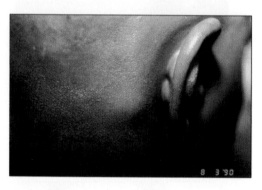

Figure 5.26
Lymphadenopathy occurs in 100% of patients.

serum half-life is 4 hours. Kratka et al. [252], Stobel and Rohrborn [253], and Summer and Goggelman [254] found DNCB to be mutagenic in *Salmonella typhimurium* in the bacterial plate incorporation assay (Ames assay). Therefore, extreme caution must be used with DNCB. The issue of DNCB safety is controversial. Weisburger et al. [255] found DNCB to be noncarcinogenic when fed in large doses to mice and rats up to 4 months. The purity of DNCB samples is also an issue. Certain chloronitrobenzenes that are known mutagens are possible contaminants in preparations of DNCB [256].

Side effects of DNCB include a marked blistering reaction, autoeczematization, adenopathy, urticaria, and tolerance. Tolerance can sometimes be reversed with cimetidine 300 mg orally three times a day for 3–4 weeks [169].

Squaric acid dibutyl ester

Happle achieved good results in 70% of patients treated with topical SADBE [215]. Flowers et al. [257] found SADBE to be effective in 4/8 cases. Case et al. [258] showed excellent responses in 11/26 (52%) of cases.

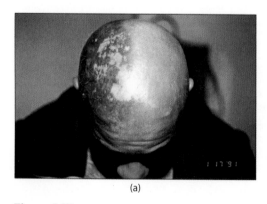

(a)

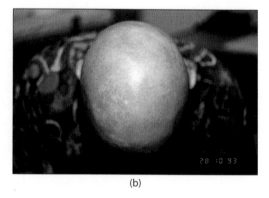

(b)

Figure 5.27
Pigmentary changes with diphenylcyclopropenone (DPCP): (a) hypo- and hyperpigmentation ("dychromia in confetti") after 24 weeks of treatment in an East Indian patient; (b) the same patient, with most pigmentary changes resolved.

(Continued)

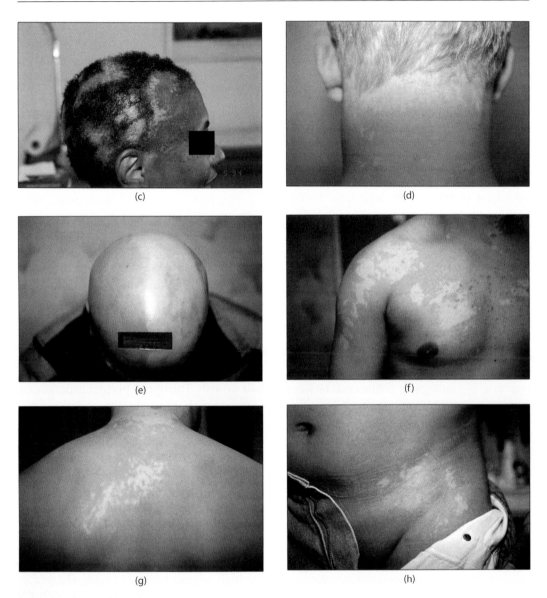

Figure 5.27 (*Continued*)
(c) Hypo- and hyperpigmentation in an African American patient; (d) vitiligo on the back of the neck; (e) vitiligo on half of the scalp in a patient who had been applying DPCP at home; (f–h) vitiliginous patches on areas remote to the scalp.

Caserio [259] showed a success rate of 28% (4/14 cases). Giannetti and Orecchia [260] reported a good response in 5/26 cases. Micali et al. [261] showed a 49% success rate in 73 cases with over 50% scalp involvement. Chua et al. [262] reported a 68% (13/19) success rate in a half-head study. Orecchia [263] has used SADBE in children under 13 and showed a 32% (9/28) chance of cosmetically acceptable regrowth. Tosti et al. [264] also treated children, with an initial success rate of 30% (10/33). Two-thirds of the initial responders no longer responded to the SADBE, with subsequent relapses over the long term. Barth et al. [265] showed only minimal signs of terminal hair regrowth in 3/17 patients and do not recommend the use of SADBE in AA.

Orecchia et al. [266] used SADBE in combination with photochemotherapy (PUVA) on three patients and did not find increased efficacy with combined treatment. They concluded that the two associated therapies showed an impaired efficacy because of the inhibition of the SADBE action by PUVA. PUVA impairs Langerhans cells, and thus inhibits induction and elicitation of allergic contact dermatitis. PUVA also results in a systemic immunosuppression through direct or indirect (via interleukin-1) stimulation of prostaglandins (PGE2), with the effect of an efferent lymphatic blockade. This would clearly affect any benefits of a contact allergen.

SADBE has been shown to be Ames-assay-negative. No mutagenic contaminants were detected on gas chromatography–mass spectrometry [267]. Furthermore, lifetime subcutaneous injections of squaric acid into ICR/Ha Swiss mice resulted in a low incidence of tumors at the injection site, equaling that of control animals [268]. SADBE is an ideal immunogen in that it is a strong topical sensitizer, it is used only rarely in industry, is not found in the natural environment, and does not react with other chemicals. However, it loses its stability in the presence of water.

Phototherapy

Photochemotherapy

The mechanism of action of PUVA on AA is believed to be a photoimmunologic action [269]. It may affect T cell function and antigen presentation, and possibly inhibit local immunologic attack against the hair follicle by depleting Langerhans cells [269] (see Figure 5.28). The psoralen is administered either topically or orally, and is followed

in 1 hour or 2 hours with UVA irradiation. Treatments are administered two to three times a week, with gradual increase in UVA dosage. Burns are more likely to occur with topical therapy, but ocular toxicity is avoided.

Mitchell and Douglas [269] used a combination of topical 0.1% 8-methoxypsoralen (8–MOP) and UVA, and showed excellent regrowth in 8/22 (36.3%) and good regrowth in 2/22 (9%). Mean total UVA exposure for responders was 171.1 joules/cm^2, with a mean total number of treatments of 47. Almost all the patients available for follow-up experienced relapse when PUVA was tapered. Claudy and Gagnaire [270] used systemic PUVA with total body irradiation and showed a success rate of 70%. Larko and Swanbeck [271] studied 40 patients with systemic PUVA, comparing whole body irradiation and scalp irradiation only. Whole body treatment did not produce significantly better hair growth. Thirty-five percent experienced hair regrowth, but only 20% experienced a full regrowth. Relapses were frequent, with median time to relapse being 10 weeks. Lassus et al. [272] studied 41 patients with oral 8–MOP and whole body irradiation, and local 8–MOP plus local UVA irradiation. No significant differences were seen. There was a response rate of almost 50% in each group. Only 10% relapsed after 6–12 months.

The major problem with PUVA therapy is the high relapse rate that frequently sets in after tapering the treatment [273,274]. Today's concern about PUVA and its promotion of all types of skin cancer, including melanoma [275], together with the need for long-term therapy in AA, make PUVA therapy less than satisfactory.

Excimer laser

A few case series have shown successful results with 308-nm excimer laser in treating patchy AA [276–281]. The initial fluences were less than the minimal erythema dose. The fluences were then increased by 50 mJ/cm^2 every

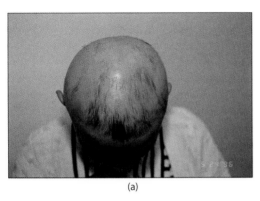

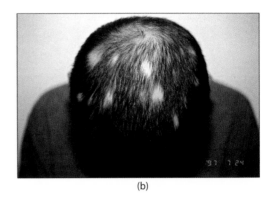

(a)   (b)

Figure 5.28
Photochemotherapy (PUVA) in alopecia areata: a 22-year-old patient with extensive alopecia affecting 95% of his scalp for 2 years. He was unresponsive to 24 weeks of topical immunotherapy with diphenylcyclopropenone. (a) Baseline before PUVA; (b) after 1 year of PUVA. He still has refractory patches that are amenable to intralesional corticosteroid therapy.

two sessions. The treatment was administered twice weekly to every patch of AA for a maximum of 24 sessions. Hair regrowth has been shown in 41.5% of patches [279].

Narrow band UVB

Bayramgürler et al. used narrow band UVB that was not effective in a retrospective analysis of 25 patients with AA [282].

Systemic therapy

Corticosteroids

Systemic corticosteroids have been used for many years in patients with rapid progressive and extensive AA. They are frequently effective in the treatment of AA, but their use is controversial. They are not routinely used because of side effects, and they do not alter the long-term prognosis. Side effects of systemic steroids include hyperglycemia, osteoporosis, cataracts, immunosuppression, obesity, dysmenorrhea, acne, weight gain, striae (Figure 5.29), mood changes/emotional lability, and Cushing syndrome [283–285].

In our clinic, we use systemic steroids only in exceptional cases. Oral corticosteroids are contraindicated in children due to their side effect profile. Different regimens have been tried, including single dose administration [286], alternating doses of prednisone as long-term treatment [283–285] or short-term treatment with high doses of intravenous methylprednisolone [287,288]; other authors suggest tapered doses over weeks [289] and some clinics use an interval therapy with tapered doses over 1 week every month for 3–6 months [75,283–296].

In general, success rates are found to be much better in multifocal AA compared to ophiasic, totalis, and universalis AA [283–285]. Pulse therapy, especially those with long corticosteroid free intervals and high-dose ultra-short-term treatments seem to have less of a side effect profile than daily or alternate day oral regimens with a reasonable treatment outcome [75,295,297,298].

Kar et al. performed a placebo-controlled randomized study on oral prednisone in 43 patients [284]. Out of the 43 patients, 23 patients received 200 mg prednisone weekly over 3 months followed by a 3-month observation period. Sixty percent of the treated patients showed regrowth, and 30% experienced moderate to significant hair regrowth (31%–60%) compared

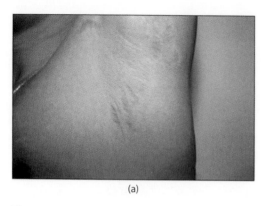

(a)

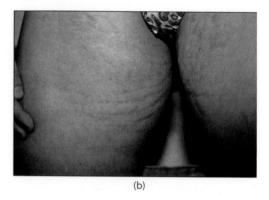

(b)

Figure 5.29
The chronic use of systemic steroids for alopecia areata can have significant side effects.
(a, b) Striae in a patient with alopecia universalis who had been on systemic steroids for 1 year.

to no regrowth in the placebo arm. Ait Ourhroui et al. administered 300 mg oral prednisone once monthly over 3 to 6 months in a prospective open label study on 34 patients with progressive AA affecting more than 40% of the scalp. An incomplete or cosmetically acceptable response was noted in 82% of the patients [283]. Sharma et al. used pulsed oral prednisolone 300 mg once monthly for a minimum of 4 months in patients with extensive AA and AT/AU. Cosmetically acceptable regrowth was found in 58% of patients [286]. Winter et al. in 1976 used alternate-day prednisone. The treatment was not found to be substantially effective and showed no obvious beneficial change in the natural course of AA after a 15-month follow-up period [285]. Price recommended oral prednisone at a dose of 40 mg daily for 1 week, tapered down by 5 mg every week for 3 weeks followed by 15 mg for 3 days, 10 mg for 3 days, and 5 mg for 3 days in combination with topical minoxidil daily and intralesional corticosteroids in patients with extensive and rapidly spreading AA [289]. A similar treatment concept was suggested by Olsen et al. for patients with mild to extensive AA. The treatment was combined with either topical minoxidil or vehicle. The topical treatment was continued for 14 additional weeks.

A total of 47% of patients responded to the prednisone treatment with more than 25% of regrowth. Topical minoxidil was found to be helpful to prevent relapse after discontinuation of the corticosteroid treatment [75].

Unger and Schlemmer in 1978 [295] suggested low dose oral prednisone in combination with intralesional and topical corticosteroids. Friedli et al. used pulse therapy with intravenous methylprednisolone, 250 mg, twice daily on 3 consecutive days. Twelve out of 20 patients with multifocal, patchy AA showed 50%–100% regrowth. The regimen appeared ineffective in patients with AT, AU, or ophiasic AA [288]. Burton and Shuster in 1975 used intravenous prednisolone at 2000 mg as a single dose in 22 patients with AT and 500 mg oral prednisolone in 13 patients with AT with an overall unsatisfactory response rate [287].

Kurosawa et al. compared different treatment modalities. They used dexamethason 0.5 mg/day for 6 months or intramuscular triamcinolone acetonide 40 mg once a month for 6 months followed by 40 mg once every 1.5 months for 1 year or pulse therapy with oral prednisolone at 80 mg for 3 consecutive days once every 3 months. Response rates were found to be best with intramuscular triamcinolone acetonide in patients with multifocal AA, and relapse rates in patients with AT/AU were found to be the lowest in the patients who received pulse therapy with oral prednisolone [292,299].

Cyclosporine

Cyclosporine is an immunosuppressant that was originally isolated from the Norwegian fungus *Tolypocladium inflate*. It is widely used in post-allogeneic organ transplant patients and in the treatment of autoimmune diseases and has shown some benefit in the treatment of AA [74,294,300,301]. However, the occurrence of AA has also been reported in organ transplant patients who were taking cyclosporine [302–305]. Cyclosporine inhibits helper T cell activation and suppresses IFN-γ production. Drawbacks of systemic cyclosporine are the side effect profile, which includes, among other things, nephrotoxicity, immune suppression, hypertension, hypertrichosis of body hair, growth of extra tissue on the gums, depression, and high relapse rates after discontinuation and therefore a need for long-term treatment.

Due to the side effect profile, the high recurrence rate following discontinuation of the treatment, the long treatment periods, and the inability to change the ultimate prognosis of the disease, this treatment should be reserved for exceptional AA cases.

Gupta et al. treated 6 patients at 6 mg/kg/day for 12 weeks. Cosmetically acceptable terminal hair regrowth was found in 50% of the patients. However, high relapse rates occurred in all patients within 3 months of discontinuation of the treatment [306]. Shapiro et al. combined oral cyclosporine at 4 mg/kg/day with low dose prednisone at 5 mg/day. Reasonable regrowth was seen in 25% of patients, but again high recurrence rates were noted after discontinuation of cyclosporine (Figure 5.30) [74]. Kim at al. achieved success rates of up to 76.7% with a combination therapy of oral cyclosporine and oral methylprednisolone [300]. Shaheedi-Dadras et al. treated patients with AT and AU with monthly intravenous methylprednisolone at 500 mg for 3 days and oral cyclosporine (2.5 mg/kg/day) for 5 to 8 months. Hair regrowth of >70% was seen in 33% of patients [294].

Topical cyclosporine at concentrations of 10% has not yet shown to be effective in patients with AA [307,308]. However, Verma et al. used the Dundee bald rat as an animal model and were able to show hair regrowth and reduced inflammation after application of topical cyclosporine in a lipid vehicle [309].

Sulfasalazine

Sulfasalazine is a sulfa-drug and is widely used as an anti-inflammatory agent in the treatment of inflammatory bowel disease, rheumatoid arthritis, and juvenile spondyloarthropathies. Sulfasalazine is a derivative of mesalazine (5-aminosalicylic acid, or 5-ASA); it is primarily used for both its immunomodulatory and immunosuppressive actions, including inhibition of T cell proliferation, natural killer cell activity, and antibody production. Sulfasalazine also inhibits the T cell cytokines IL-2 and IFN-γ and the monocyte/macrophage cytokines IL-1, TNF-α, and IL-6 [301].

Very little is published on the use of sulfasalazines in AA. Ellis at al. reported a response rate of 23% in patients with severe AA [310]. Aghaei treated 22 patients with sulfasalazine starting with 500 mg twice daily for 4 weeks, followed by 1000 mg twice daily for 4 weeks and 1500 mg twice daily for 4 months. Complete hair regrowth was noted in 27.3% of patients. However, relapse occurred in 45.5% of patients. Adverse effects included gastrointestinal distress, rash, headache, and laboratory abnormalities in 31.8% [311]. Rashidi and Mahd treated 39 patients with 1500 mg sulfasalzine twice daily for 6 months. A total of 25.6% of the patients

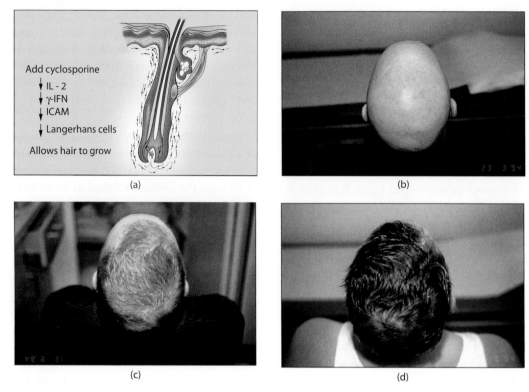

Figure 5.30

Cyclosporin in alopecia areata. (a) Mechanism of action by inhibiting the Th$_1$ response to the hair follicle. (b) A 28-year-old male with alopecia universalis for 2 years; (c) 3 months of systemic cyclosporin (4 mg/kg/day) and prednisone 5 mg/day; (d) 5 months of therapy. The patient had to discontinue therapy owing to serum transaminase changes and cholesterol elevation.

responded with full regrowth, whereas 30.7% showed mild to moderate regrowth [299,312].

Methotrexate

Methotrexate (MTX), formerly known as amethopterin, is an antimetabolite and antifolate drug. It inhibits the metabolism of folic acid. MTX is mainly used in the treatment of cancer and autoimmune diseases [313].

Droitcourt et al. reported a 50% success rate with complete regrowth with a combination therapy of MTX and intravenous 500 mg methylprednisolone per day for 3 consecutive days monthly [314]. Chartaux and Joly showed success rates of 63%–64% with a combination of MTX at 15 mg weekly and prednisone at 10 mg or 20 mg daily [315,316] and hair regrowth in 57% of patients with AT and AU with MTX alone. The onset of hair regrowth was noted after a median delay of 3 months. Adverse events consisting of transient elevated transaminases, persistent nausea, and lymphocytopenia occurred in 21% of patients [316]. Royer et al. treated 14 children aged 8–18 years with MTX at doses between 15 and 25 mg/week. Five children showed more than 50% regrowth, the others were considered treatment failures [317].

Biologics

Modern immunosuppressant drugs, mainly developed for the treatment of psoriasis, such as infliximab and adalimumab, bind to TNF-α, preventing it from activating TNF receptors or like efalizumab, which binds to the CD11a subunit of lymphocyte function-associated antigen 1 have been tried for the treatment of AA. Unfortunately, all studies failed to show effectiveness [318,319]. Some studies show the occurrence or worsening of AA under treatment with these biologics [320–324]. Further studies are necessary to determine whether these or other biologics are of any use for the systemic treatment of AA [299].

Treatment plan

Therapeutic selection for AA depends on patient age, extent of alopecia, and motivation for treatment. The dermatologist should first discuss all therapeutic options and outcomes, allowing the patient to become an active member of the therapeutic team. Topical therapies with minoxidil, corticosteroids, and anthralin can be considered for children of less than 10 years of age, whereas in adults other options to be considered include intralesional corticosteroids or immunotherapy. Systemic therapy should only be carefully considered in adults with rapid progressive AA or therapy refractory AA.

A practical treatment algorithm for the treatment of AA is the University of California, San Francisco–University of British Columbia alopecia areata treatment protocol (see Figure 5.31). Patients are divided into those less than 10 years of age and those over 10 years of age. Patients over 10 are then subdivided into those with less than 50% scalp hair loss and those with more than 50% scalp hair loss.

For those with less than 50% scalp hair loss, the following options are offered. First, we always offer the patient the option of no treatment, as many AA patients will regrow their hair without treatment. However, most of our patients are well motivated and want treatment. First line therapy for scalp AA is intralesional corticosteroid injections into the alopecic patches. If there is no response after 3–4 months, we will add a minoxidil 5% solution twice daily and a superpotent corticosteroid cream such as clobetasol propionate applied 30 minutes after the minoxidil in addition to the monthly injections. If there is no benefit, another option is short-contact anthralin therapy with anthralin 1.0% cream applied for up to 1 hour daily combined with topical minoxidil 5% solution applied twice daily.

For those patients with more than 50% scalp involvement, our first line is topical immunotherapy with DPCP. If there is no response by 52 weeks, topical immunotherapy is discontinued. Other options that can be offered to the patient are systemic PUVA, minoxidil 5% solution, short-contact anthralin, and superpotent topical steroids. A scalp prosthesis should be available to all patients with more than 50% scalp involvement, and can give great satisfaction to a majority of patients (see Chapter 8).

For children, therapeutic modality choices depend on patient age. Those older than 10 years are treated with the same protocols as adults. In those younger than 10 years, intralesional corticosteroids are avoided and topical immunotherapy is not implemented, although several European studies have demonstrated efficacy and safety in children as young as 5 years [263,264]. For those under 10 years of age, therapeutic options include minoxidil alone or in combination with a mid-potency topical corticosteroid or anthralin.

Ultimately, the therapeutic plan is developed through team interaction between the patient, the patient's family, and the physician. For some patients, support groups play an important role in the overall therapeutic strategy, and the dermatologist needs to become familiar with support groups and

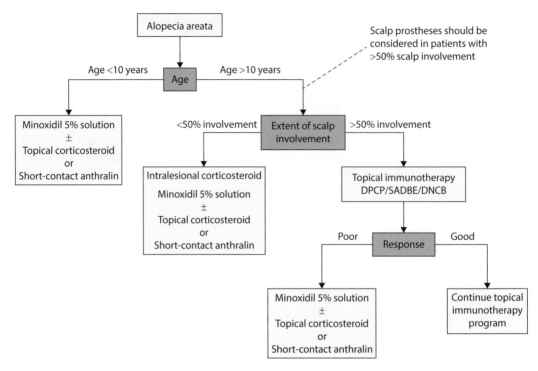

Figure 5.31
University of California at San Francisco–University of British Columbia treatment protocol for alopecia areata. (Permission granted by Drs. Jerry Shapiro, Vera H. Price, and Harvey Lui.)

suppliers of hairpieces. Physicians need to take time to address the psychological needs of their patients, exploring the impact of alopecia on the patient's emotional well-being. It is the role of the dermatologist to explain the diagnosis and inform the patient of all the therapeutic options, safety profiles, and outcomes. It is imperative that the physician spend sufficient time with the patient, just as one would with a patient who had recently been diagnosed as diabetic. The National Alopecia Areata Foundation (NAAF) (www .alopeciaareata.org) offers patients and physicians information, including brochures, bimonthly newsletters, research updates, sources for scalp prostheses, pen pals for children, videos for children to take to school, and information about support groups, which are present in many large cities in the United States and Canada. The

NAAF has an annual convention for patients and their families, and this is often the turning point for them in terms of coping with the condition. Physicians are welcome to attend.

REFERENCES

1. Safavi K, Prevalence of alopecia areata in the First National Health and Nutrition Examination Survey [letter]. *Arch Dermatol*, 1992. **128**(5): 702.
2. Safavi KH et al., Incidence of alopecia areata in Olmsted County, Minnesota, 1975 through 1989. *Mayo Clin Proc*, 1995. **70**(7): 628–33.
3. Nanda A, Al-Fouzan AS, and Al-Hasawi F, Alopecia areata in children: A clinical profile. *Pediatr Dermatol*, 2002. **19**(6): 482–5.
4. Price VH, Alopecia areata: Clinical aspects. *J Invest Dermatol*, 1991. **96**(5): 68S.

5. Colombe BW et al., HLA class II antigen associations help to define two types of alopecia areata. *J Am Acad Dermatol*, 1995. **33**(5 Pt 1): 757–64.

6. Alkhalifah A, Alopecia areata update. *Dermatol Clin*, 2013. **31**(1): 93–108.

7. Elenkov IJ and Chrousos GP, Stress hormones, proinflammatory and antiinflammatory cytokines, and autoimmunity. *Ann NY Acad Sci*, 2002. **966**: 290–303.

8. Ikeda T, Produced alopecia areata based on the focal infection theory and mental motive theory. *Dermatologica*, 1967. **134**(1): 1–11.

9. McDonagh AJ and Messenger AG, The aetiology and pathogenesis of alopecia areata. *J Dermatol Sci*, 1994. **7 Suppl**: S125–35.

10. McElwee K et al., Genetic susceptibility and severity of alopecia areata in human and animal models. *Eur J Dermatol*, 2001. **11**(1): 11–6.

11. McElwee KJ et al., Melanocyte and gonad activity as potential severity modifying factors in C3H/HeJ mouse alopecia areata. *Exp Dermatol*, 2001. **10**(6): 420–9.

12. Petukhova L et al., The genetics of alopecia areata: What's new and how will it help our patients? *Dermatol Ther*, 2011. **24**(3): 326–36.

13. Rodriguez TA and Duvic M, Onset of alopecia areata after Epstein-Barr virus infectious mononucleosis. *J Am Acad Dermatol*, 2008. **59**(1): 137–9.

14. Alkhalifah A et al., Alopecia areata update: Part I. Clinical picture, histopathology, and pathogenesis. *J Am Acad Dermatol*, 2010. **62**(2): 177–88.

15. Alkhalifah A et al., Alopecia areata update: Part II. Treatment. *J Am Acad Dermatol*, 2010. **62**(2): 191–202.

16. Wang E and McElwee KJ, Etiopathogenesis of alopecia areata: Why do our patients get it? *Dermatol Ther*, 2011. **24**(3): 337–47.

17. Muller RWS, Alopecia areata: An evaluation of 736 patients. *Arch Dermatol*, 1963. **88**: 290–7.

18. Shellow WV, Edwards JE, and Koo JY, Profile of alopecia areata: A questionnaire analysis of patient and family. *Int J Dermatol*, 1992. **31**(3): 186–9.

19. Price VH and Colombe BW, Heritable factors distinguish two types of alopecia areata. *Dermatol Clin*, 1996. **14**(4): 679–89.

20. Colombe BW, Lou CD, and Price VH, The genetic basis of alopecia areata: HLA associations with patchy alopecia areata versus alopecia totalis and alopecia universalis. *J Invest Dermatol Symp Proc*, 1999. **4**(3): 216–9.

21. Colombe BW et al., HLA class II alleles in long-standing alopecia totalis/alopecia universalis and long-standing patchy alopecia areata differentiate these two clinical groups. *J Invest Dermatol*, 1995. **104**(5 Suppl): 4S–5S.

22. Cole JP, *The Optimal Holding Solution and Temperature for Hair Follicle*. Accessed Feb. 28, 2005, http://www.forhair.com/optimal-holding-solution-and-temperature-for-hair-follicle.

23. Dmitrienko LP and Shakhnes IE, Familial alopecia in twins. *Vestn Dermatol Venerol*, 1977. **9**: 59–61.

24. Goldstein LM and Chipizhenko VA, Familial alopecia areata. *Vestn Dermatol Venerol*, 1978. **10**: 36–8.

25. Jackow C, Puffer N, and Hordinsky M, Alopecia areata and cytomegalovirus infection in twins: Genes versus environment? *J Am Acad Dermatol*, 1998. **38**(3): 418–25.

26. Scerri L and Pace JL, Identical twins with identical alopecia areata. *J Am Acad Dermatol*, 1992. **27**(5 Pt 1): 766–7.

27. Jabbari A et al., Genetic basis of alopecia areata: A roadmap for translational research. *Dermatol Clin*, 2013. **31**(1): 109–17.

28. So A, Genetics, polymorphism and regulation of expression of HLA region genes. In *HLA and Disease*, Lechler R, Editor. 1994. San Diego: Academic Press. p. 1.

29. Kuntz BM, Selzle D, and Braun-Falco O, HLA antigens in alopecia areata. *Arch Dermatol*, 1977. **113**(12): 1717.

30. Kianto U et al., HLA-B12 in alopecia areata. *Arch Dermatol*, 1977. **113**(12): 1716.

31. Hacham-Zadeh S et al., HLA and alopecia areata in Jerusalem. *Tissue Antigens*, 1981. **18**(1): 71–4.

32. Averbakh EV and Pospelov LE, HLA antigens of patients with alopecia areata. *Vestn Dermatol Venerol*, 1986. **1**: 24–6.

33. Lutz G, Kessler M, and Bauer R, Class I alloantigens in alopecia areata. *Z Hautkr*, 1986. **61**(14): 1014, 1019–22.

34. Zlotogorski A, Weinrauch L, and Brautbar C, Familial alopecia areata: No linkage with HLA. *Tissue Antigens*, 1990. **36**(1): 40–1.

35. Duvic M, Welsh EA, and Jackow C, Analysis of HLA-D locus alleles in alopecia areata patients and families. *J Invest Dermatol*, 1995. **104**(5 Suppl): 5S–6S.

36. Mikesell JF, Bergfeld WF, and Braun WE, HLA-DR antigens in alopecia areata. Preliminary report. *Cleve Clin Q*, 1986. **53**(2): 189–91.

37. Morling N, Frentz G, and Fugger L, DNA polymorphism of HLA class II genes in alopecia areata. *Dis Markers*, 1991. **9**(1): 35–42.

38. Orecchia G, Belvedere MC, and Martinetti M, Human leukocyte antigen region involvement in the genetic predisposition to alopecia areata. *Dermatologica*, 1987. **175**(1): 10–14.

39. Welsh EA, Clark HH, and Epstein SZ, Human leukocyte antigen-DQB1*03 alleles are associated with alopecia areata. *J Invest Dermatol*, 1994. **103**(6): 758–63.

40. Zhang L et al., HLA associations with alopecia areata. *Tissue Antigens*, 1991. **38**(2): 89–91.

41. Ramot Y et al., Alopecia areata and Down syndrome: A true association or a coincidence. *Int J Trichology*, 2013. **5**(4): 227–8.

42. Du Vivier A and Munro DD, Alopecia areata, autoimmunity, and Down's syndrome. *Br Med J*, 1975. **1**(5951): 191–2.

43. Betterle C, Greggio NA, and Volpato M, Clinical review 93: Autoimmune polyglandular syndrome type 1. *J Clin Endocrinol Metab*, 1998. **83**(4): 1049–55.

44. Tarlow JK et al., Severity of alopecia areata is associated with a polymorphism in the interleukin-1 receptor antagonist gene. *J Invest Dermatol*, 1994. **103**(3): 387–90.

45. Harmon CS and Nevins TD, IL-1 alpha inhibits human hair follicle growth and hair fiber production in whole-organ cultures. *Lymphokine Cytokine Res*, 1993. **12**(4): 197–203.

46. Philpott MP et al., Effects of interleukins, colony-stimulating factor and tumour necrosis factor on human hair follicle growth in vitro: A possible role for interleukin-1 and tumour necrosis factor-α in alopecia areata. *Br J Dermatol*, 1996. **135**(6): 942–8.

47. 2nd International Research Workshop on alopecia areata. Bethesda, Maryland, November 7–8, 1994. *J Invest Dermatol*, 1995. **104**(5 Suppl): 1S–45S.

48. McElwee KJ, Third International Research Workshop on alopecia areata. *J Invest Dermatol*, 1999. **4**(3): 197–254.

49. Bergfeld W, Alopecia areata and thyroid disease. *J Invest Dermatol*, 1999. **4**(3): 252.

50. Puavilai S et al., Prevalence of thyroid diseases in patients with alopecia areata. *Int J Dermatol*, 1994. **33**(9): 632–3.

51. Kenney Jr. JA, Vitiligo. *Dermatol Clin*, 1988. **6**(3): 425–34.

52. Shong YK and Kim JA, Vitiligo in autoimmune thyroid disease. *Thyroidology*, 1991. **3**(2): 89–91.

53. Friedmann PS, Decreased lymphocyte reactivity and auto-immunity in alopecia areata. *Br J Dermatol*, 1981. **105**(2): 145–51.

54. Kumar B, Sharma VK, and Sehgal S, Antismooth muscle and antiparietal cell antibodies in Indians with alopecia areata. *Int J Dermatol*, 1995. **34**(8): 542–5.

55. Werth VP, Incidence of alopecia areata in lupus erythematosus. *Arch Dermatol*, 1992. **128**(3): 368–71.

56. Kamada N, Hatamochi A, and Shinkai H, Alopecia areata associated with myasthenia gravis and thymoma: A case of alopecia with marked improvement following thymectomy and high level prednisolone administration. *J Dermatol*, 1997. **24**(12): 769–72.

57. Korn-Lubetzki I, Virozov Y, and Klar A, Myasthenia gravis and alopecia areata [letter; comment]. *Neurology*, 1998. **50**(2): 578.

58. Kubota A, Komiyama A, and Hasegawa O, Myasthenia gravis and alopecia areata [see comments]. *Neurology*, 1997. **48**(3): 774–5.

59. Noguchi Y et al., Myasthenia gravis with alopecia totalis. *Acta Paediatr Jap*, 1998. **40**(1): 99–101.

60. Tan RS, Ulcerative colitis, myasthenia gravis, atypical lichen planus, alopecia areata, vitiligo. *Proc R Soc Med*, 1974. **67**(3): 195–6.

61. Faergemann J, Lichen sclerosus et atrophicus generalisatus, alopecia areata, and polymyalgia rheumatica found in the same patient. *Cutis*, 1979. **23**(6): 757–8.

62. Thompson DM, Robinson TW, and Lennard-Jones J, Alopecia areata, vitiligo, scleroderma and ulcerative colitis. *Proc R Soc Med*, 1974. **67**(10): 1010–2.

63. Treem WR, Veligati LN, and Rotter JL, Ulcerative colitis and total alopecia in a mother and her son. *Gastroenterology*, 1993. **104**(4): 1187–91.

64. Ertekin V, Tosun MS, and Erdem T, Screening of celiac disease in children with alopecia areata. *Indian J Dermatol*, 2014. **59**(3): 317.

65. Aloi PG, Colonna SM, and Manzoni R, Association of lichen ruber planus, alopecia areata and vitiligo. *G Ital Dermatol Venereol*, 1987. **122**(4): 197–200.

66. Brenner W, Diem E, and Gschnait F, Coincidence of vitiligo, alopecia areata, onychodystrophy, localized scleroderma and lichen planus. *Dermatologica*, 1979. **159**(4): 356–60.

67. Conte A, Inverardi D, and Loconsole F, A retrospective study of 200 cases of lichen. *G Ital Dermatol Venereol*, 1990. **125**(3): 85–9.

68. Dhar S, Colocalization of alopecia areata and lichen planus [letter]. *Pediatr Dermatol*, 1996. **13**(3): 258–9.

69. Mann RJ, Wallington TB, and Warin RP, Lichen planus with late onset hypogamma-globulinaemia: A causal relationship? *Br J Dermatol*, 1982. **106**(3): 357–60.

70. Boni R, Trueb RM, and Wuthrich B, Alopecia areata in a patient with candidiasis-endocrinopathy syndrome: Unsuccessful treatment trial with diphenylcyclopropenone. *Dermatology*, 1995. **191**(1): 68–71.

71. Bunnag P and Rajatanavin R, Polyglandular autoimmune (PGA) syndromes: Report of three cases and review of the literature. *J Med Assoc Thai*, 1994. **77**(6): 327–33.

72. Delambre C et al., Autoimmune polyen-docrinopathy and chronic mucocutaneous candidiasis. *Ann Dermatol Venereol*, 1989. **116**(2): 117–21.

73. Gupta AK, Ellis CN, and Cooper KD, Oral cyclosporine for the treatment of alopecia areata. A clinical and immunohistochemical analysis. *J Am Acad Dermatol*, 1990. **22**(2 Pt 1): 242–50.

74. Shapiro J et al., Systemic cyclosporine and low dose prednisone in the treatment of chronic severe alopecia areata: A clinical and immunopathologic evaluation. *J Am Acad Dermatol*, 1997. **36**: 114–7.

75. Olsen EA, Carson SC, and Turney EA, Systemic steroids with or without 2% topical minoxidil in the treatment of alopecia areata. *Arch Dermatol*, 1992. **128**: 1467–73.

76. Muller HK, Rook AJ, and Kubba R, Immunohistology and autoantibody studies in alopecia areata. *Br J Dermatol*, 1980. **102**(5): 609–10.

77. Gilhar A et al., Failure of passive transfer of serum from patients with alopecia areata and alopecia universalis to inhibit hair growth in transplants of human scalp skin grafted onto nude mice. *Br J Dermatol*, 1992. **126**(2): 166–71.

78. Tobin DJ et al., Antibodies to hair follicles in alopecia areata. *J Invest Dermatol*, 1994. **102**(5): 721–4.

79. Tobin DJ et al., Hair follicle structures tar-geted by antibodies in patients with alopecia areata. *Arch Dermatol*, 1997. **133**(1): 57–61.

80. Bertolini M et al., Abnormal interactions between perifollicular mast cells and CD8+ T-cells may contribute to the pathogenesis of alopecia areata. *PLoS One*, 2014. **9**(5): e94260.

81. Majewski BB, Koh MS, and Taylor DR, Increased ratio of helper to suppressor T cells in alopecia areata. *Br J Dermatol*, 1984. **110**(2): 171–5.

82. Hordinsky MK et al., Suppressor cell num-ber and function in alopecia areata. *Arch Dermatol*, 1984. **120**(2): 188–94.

83. Gilhar A, Etzioni A, and Paus R, Alopecia areata. *N Engl J Med*, 2012. **366**: 1515–25.

84. McElwee KJ et al., Transfer of CD8(+) cells induces localized hair loss whereas CD4(+)/CD25(−) cells promote systemic alopecia areata and CD4(+)/CD25(+) cells blockade disease onset in the C3H/HeJ mouse model. *J Invest Dermatol*, 2005. **124**: 947–57.

85. McElwee KJ, Spiers EM, and Oliver RF, In vivo depletion of CD8+ T cells restores hair growth in the DEBR model for alopecia areata. *Br J Dermatol*, 1996. **135**: 211–7.

86. Gilhar A, Ullmann Y, and Berkutzki T, Autoimmune hair loss (alopecia areata) transferred by T lymphocytes to human scalp explants on SCID mice. *J Clin Invest*, 1998. **101**(1): 62–7.

87. Tsuboi H, Tanei R, and Fujimura T, Characterization of infiltrating T cells in human scalp explants from alopecia areata to SCID nude mice: Possible role of the disappearance of CD8+ T lymphocytes in the process of hair regrowth. *J Dermatol*, 1999. **26**(12): 797–802.

88. Gilhar A et al., Autoimmune disease induction in a healthy human organ: A humanized mouse model of alopecia areata. *J Invest Dermatol*, 2013. **133**: 844–7.

89. Christoph T, Muller-Rover S, and Audring H, The human hair follicle immune system: Cellular composition and immune privilege. *Br J Dermatol*, 2000. **142**(5): 862–73.

90. Paus R, Christoph T, and Muller-Rover S, Immunology of the hair follicle: A short journey into terra incognita. *J Invest Dermatol Symp Proc*, 1999. **4**(3): 226–34.

91. Mosmann TR and Coffman RL, TH1 and TH2 cells: Different patterns of lymphokine secretion lead to different functional properties. *Annu Rev Immunol*, 1989. **7**: 145–73.

92. Hoffmann R, Eicheler W, and Huth A, Cytokines and growth factors influence hair growth in vitro. Possible implications for the pathogenesis and treatment of alopecia areata. *Arch Dermatol Res*, 1996. **288**(3): 153–6.

93. Sato-Kawamura M, Aiba S, and Tagami H, Strong expression of CD40, CD54 and HLA-DR antigen and lack of evidence for direct cellular cytotoxicity are unique immunohistopathological features in alopecia areata. *Arch Dermatol Res*, 2003. **294**(12): 536–43.

94. Arca E et al., Interferon-gamma in alopecia areata. *Eur J Dermatol*, 2004. **14**(1): 33–6.

95. Deeths MJ et al., Phenotypic analysis of T-cells in extensive alopecia areata scalp suggests partial tolerance. *J Invest Dermatol*, 2006. **126**(2): 366–73.

96. Kuwano Y et al., Serum chemokine profiles in patients with alopecia areata. *Br J Dermatol*, 2007. **157**(3): 466–473.

97. Stamatis Gregoriou et al., Cytokines and other mediators in alopecia areata. *Mediators Inflamm*, 2010. **2010**: 928030. doi: 10.1155/2010/928030.

98. Hoffmann R et al., Cytokine mRNA levels in alopecia areata before and after treatment with the contact allergen diphenylcyclopropenone. *J Invest Dermatol*, 1994. **103**(4): 530–3.

99. Groves RW et al., Analysis of epidermal IL-1 family members in vivo using transgenic mouse models. *J Invest Dermatol*, 1994. **102**: 556.

100. Galbraith GMP et al., Contribution of interleukin 1β and KM loci to alopecia areata. *Hum Hered*, 1999. **49**(2): 85–9.

101. Pociot F et al., A TaqI polymorphism in the human interleukin-1β (IL-1β) gene correlates with IL-1β secretion in vitro. *Eur J Clin Invest*, 1992. **22**(6): 396–402.

102. Teraki Y, Imanishi K, and Shiohara T, Cytokines in alopecia areata: Contrasting cytokine profiles in localized form and extensive form (alopecia universalis). *Acta Derm Venereol*, 1996. **76**(6): 421–3.

103. Bodemer C et al., Role of cytotoxic T cells in chronic alopecia areata. *J Invest Dermatol*, 2000. **114**(1): 112–6.

104. Hoffmann R et al., Growth factor mRNA levels in alopecia areata before and after treatment with the contact allergen diphenylcyclopropenone. *Acta Derm Venereol*, 1996. **76**(1): 17–20.

105. Ansel J et al., Cytokine modulation of keratinocyte cytokines. *J Invest Dermatol*, 1990. **94**(6 Suppl): 101S–7S.

106. Symington FW, Lymphotoxin, tumor necrosis factor, and gamma interferon are cytostatic for normal human keratinocytes. *J Invest Dermatol*, 1989. **92**(6): 798–805.

107. Kim HS et al., Immunoreactivity of corticotropin-releasing hormone, adrenocorticotropic hormone and α-melanocyte-stimulating hormone in alopecia areata. *Exp Dermatol*, 2006. **15**(7): 515–22.

108. Kuwano Y et al., Serum BAFF and APRIL levels in patients with alopecia areata. *J Dermatol Sci*, 2008. **50**(3): 236–9.

109. Mackay F et al., BAFF and APRIL: A tutorial on B cell survival. *Annu Rev Immunol*, 2003. **21**: 231–64.

110. Mackay F and Leung H, The role of the BAFF/APRIL system on T cell function. *Semin Immunol*, 2006. **18**(5): 284–9.

111. Skinner Jr RB, Light WH, and Bale GF, Alopecia areata and presence of cytomegalovirus DNA [letter]. *JAMA*, 1995. **273**(18): 1419–20.

112. Garcia-Hernandez MJ, Torres MJ, and Palomares JC, No evidence of cytomegalovirus DNA in alopecia areata [letter]. *J Invest Dermatol*, 1998. **110**(2): 185.

113. McElwee KJ, Boggess D, and Burgett B, Murine cytomegalovirus is not associated with alopecia areata in C3H/HeJ mice [letter]. *J Invest Dermatol*, 1998. **110**(6): 986–7.

114. Tosti A, La Placa M, and Placucci F, No correlation between cytomegalovirus and alopecia areata [letter]. *J Invest Dermatol*, 1996. **107**(3): 443.

115. Baker GH, Psychological factors and immunity. *J Psychosom Res*, 1987. **31**(1): 1–10.

116. Perini GI, Veller Fornasa C, and Cipriani R, Life events and alopecia areata. *Psychother Psychosom*, 1984. **41**(1): 48–52.

117. Colon EA, Popkin MA, and Callies AL, Lifetime prevalence of psychiatric disorders in patients with alopecia areata. *Compr Psychiatry*, 1991. **32**(3): 245–51.

118. De Waard-van der Spek FB et al., Juvenile versus maturity-onset alopecia areata—A comparative retrospective clinical study. *Clin Exp Dermatol*, 1989. **14**(6): 429–33.

119. van der Steen P et al., Can alopecia areata be triggered by emotional stress? An uncontrolled evaluation of 178 patients with extensive hair loss. *Acta Derm Venereol*, 1992. **72**(4): 279–80.

120. Nutbrown M et al., Abnormalities in the ultrastructure of melanocytes and the outer root sheath of clinically normal hair follicles from alopecia areata scalps. *J Invest Dermatol*, 1995. **104**(5 Suppl): 12S–3S.

121. Tobin DJ, Fenton DA, and Kendall MD, Ultrastructural observations on the hair bulb melanocytes and melanosomes in acute alopecia areata. *J Invest Dermatol*, 1990. **94**(6): p. 803–7.

122. Tobin SJ, Morphological analysis of hair follicles in alopecia areata. *Microsc Res Tech*, 1997. **38**(4): 443–51.

123. Hosoi J, Murphy GF, and Egan CL, Regulation of Langerhans cell function by nerves containing calcitonin gene-related peptide. *Nature*, 1993. **363**(6425): 159–63.

124. Hordinsky MK et al., Structure and function of cutaneous nerves in alopecia areata. *J Invest Dermatol*, 1995. **104**(5 Suppl): 28S–9S.

125. Raud J, Lundeberg T, and Brodda-Jansen G, Potent anti-inflammatory action of calcitonin gene-related peptide. *Biochem Biophys Res Commun*, 1991. **180**(3): 1429–35.

126. Paus R, Heinzelmann T, and Schultz KD, Hair growth induction by substance P. *Lab Invest*, 1994. **71**(1): 134–40.

127. Ericson M, Differential expression of substance P in perifollicular scalp blood vessels and nerves after topical therapy with capsaicin 0.075% (Zostrix) in controls and patients with alopecia areata. *J Invest Dermatol*, 1999. **112**: 653.

128. Sundberg JP, Cordy WR, and King Jr LE, Alopecia areata in aging C3H/HeJ mice. *J Invest Dermatol*, 1994. **102**(6): 847–56.

129. Michie HJ et al., The DEBR rat: An animal model of human alopecia areata. *Br J Dermatol*, 1991. **125**(2): 94–100.

130. Smyth JR Jr and McNeil M, Alopecia areata and universalis in the Smyth chicken model for spontaneous autoimmune vitiligo. *J Investig Dermatol Symp Proc*, 1999. **4**(3): 211–5.

131. McElwee KJ et al., Experimental induction of alopecia areata-like hair loss in C3H/HeJ mice using full-thickness skin grafts. *J Invest Dermatol*, 1998. **111**(5): 797–803.

132. Liu H, Tang L, and McLean D, Leflunomide in the alopecia areata DEBR rat. *J Invest Dermatol*, 1999. **4**(3): 249.

133. Shapiro J, Sundberg JP, and Bissonette R, Alopecia areata-like hair loss in C3H/HeJ mice and DEBR rats can be reversed using topical diphencyprone. *J Invest Dermatol Symp Proc*, 1999. **4**(3): 239.

134. Freyschmidt-Paul P, Sundberg JP, and Happle R, Successful treatment of alopecia areata-like hair loss with the contact

sensitizer squaric acid dibutylester (SADBE) in C3H/HeJ mice. *J Invest Dermatol*, 1999. **113**(1): 61–8.

135. Green M, Catalog of mutant genes and polymorphic loci. In *Genetic Variants and Strains of the Laboratory Mouse*, Lyon M, Editor. 1989. Oxford: Oxford University Press.

136. Godwin AR and Capecchi MR, Hair defects in Hoxc13 mutant mice. *J Invest Dermatol Symp Proc*, 1999. **4**(3): 244–7.

137. Tong X and Coulombe PA, Mouse models of alopecia: Identifying structural genes that are baldly needed. *Trends Mol Med*, 2003. **9**(2): 79–84.

138. Messenger AG, Slater DN, and Bleehen SS, Alopecia areata: Alterations in the hair growth cycle and correlation with the follicular pathology. *Br J Dermatol*, 1986. **114**(3): 337–47.

139. Whiting DA, Histopathologic features of alopecia areata: A new look. *Arch Dermatol*, 2003. **139**(12): 1555–9.

140. Headington J, The histology of alopecia areata. *J Invest Dermatol*, 1991. **96**: 69S.

141. Perret C, Wiesner-Menzel L, and Happle R, Immunohistochemical analysis of T-cell subsets in the peribulbar and intrabulbar infiltrates of alopecia areata. *Acta Derm Venereol*, 1984. **64**(1): 26–30.

142. Wiesner-Menzel L and Happle R, Intrabulbar and peribulbar accumulation of dendritic OKT 6-positive cells in alopecia areata. *Arch Dermatol Res*, 1984. **276**(5): 333–4.

143. Whiting DA, Histopathologic features of alopecia areata: A new look. *Arch Dermatol*, 2003. **139**: 1555–9.

144. Kohchiyama A, Hatamochi A, and Ueki H, Increased number of OKT6-positive dendritic cells in the hair follicles of patients with alopecia areata. *Dermatologica*, 1985. **171**(5): 327–31.

145. Elston DM, McCollough ML, and Bergfeld WF, Eosinophils in fibrous tracts and near hair bulbs: A helpful diagnostic feature of alopecia areata [see comments]. *J Am Acad Dermatol*, 1997. **37**(1): 101–6.

146. El Darouti M, Marzouk SA, and Sharawi E, Eosinophils in fibrous tracts and near hair bulbs: A helpful diagnostic feature of alopecia areata [letter; comment]. *J Am Acad Dermatol*, 2000. **42**(2 Pt 1): 305–7.

147. Nutbrown M, MacDonald Hull SP, and Baker TG, Ultrastructural abnormalities in the dermal papillae of both lesional and clinically normal follicles from alopecia areata scalps. *Br J Dermatol*, 1996. **135**(2): 204–10.

148. McDonagh AJ, Snowden JA, and Stierle C, HLA and ICAM-1 expression in alopecia areata in vivo and in vitro: The role of cytokines. *Br J Dermatol*, 1993. **129**(3): 250–6.

149. Lee JY and Hsu ML, Alopecia syphilitica, a simulator of alopecia areata: Histopathology and differential diagnosis. *J Cutan Pathol*, 1991. **18**(2): 87–92.

150. Peereboom-Wynia JD et al., Scanning electron microscopy comparing exclamation mark hairs in alopecia areata with normal hair fibres, mechanically broken by traction. *Clin Exp Dermatol*, 1989. **14**(1): 47–50.

151. Camacho F, Alopecia areata clinical features. In *Trichology: Diseases of the Pilosebaceous Follicle*, Camacho F, Editor. 1997. Madrid: Aula Medica Group. p. 417–50.

152. Muralidhar S, Sharma VK, and Kaur S, Ophiasis inversus: A rare pattern of alopecia areata [letter] [see comments]. *Pediatr Dermatol*, 1998. **15**(4): 326–7.

153. De Berker D, Baran R, and Dawber RP, *Handbook of the Diseases of the Nails and Their Management*. 1995. Oxford: Blackwell Science.

154. Tosti A, Idiopathic trachyonychia (twenty-nail dystrophy): A pathological study of 23 patients. *Br J Dermatol*, 1994. **131**(6): 866–72.

155. Tosti A, Barclazzi F, and Piraccini BM, Is trachyonychia, a variety of alopecia areata, limited to the nails? *J Invest Dermatol*, 1995. **104**(5 Suppl): 27S–28S.

156. Tosti A et al., Nail changes and alopecia areata. *G Ital Dermatol Venereol*, 1985. **120**(3): 169–71.

157. Tosti A et al., Trachyonychia associated with alopecia areata: A clinical and pathologic study. *J Am Acad Dermatol*, 1991. **25**(2 Pt 1): 266–70.

158. Tosti A, Palmerio B, and Veronesi S, 20 nail dystrophy, alopecia areata, lichen planus. *G Ital Dermatol Venereol*, 1985. **120**(2): 131–2.

159. Miteva M and Tosti A, Hair and scalp dermatoscopy. *J Am Acad Dermatol*, 2012. **67**(5): 1040–8.

160. Rudnicka L et al., Trichoscopy update 2011. *J Dermatol Case Rep*, 2011. **5**(4): 82–8.

161. Kibar M et al., Trichoscopic findings in alopecia areata and their relation to disease activity, severity and clinical subtype in Turkish patients. *Australas J Dermatol*, 2013. doi: 10.1111/ajd.

162. Madani S and Shapiro J, The scalp biopsy: Making it more efficient. *Dermatol Surg*, 1999. **25**(7): 537–8.

163. Broniarczyk-Dyła G et al., Abnormalities of structure and function of the thyroid in patients with alopecia areata. *Przegl Dermatol*, 1989. **76**(5–6): 416–21.

164. Salamon T, Musafija A, and Milicević M, Alopecia areata and diseases of the thyroid gland. *Dermatologica*, 1971. **142**(1): 62–3.

165. Klein U, Weinheimer B, and Zaun H, Simultaneous occurrence of areata alopecia and immunothyroiditis. *Int J Dermatol*, 1974. **13**(3): 116–8.

166. Bakry OA et al., Thyroid disorders associated with alopecia areata in Egyptian patients. *Indian J Dermatol*, 2014. **59**(1): 49–55.

167. Hordinsky MK, Overview of alopecia areata. *J Investig Dermatol Symp Proc*, 2013. **16**(1): S13–5.

168. Tasaki M, Hanada K, and Hashimoto I, Analyses of serum copper and zinc levels and copper/zinc ratios in skin diseases. *J Dermatol*, 1993. **20**(1): 21–4.

169. Mitchell AJ and Krull EA, Alopecia areata: Pathogenesis and treatment. *J Am Acad Dermatol*, 1984. **11**(5 Pt 1): 763–75.

170. Garcia-Hernandez MJ, Rodriguez-Pichardo A, and Camacho F, Congenital triangular alopecia (Brauer nevus). *Pediatr Dermatol*, 1995. **12**(4): 301–3.

171. Dominguez E, Eslinger MR, and McCord SV, Postoperative (pressure) alopecia: Report of a case after elective cosmetic surgery. *Anesth Analg*, 1999. **89**(4): 1062–3.

172. Kosanin RM, Riefkohl R, and Barwick WJ, Postoperative alopecia in a woman after a lengthy plastic surgical procedure. *Plast Reconstr Surg*, 1984. **73**(2): 308–9.

173. Poma PA, Pressure-induced alopecia. Report of a case after gynecologic surgery. *J Reprod Med*, 1979. **22**(4): 219–21.

174. Wiles JC and Hansen RC, Postoperative (pressure) alopecia. *J Am Acad Dermatol*, 1985. **12**(1 Pt 2): 195–8.

175. Bateman T, *Practical Synopsis of Cutaneous Diseases*. 4th edition. 1817.

176. Olsen E, Hordinsky M, and McDonald-Hull S, Alopecia areata investigational assessment guidelines. National Alopecia Areata Foundation. *J Am Acad Dermatol*, 1999. **40**(2 Pt 1): 242–6.

177. Drake LA, Dinehart SM, and Farmer ER, Guidelines of care for alopecia areata. *J Am Acad Dermatol*, 1992. **26**(2 Pt 1): 247–50.

178. Sawaya ME and Hordinsky MK, Glucocorticoid regulation of hair growth in alopecia areata. *J Invest Dermatol*, 1995. **104**(5 Suppl): 30S.

179. Price VH, Treatment of hair loss. *New Engl J Med*, 1999. **341**(13): 964–73.

180. Shapiro J and Price VH, Hair regrowth. Therapeutic agents. *Dermatol Clin*, 1998. **16**(2): 341–56.

181. Porter D and Burton JL, A comparison of intra-lesional triamcinolone hexacetonide and triamcinolone acetonide in alopecia areata. *Br J Dermatol*, 1971. **85**(3): 272–3.

182. Shapiro J, Alopecia areata. Update on therapy. *Dermatol Clin*, 1993. **11**(1): 35–46.

183. Whiting DA, The treatment of alopecia areata. *Cutis*, 1987. **40**(3): 247–50.

184. Bergfeld W, Alopecia areata symposium. *Pediat Dermatol*, 1987. **4**: 144.

185. Thiers B, Alopecia areata symposium. *Pediat Dermatol*, 1987. **4**: 136.

186. Tosti A et al., Clobetasol propionate 0.05% under occlusion in the treatment of alopecia totalis/universalis. *J Am Acad Dermatol*, 2003. **49**(1): 96–8.

187. Tosti A et al., Efficacy and safety of a new clobetasol propionate 0.05% foam in alopecia areata: A randomized, doubleblind placebo-controlled trial. *J Eur Acad Dermatol Venereol*, 2006. **20**(10): 1243–7.

188. Mancuso G et al., Efficacy of betamethasone valerate foam formulation in comparison with betamethasone dipropionate lotion in

the treatment of mild-to-moderate alopecia areata: A multicenter, prospective, randomized, controlled, investigator-blinded trial. *Int J Dermatol*, 2003. **42**(7): 572–5.

189. Gill K, Alopecia totalis—Treatment with fluocinolone acetonide. *Arch Dermatol*, 1963. **87**: 384.

190. Pascher F, Kurtin S, and Andrade R, Assay of 0.2 percent fluocinolone acetonide cream for alopecia areata and totalis. Efficacy and side effects including histologic study of the ensuing localized acneform response. *Dermatologica*, 1970. **141**(3): 193–202.

191. Montes LF, Topical halcinonide in alopecia areata and in alopecia totalis. *J Cutan Pathol*, 1977. **4**(2): 47–50.

192. Charuwichitratana S, Wattanakrai P, and Tanrattanakorn S, Randomized double-blind placebo-controlled trial in the treatment of alopecia areatawith 0.25% desoximetasone cream. *Arch Dermatol*, 2000. **136**(10): 1276–7.

193. Leyden JL and Kligman AM, Treatment of alopecia areata with steroid solution. *Arch Dermatol*, 1972. **106**(6): 924.

194. Fiedler VC, Alopecia areata: Current therapy. *J Invest Dermatol*, 1991. **96**(5): 69S–70S.

195. Buhl AE, Minoxidil's action in hair follicles. *J Invest Dermatol*, 1991. **96**(5): 73S–74S.

196. Price V, Progress in dermatology. *Bull Dermatol Foundation*, 1991. **25**: 1.

197. Khoury EL, Price VH, and Abdel-Salam MM, Topical minoxidil in alopecia areata: No effect on the perifollicular lymphoid infiltration. *J Invest Dermatol*, 1992. **99**(1): 40–7.

198. Fiedler VC, Alopecia areata. A review of therapy, efficacy, safety, and mechanism [editorial] [see comments]. *Arch Dermatol*, 1992. **128**(11): 1519–29.

199. Fiedler-Weiss VC, Topical minoxidil solution (1% and 5%) in the treatment of alopecia areata. *J Am Acad Dermatol*, 1987. **16**(3 Pt 2): 745–8.

200. Fiedler-Weiss VC et al., Topical minoxidil dose-response effect in alopecia areata. *Arch Dermatol*, 1986. **122**(2): 180–2.

201. Price VH, Topical minoxidil in extensive alopecia areata, including 3-year follow-up. *Dermatologica*, 1987. **175**(Suppl 2): 36–41.

202. Price VH, Topical minoxidil (3%) in extensive alopecia areata, including long-term efficacy. *J Am Acad Dermatol*, 1987. **16**(3 Pt 2): 737–44.

203. Fransway AF and Muller SA, 3 percent topical minoxidil compared with placebo for the treatment of chronic severe alopecia areata. *Cutis*, 1988. **41**(6): 431–5.

204. Ranchoff RE et al., Extensive alopecia areata. Results of treatment with 3% topical minoxidil. *Cleve Clin J Med*, 1989. **56**(2): 149–54.

205. Vestey JP and Savin JA, A trial of 1% minoxidil used topically for severe alopecia areata. *Acta Derm Venereol*, 1986. **66**(2): 179–80.

206. Morhenn VB, Orenberg EK, and Kaplan J, Inhibition of a Langerhans cell-mediated immune response by treatment modalities useful in psoriasis. *J Invest Dermatol*, 1983. **81**(1): 23–7.

207. Buchner U, Irritant versus allergic contact dermatitis for the treatment of alopecia areata. *Arch Dermatol Res*, 1979. **264**: 123.

208. Swanson NA, Mitchell AJ, and Leahy MS, Topical treatment of alopecia areata. *Arch Dermatol*, 1981. **117**(7): 384–7.

209. Fiedler-Weiss VC and Buys CM, Evaluation of anthralin in the treatment of alopecia areata. *Arch Dermatol*, 1987. **123**(11): 1491–3.

210. Schmoeckel C et al., Treatment of alopecia areata by anthralin-induced dermatitis. *Arch Dermatol*, 1979. **115**(10): 1254–5.

211. Shapiro J and Price VH, Hair regrowth. Therapeutic agents. *Dermatol Clin*, 1998. **16**(2): 341–56.

212. Fiedler VC, Wendraw A, and Szpunar GJ, Treatment-resistant alopecia areata. Response to combination therapy with minoxidil plus anthralin. *Arch Dermatol*, 1990. **126**(6): 756–9.

213. Nelson DA and Spielvogel RL, Anthralin therapy for alopecia areata. *Int J Dermatol*, 1985. **24**(9): 606–7.

214. Happle R, Klein HM, and Macher E, Topical immunotherapy changes the composition of the peribulbar infiltrate in alopecia areata. *Arch Dermatol Res*, 1986. **278**(3): 214–8.

215. Happle R, Kalveram KJ, and Buchner U, Contact allergy as a therapeutic tool for alopecia areata: Application of squaric acid dibutylester. *Dermatologica*, 1980. **161**(5): 289–97.

216. Harland CC and Saihan EM, Regression of cutaneous metastatic malignant melanoma with topical diphencyprone and oral cimetidine [letter]. *Lancet*, 1989. **2**(8660): 445.

217. Lane PR and Hogan DJ, Diphencyprone [letter]. *J Am Acad Dermatol*, 1988. **19**(2 Pt 1): 364–5.

218. Van der Steen PH, Boezeman JB, and Happle R, Topical immunotherapy for alopecia areata: Re-evaluation of 139 cases after an additional follow-up period of 19 months. *Dermatology*, 1992. **184**(3): 198–201.

219. Hull SM and Norris JF, Diphencyprone in the treatment of long-standing alopecia areata. *Br J Dermatol*, 1988. **119**(3): 367–74.

220. MacDonald-Hull S, Post therapy relapse rate in alopecia areata after successful treatment with diphencyprone. *J Dermatol Treat*, 1989. **1**: 71.

221. Hull SM and Cunliffe WJ, Successful treatment of alopecia areata using the contact allergen diphencyprone [letter]. *Br J Dermatol*, 1991. **124**(2): 212–3.

222. Wiseman M et al., Predictive model for immunotherapy of alopecia areata with diphencyprone. *Arch Dermatol*, 2001. **137**(8): 1063–8.

223. Gordon PM et al., Topical diphencyprone for alopecia areata: Evaluation of 48 cases after 30 months' follow-up. *Br J Dermatol*, 1996. **134**(5): 869–71.

224. Monk B, Induction of hair growth in alopecia totalis with diphencyprone sensitization. *Clin Exp Dermatol*, 1989. **14**(2): 154–7.

225. Hatzis J, Georgiotono K, and Kostakis P, Treatment of alopecia areata with diphencyprone. *Australas J Dermatol*, 1988. **29**(1): 33–6.

226. Ashworth J, Tuyp E, and Mackie RM, Allergic and irritant contact dermatitis compared in the treatment of alopecia totalis and universalis. A comparison of the value of topical diphencyprone and tretinoin gel. *Br J Dermatol*, 1989. **120**(3): 397–401.

227. Orecchia G and Rabbiosi G. Treatment of alopecia areata with diphencyprone. *Dermatologica*, 1985. **171**(3): 193–6.

228. Berth-Jones J and Hutchinson PE, Treatment of alopecia totalis with a combination of inosine pranobex and diphencyprone compared to each treatment alone. *Clin Exp Dermatol*, 1991. **16**(3): 172–5.

229. Shapiro J et al., Treatment of severe alopecia areata with topical diphenylcyclopropenone and 5% minoxidil: A clinical and immunopathologic evaluation. *J Invest Dermatol*, 1995. **104**(5 Suppl): 36S.

230. Hull SM, Pepall L, and Cunliffe WJ, Alopecia areata in children: Response to treatment with diphencyprone. *Br J Dermatol*, 1991. **125**(2): 164–8.

231. van der Steen PH et al., Treatment of alopecia areata with diphenylcyclopropenone. *J Am Acad Dermatol*, 1991. **24**(2 Pt 1): 253–7.

232. Berth-Jones J, Mc Burney A, and Hutchinson PE, Diphencyprone is not detectable in serum or urine following topical application. *Acta Derm Venereol*, 1994. **74**(4): 312–3.

233. Wilkerson MG, Connor TH, and Henkin J, Assessment of diphenylcyclopropenone for photochemically induced mutagenicity in the Ames assay. *J Am Acad Dermatol*, 1987. **17**(4): 606–11.

234. Wilkerson MG, Henkin J, and Wilkin JK, Diphenylcyclopropenone: Examination for potential contaminants, mechanisms of sensitization, and photochemical stability. *J Am Acad Dermatol*, 1984. **11**(5 Pt 1): 802–7.

235. Perret C, Treatment of alopecia areata. In *Hair and Hair Diseases*, Happle R, Orfanos CE, Editors. 1990. New York: Springer Verlag. p. 529.

236. Perret CM, Steijlen PM, and Happle R, Alopecia areata: pathogenesis and topical immunotherapy. *Ned Tijdschr Geneeskd*, 1989. **133**(25): 1256–60.

237. Shah M, Lewis FM, and Messenger AG, Hazards in the use of diphencyprone [letter] [see comments]. *Br J Dermatol*, 1996. **134**(6).

238. Fernandez-Redondo V et al., Hazards in the use of diphencyprone. *Allergy*, 2000. **55**(2): 202–3.

239. Orecchia G and Stock J, Diphenylcyclopropenone: An important agent known to cause depigmentation [letter; comment]. *Dermatology*, 1999. **199**(2): 198.

240. van der Steen P and Happle R, "Dyschromia in confetti" as a side effect of topical immunotherapy with diphenylcyclopropenone. *Arch Dermatol*, 1992. **128**(4): 518–20.

241. Duhra P and Foulds IS, Persistent vitiligo induced by diphencyprone [letter]. *Br J Dermatol*, 1990. **123**(3): 415–16.

242. Hatzis J, Gourgiotou K, and Tosca A, Vitiligo as a reaction to topical treatment with diphencyprone [see comments]. *Dermatologica*, 1988. **177**(3): 146–8.

243. Henderson CA and Ilchyshyn A, Vitiligo complicating diphencyprone sensitization therapy for alopecia universalis [letter]. *Br J Dermatol*, 1995. **133**(3): 496–7.

244. Orecchia G and Perfetti L, Vitiligo and topical allergens [letter; comment]. *Dermatologica*, 1989. **179**(3): 137–8.

245. Alam M, Gross EA, and Savin RC, Severe urticarial reaction to diphenylcyclopropenone therapy for alopecia areata. *J Am Acad Dermatol*, 1999. **40**(1): 110–2.

246. Tosti A, Guerra L, and Bardazzi F, Contact urticaria during topical immunotherapy. *Contact Dermatitis*, 1989. **21**(3): 196–7.

247. Skrebova N et al., Severe dermographism after topical therapy with diphenylcyclopropenone for alopecia universalis. *Contact Dermatitis*, 2000. **42**(4): 212–5.

248. Perret CM et al., Erythema multiforme-like eruptions: A rare side effect of topical immunotherapy with diphenylcyclopropenone. *Dermatologica*, 1990. **180**(1): 5–7.

249. Daman LA, Rosenberg EW, and Drake L, Treatment of alopecia areata with dinitrochlorobenzene. *Arch Dermatol*, 1978. **114**(7): 1036–8.

250. Happle R, Antigenic competition as a therapeutic concept for alopecia areata. *Arch Dermatol Res*, 1980. **267**(1): 109–14.

251. Hehir ME and du Vivier A, Alopecia areata treated with DNCB. *Clin Exp Dermatol*, 1979. **4**(3): 385–7.

252. Kratka J et al., Dinitrochlorobenzene: Influence on the cytochrome P-450 system and mutagenic effects. *Arch Dermatol Res*, 1979. **266**(3): 315–8.

253. Strobel R and Rohrborn G, Mutagenic and cell transforming activities of 1-chlor-2,4-dinitrobenzene (DNCB) and squaric-acid dibutylester (SADBE). *Arch Toxicol*, 1980. **45**(4): 307–14.

254. Summer KH and Goggelmann W, 1-chloro-2,4-dinitrobenzene depletes glutathione in rat skin and is mutagenic in *Salmonella typhimurium*. *Mutat Res*, 1980. **77**(1): 91–3.

255. Weisburger EK, Russfield AB, and Homburger F, Testing of twenty-one environmental aromatic amines or derivatives for long-term toxicity or carcinogenicity. *J Environ Pathol Toxicol*, 1978. **2**(2): 325–56.

256. Wilkerson MG, Wilkin JK, and Smith RG, Contaminants of dinitrochlorobenzene. *J Am Acad Dermatol*, 1983. **9**(4): 554–7.

257. Flowers FP et al., Topical squaric acid dibutylester therapy for alopecia areata. *Cutis*, 1982. **30**(6): 733–6.

258. Case PC, Mitchell AJ, and Swanson NA, Topical therapy of alopecia areata with squaric acid dibutylester. *J Am Acad Dermatol*, 1984. **10**(3): 447–50.

259. Caserio RJ, Treatment of alopecia areata with squaric acid dibutylester. *Arch Dermatol*, 1987. **123**(8): 1036–41.

260. Giannetti A and Orecchia G, Clinical experience on the treatment of alopecia areata with squaric acid dibutyl ester. *Dermatologica*, 1983. **167**(5): 280–2.

261. Micali G et al., Treatment of alopecia areata with squaric acid dibutylester. *Int J Dermatol*, 1996. **35**(1): 52–6.

262. Chua SH, Goh CL, and Ang CB, Topical squaric acid dibutylester therapy for alopecia areata: A double-sided patient-controlled study. *Ann Acad Med Singapore*, 1996. **25**(6): 842–7.

263. Orecchia G, Malagoli P, and Santagostino L, Treatment of severe alopecia areata with squaric acid dibutylester in pediatric patients. *Pediatr Dermatol*, 1994. **11**(1): 65–8.

264. Tosti A et al., Long-term results of topical immunotherapy in children with alopecia totalis or alopecia universalis. *J Am Acad Dermatol*, 1996. **35**(2 Pt 1): 199–201.

265. Barth JH, Darley CR, and Gibson JR, Squaric acid dibutyl ester in the treatment of alopecia areata. *Dermatologica*, 1985. **170**(1): 40–2.

266. Orecchia G et al., Photochemotherapy plus squaric acid dibutylester in alopecia areata treatment [letter]. *Dermatologica*, 1990. **181**(2): 167–9.

267. Wilkerson MG et al., Squaric acid and esters: Analysis for contaminants and stability in solvents. *J Am Acad Dermatol*, 1985. **13**(2 Pt 1): 229–34.

268. Van Duuren BL, Melchionne S, and Blair R, Carcinogenicity of isosters of epoxides and lactones: Aziridine ethanol, propane sultone, and related compounds. *J Natl Cancer Inst*, 1971. **46**(1): 143–9.

269. Mitchell AJ and Douglass MC, Topical photo-chemotherapy for alopecia areata. *J Am Acad Dermatol*, 1985. **12**(4): 644–9.

270. Claudy AL and Gagnaire D, Photochemo-therapy for alopecia areata. *Acta Derm Venereol*, 1980. **60**(2): 171–2.

271. Larko O and Swanbeck G, PUVA treatment of alopecia totalis. *Acta Derm Venereol*, 1983. **63**(6): 546–9.

272. Lassus A et al., PUVA treatment for alo-pecia areata. *Dermatologica*, 1980. **161**(5): 298–304.

273. Healy E and Rogers S, PUVA treatment for alopecia areata—Does it work? A retrospec-tive review of 102 cases. *Br J Dermatol*, 1993. **129**(1): 42–4.

274. Taylor CR and Hawk JL, PUVA treatment of alopecia areata partialis, totalis, and universalis: Audit of 10 years' experience at St John's Institute of Dermatology. *Br J Dermatol*, 1995. **133**(6): 914–8.

275. Stern RS, Nichols KT, and Vakeva LH, Malignant melanoma in patients treated for psoriasis with methoxsalen (psoralen) and ultraviolet A radiation (PUVA). The PUVA Follow-Up Study [see comments]. *New Engl J Med*, 1997. **336**(15): 1041–5.

276. Zakaria W et al., 308-nm excimer laser ther-apy in alopecia areata. *J Am Acad Dermatol*, 2004. **51**(5): 837–8.

277. Raulin C et al., Excimer laser therapy of alopecia areata-side-by-side evaluation of a representative area. *J Dtsch Dermatol Ges*, 2005. **3**(7): 524–6.

278. Gundogan C, Greve B, and Raulin C, Treatment of alopecia areata with the 308-nm xenon chloride excimer laser: Case report of two successful treatments with the excimer laser. *Lasers Surg Med*, 2004. **34**(2): 86–90.

279. Al-Mutairi N, 308-nm excimer laser for the treatment of alopecia areata. *Dermatol Surg*, 2007. **33**(12): 1483–7.

280. Al-Mutairi N, 308-nm excimer laser for the treatment of alopecia areata in children. *Pediatr Dermatol*, 2009. **26**(5): 547–50.

281. McMichael AJ, Excimer laser: A module of the alopecia areata common protocol. *J Investig Dermatol Symp Proc*, 2013. **16**(1): S77–9.

282. Bayramgürler D et al., Narrowband ultra-violet B phototherapy for alopecia areata. *Photodermatol Photoimmunol Photomed*, 2011. **27**(6): 325–7.

283. Ait Ourhroui M, Hassam B, and Khoudri I, Treatment of alopecia areata with prednisone in a once-monthly oral pulse. *Ann Dermatol Venereol*, 2010. **137**(8–9): 514–8.

284. Kar BR et al., Placebo-controlled oral pulse prednisolone therapy in alopecia areata. *J Am Acad Dermatol*, 2005. **52**: 287–90.

285. Winter RJ, Kern F, and Blizzard RM, Prednisone therapy for alopecia areata. A follow-up report. *Arch Dermatol*, 1976. **112**: 1549–52.

286. Sharma VK, Pulsed administration of corti-costeroids in the treatment of alopecia areata. *Int J Dermatol*, 1996. **35**: 133–6.

287. Burton JL and Shuster S, Large doses of glucocorticoid in the treatment of alopecia areata. *Acta Derm Venereol*, 1975. **55**: 493–6.

288. Friedli A et al., Pulse methylprednisolone therapy for severe alopecia areata: An open prospective study of 45 patients. *J Am Acad Dermatol*, 1998. **39**: 597–602.

289. Price VH, Treatment of hair loss. *N Engl J Med*, 1999. **341**(13): 964–73.

290. Alkhalifah A et al., Alopecia areata update: Part I. Clinical picture, histopathology, and pathogenesis. *J Am Acad Dermatol*, 2010. **62**(2): 177–88; quiz 189–90.

291. Alkhalifah A et al., Alopecia areata update: Part II. Treatment. *J Am Acad Dermatol*, 2010. **62**(2): 191–202; quiz 203–4.

292. Kurosawa M et al., A comparison of the efficacy, relapse rate and side effects among three modalities of systemic corticosteroid therapy for alopecia areata. *Dermatology*, 2006. **212**(4): 361–5.

293. Lester RS, Knowles SR, and Shear NH, The risks of systemic corticosteroid use. *Dermatol Clin*, 1998. **16**: 277–88.

294. Shaheedi-Dadras M et al., The effect of methylprednisolone pulse-therapy plus oral cyclosporine in the treatment of alopecia totalis and universalis. *Arch Iran Med*, 2008. **11**(1): 90–3.

295. Unger WP and Schemmer RJ, Corticosteroids in the treatment of alopecia totalis. Systemic effects. *Arch Dermatol*, 1978. **114**(10): 1486–90.

296. Yang CC et al., Early intervention with high-dose steroid pulse therapy prolongs disease-free interval of severe alopecia areata: A retrospective study. *Ann Dermatol Venereol*, 2013. **25**(4): 471–4.

297. Price VH, Treatment of hair loss. *N Engl J Med*, 1999. **341**(13): 964–73.

298. Yang CC et al., Early intervention with high-dose steroid pulse therapy prolongs disease-free interval of severe alopecia areata: A retrospective study. *Ann Dermatol*, 2013. **25**(4): 471–4.

299. Otberg N, Systemic treatment for alopecia areata. *Dermatol Ther*, 2011. **24**(3): 320–5.

300. Kim BJ et al., Combination therapy of cyclosporine and methylprednisolone on severe alopecia areata. *J Dermatolog Treat*, 2008. **19**(4): 216–20.

301. Ranganath VK and Furst DE, Disease-modifying antirheumatic drug use in the elderly rheumatoid arthritis patient. *Rheum Dis Clin North Am*, 2007. **33**: 197–217.

302. Phillips MA, Graves JE, and Nunley JR, Alopecia areata presenting in 2 kidney-pancreas transplant recipients taking cyclosporine. *J Am Acad Dermatol*, 2005. **53**(5 suppl. 1): S252–5.

303. Cerottini JP, Panizzon RG, and de Viragh PA, Multifocal alopecia areata during systemic cyclosporine A therapy. *Dermatology*, 1999. **198**: 415–7.

304. Davies MG and Bowers PW, Alopecia areata arising in patients receiving cyclosporin immunosuppression. *Br J Dermatol*, 1995. **132**: 835–6.

305. Dyall-Smith D, Alopecia areata in a renal transplant recipient on cyclosporin. *Australas J Dermatol*, 1996. **37**: 226–7.

306. Gupta AK and Charrette A, The efficacy and safety of 5α-reductase inhibitors in androgenetic alopecia: A network meta-analysis and benefit-risk assessment of finasteride and dutasteride. *J Dermatolog Treat*, 2014. **25**(2): 156–61.

307. de Prost Y et al., Treatment of severe alopecia areata by topical applications of cyclosporine: Comparative trial versus placebo in 43 patients. *Transplant Proc*, 1988. **20**(3 Suppl 4): 112–3.

308. Mauduit G et al., Treatment of severe alopecia areata with topical applications of cyclosporin A [in French]. *Ann Dermatol Venereol*, 1987. **114**: 507–10.

309. Verma DD et al., Treatment of alopecia areata in the DEBR model using cyclosporin A lipid vesicles. *Eur J Dermatol*, 2004. **14**: 332–8.

310. Ellis CN, Brown MF, and Voorhees JJ, Sulfasalazine for alopecia areata. *J Am Acad Dermatol*, 2002. **46**(4): 541–4.

311. Aghaei S, An uncontrolled, open label study of sulfasalazine in severe alopecia areata. *Indian J Dermatol Venereol Leprol*, 2008. **74**(6): 611–3.

312. Rashidi T and Mahd AA, Treatment of persistent alopecia areata with sulfasalazine. *Int J Dermatol*, 2008. **47**(8): 850–2.

313. Bannwarth B et al., Methotrexate in rheumatoid arthritis. An update. *Drugs*, 1994. **47**(1): 25–50.

314. Droitcourt C et al., Interest of high-dose pulse corticosteroid therapy combined with methotrexate for severe alopecia areata: A retrospective case series. *Dermatology*, 2012. **224**(4): 369–73.

315. Chartaux E and Joly P, Long-term follow-up of the efficacy of methotrexate alone or in combination with low doses of oral corticosteroids in the treatment of alopecia areata totalis or universalis. [Article in French]. *Ann Dermatol Venereol*, 2010. **137**(8–9): 507–13.

316. Joly P, The use of methotrexate alone or in combination with low doses of oral corticosteroids in the treatment of alopecia totalis or universalis. *J Am Acad Dermatol*, 2006. **55**(4): 632–6.

317. Royer M et al., Efficacy and tolerability of methotrexate in severe childhood alopecia areata. *Br J Dermatol*, 2011. **165**(2): 407–10.

318. Price VH et al., Subcutaneous efalizumab is not effective in the treatment of alopecia areata. *J Am Acad Dermatol*, 2008. **58**(3): 395–402.

319. Strober BE et al., Etanercept does not effectively treat moderate to severe alopecia areata: An open-label study. *J Am Acad Dermatol*, 2005. **52**: 1082–4.

320. Le Bidre E et al., Alopecia areata during anti-TNF alpha therapy: Nine cases. *Ann Dermatol Venereol*, 2011. **138**(4): 285–93.

321. Kirshen C and Kanigsberg N, Alopecia areata following adalimumab. *J Cutan Med Surg*, 2009. **13**: 48–50.

322. Pan Y and Rao NA, Alopecia areata during etanercept therapy. *Ocul Immunol Inflamm*, 2009. **17**: 127–9.

323. Pelivani N et al., Alopecia areata universalis elicited during treatment with adalimumab. *Dermatology*, 2008. **216**: 320–3.

324. Posten W and Swan J, Recurrence of alopecia areata in a patient receiving etanercept injections. *Arch Dermatol*, 2005. **141**: 759–60.

6 Cicatricial alopecias: Pathogenesis, classification, clinical features, diagnosis, and management

Introduction

Cicatricial or scarring alopecias comprise a diverse group of scalp disorders that result in irreversible hair loss. All scarring alopecias are characterized clinically by a loss of follicular ostia and pathologically by a replacement of hair follicles with fibrous tissue. The terms "cicatricial" and "scarring" are used interchangeably. The destructive process can occur as a primary or secondary cicatricial alopecia.

A basic knowledge of follicular anatomy is important in the understanding of cicatricial alopecias, because the location of the destructive process is crucial in determining the irreversibility of alopecia. Follicular stem cells are located in the bulge area where the arrector pili muscle inserts into the follicles. These cells migrate down into the hair follicle, and subsequently differentiate into the various layers of the hair follicle. As the hair cycles through anagen, catagen, and telogen, there is a permanent upper portion of the hair follicle and a nonpermanent lower portion. When the inflammation is located deep, in the vicinity of the nonpermanent portion, a scarring alopecia is unlikely to develop. If the inflammation is located within the permanent portion, then a cicatrizing alopecia is more likely to occur.

Primary cicatricial alopecia refers to a group of idiopathic inflammatory diseases, characterized by a folliculocentric inflammatory process that ultimately destroys the hair follicle. Follicles can be saved from irreversible damage if this peri-bulge infiltrate can be controlled. Secondary cicatricial alopecias can be caused by almost any cutaneous inflammatory process of the scalp skin or by physical trauma, which injures the skin and skin appendages.

Scarring alopecias represent trichologic emergencies since hair follicles are permanently destroyed and therefore the patient may suffer from disfiguration, psychosocial embarrassment, and a lack of self-esteem. Cicatricial alopecias are always psychosocially distressing for the affected patient and challenging for the treating physician. A fast and confident diagnosis as well as an aggressive treatment in case of active disease are crucial in the management of scarring alopecia.

Primary cicatricial alopecias

Pathogenesis

Primary cicatricial alopecias are characterized by an inflammatory process affecting the upper, permanent portion of the follicles, particularly around the pluripotent stem cells of the bulge area, the sebaceous gland, and the infundibulum. The bulge region is located in the isthmus where the arrector pili muscle attaches to the outer root sheath. Pluripotent hair follicle stem cells are responsible for the renewal of the upper part of the hair follicle and sebaceous glands, and for the restoration of the lower cyclical component of the follicles at the onset of a new anagen period [1,2]. Damage to the bulge area and the sebaceous gland with the isthmus may result in an incomplete hair cycle and can be associated with chronic follicular inflammation and foreign body reaction, and consequently lead to scarring hair loss [3–7].

Classification

Classification for cicatrizing alopecias can be based on clinical, histopathological, or proposed pathogenic criteria [6,8]. A classification based on the nature of the inflammatory cells observed histologically around affected hair follicles was defined by a consensus meeting on cicatricial alopecia in 2001 by the North American Hair Research Society and is widely used for the distinction of the different diseases.

Primary cicatricial alopecias were classified into three main groups: (1) lymphocytic, (2) neutrophilic, and (3) mixed (Table 6.1) [9]. Although each disease has specific clinical and histopathological characteristics, the presentation of scarring alopecia in a patient can show overlapping findings and symptoms.

Clinical features and diagnosis

Primary cicatricial alopecia most commonly affects the central and parietal scalp before progressing to other sites of the scalp.

Table 6.1

Lymphocytic primary cicatricial alopecia

- Chronic cutaneous lupus erythematosus (discoid lupus erythematosus [DLE])
- Lichen planopilaris (LPP)
  - Classic LPP
  - Frontal fibrosing alopecia
  - Graham-Little syndrome
- Classic pseudopelade of Brocq (PPB)
- Central centrifugal cicatricial alopecia (CCCA)
- Alopecia mucinosa
- Keratosis follicularis spinulosa decalvans

Neutrophilic primary cicatricial alopecia

- Folliculitis decalvans
- Dissecting cellulites/folliculits (perifolliculitis abscedens et suffodiens)

Mixed cicatricial alopecia

- Folliculitis (acne) keloidalis
- Folliculitis (acne) necrotica
- Erosive pustular dermatosis

Isolated alopecic patches showing atrophy and a lack of follicular ostia with inflammatory changes such as diffuse or perifollicular erythema, follicular hyperkeratosis, pigment changes, tufting, and pustules provide hints to the diagnosis [10,11]. However, clinically visible inflammatory change might be absent in the affected lesions and may present histologically as inflammatory infiltrates in the deep dermis and subcutaneous tissue. Diagnostic tools such as a threefold magnifying lens, a 10-fold magnifying dermatoscope, or a 60- to 200-fold magnifying videodermatoscope with and without polarized light can help to identify the presence or absence of follicular ostia, perifollicular erythema, and follicular hyperkeratosis in the affected areas.

A thorough examination of the entire scalp, a detailed clinical history, and skin biopsies of an active lesion are crucial in the correct diagnosis of cicatricial alopecia. Patient-reported symptoms such as itching or pain might be used as approximate indicators of disease activity but can also be completely absent. Presence of other indirectly related symptoms, such as sun sensitivity, can also help support a particular diagnosis (e.g., discoid lupus erythematosus [DLE]).

Biopsy for cicatrizing alopecias

Scalp biopsies are crucial to confirm the diagnosis of scarring alopecia and to identify the type and localization of the inflammatory infiltrate. The following recommendations were developed at the consensus meeting on cicatricial alopecia [9] in 2001: One 4-mm punch biopsy should be taken from a clinically active area. The punch is placed parallel to the direction of the hairs and inserted to the depth of the bevel. The biopsy should include the subcutaneous fat, because this is the location of terminal anagen hair bulbs. The biopsy site is then closed with a blue 3-0 or 4-0 nylon suture. The blue suture allows for easier recognition and differentiation from hair during suture removal 7–10 days later.

The tissue is then processed for horizontal sections and stained with hematoxylin and eosin. Elastin (acid alcoholic orcein), mucin, and periodic acid–Schiff (PAS) stains may provide additional diagnosis defining information. A second 4-mm punch biopsy from a clinically active disease-affected area should be cut vertically into two equal pieces. One half provides tissue for transverse cut routine histological sections, and the other half can be used for direct immunofluorescence (DIF) studies [12].

Lymphocytic primary cicatricial alopecia

Chronic cutaneous lupus erythematosus (discoid lupus erythematosus)

DLE, together with lichen planopilaris (LPP), is the most common cause of inflammatory cicatricial alopecia [10]. Women are more often affected than men and the disease is more common in adults (with first onset typically at the age of 20–40 years) than in children [13–15].

As high as 26%–31% of children with DLE and approximately 5%–10% of adult patients will develop systemic lupus erythematosus (SLE) [15,16]. Patients with DLE are found to have a higher incidence of concurrent alopecia areata. Moreover, DLE has also been associated with veruciform xanthoma and papulonodular dermal mucinosis [17]. Longstanding DLE lesions are prone to develop squamous cell carcinomas [18] with a high occurrence of metastasis [19]; therefore, every hyperkeratotic or ulcerated lesion in a DLE patch should be biopsied early [10].

Clinical features

DLE usually presents with one or more erythematous, atrophic, and alopecic patches on the scalp. Follicular hyperkeratosis, hyperpigmentation, hypopigmentation, and telangiectasia can be present [5,6]. Hyperpigmentation is frequently found in the center of the lesion. Active lesions can be sensitive or pruritic, and the patient might report a worsening after UV exposure (Figure 6.1).

Histology

Characteristic of DLE is a dense lymphocytic infiltrate predominantly in the upper part of the follicle but frequently also in deeper parts of the follicle; it is typically located perivascular but also in the interfollicular epidermis [20–23]. Other typical features of early, active DLE lesions are lymphocyte-mediated interface dermatitis with vacuolar degeneration of the basal cell layer and necrotic keratinocytes, a thickening of the basement membrane, and destruction of sebaceous glands. Elastic fibers are frequently destroyed throughout the reticular

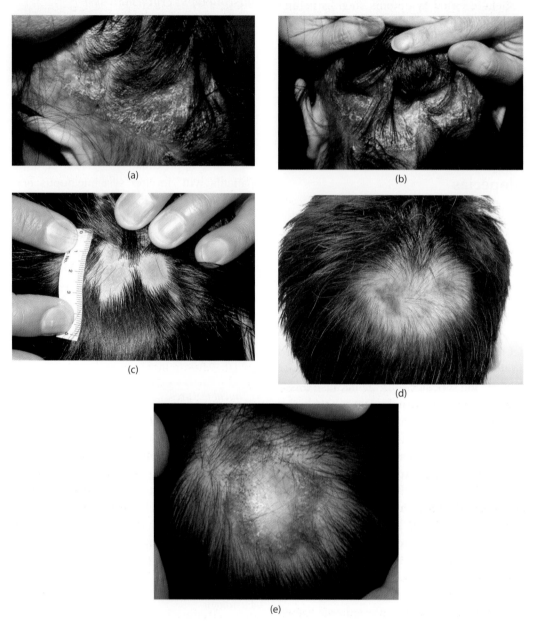

Figure 6.1

Chronic cutaneous lupus erythematosus of the scalp. (a, b) A 23-year-old female with painful erythematosus atrophic plaques; (c) a 31-year-old female with mid-scalp involvement; (d) a 39-year-old male patient with a large patch of discoid lupus erythematosus with hyperpigmentation in the occipital area; (e) a 41-year-old female patient displaying a patch of DLE with hyperkeratosis and hyperpigmentation.

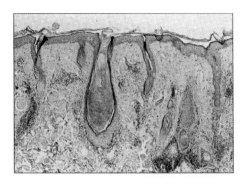

Figure 6.2
Pathology of lupus erythematosus showing periadnexal and perivascular lymphocytic infiltration with follicular hyperkeratosis.

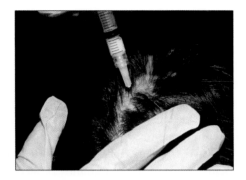

Figure 6.3
Injecting intralesional cortisone into the surrounding hairy areas of scarring alopecia. Triamcinolone 10 mg/mL, injected with a volume of 0.1 mL/injection for 20 injections, can halt further spread of the condition and reduce symptoms of itch and burning. Injections are performed once monthly.

dermis [4,12]. The hair follicle infundubula are filled with laminated keratin, which corresponds to the clinically observed follicular plugging (Figure 6.2). DIF typically shows a linear granular deposition of IgG and C3 at the dermo–epidermal junction. IgM, C1q, and rarely IgA can also be found.

Management

In limited or slowly progressive DLE, intralesional triamcinolone acetonide should be used as first-line treatment at a concentration of 10 mg/cc every 4–6 weeks, alone or in addition to oral therapy [11] (Figure 6.3). Intralesional triamcinolone acetonide can be used with or without topical class I or II corticosteroids. Topical corticosteroids alone have also been shown to be effective in milder forms of DLE [11,12,15,21].

Hydroxychloroquine at a dose of 200–400 mg daily in adults or 4–6 mg/kg in children has been shown to be highly effective. A baseline ophthalmologic examination and complete blood count is required before the therapy is started [13,15]. People taking 400 mg of hydroxychloroquine or less per day generally have a negligible risk of macular toxicity, whereas the risk begins to go up when a person takes the medication over 5 years or has a cumulative dose

of more than 1000 g [24]. Eye exams should be performed every 3 months.

Bridge therapy with oral prednisone (1 mg/ kg) tapered over the first 8 weeks of treatment might be helpful in adult patients with rapidly progressive disease [10,11]. Multimodal aggressive therapy in rapidly progressive DLE might reverse early alopecic patches and save hair follicles from the destructive process. Oral acitretin and isotretinoin have also shown some effectiveness [25,26]. Immunosuppressive therapies such as mycophenolate mofetil, methotrexate, and azathioprine should only be considered if the above therapies fail. Hair restoration surgery may be considered for burnt-out stages (Figure 6.4).

Lichen planopilaris

The term "lichen planopilaris" (LPP) was first introduced in 1895 by Pringle, who described the association of lichen planus with follicular keratotic lesions [27]. LPP is a follicular variant of lichen planus. LPP accounts for 30%–40% of scarring alopecias and is, together with DLE, the most common cause of primary cicatricial alopecia.

LPP can be subdivided into classic LPP, frontal fibrosing alopecia (FFA), and Graham-Little–Piccardi–Lassueur syndrome. Classic LPP typically starts at the crown and vertex area. The typical age of onset is around the fifth decade, and women are more often affected than men. Extracranial lichen planus may occur in up to 28% of patients [28–30].

FFA was first described by Kossard as a scarring alopecia predominantly affecting women after menopause [31–33]. It is characterized by a frontal, band-like, or circumferential scarring alopecia [4,34]. In recent years, the number of patients with FFA has markedly increased. As a consequence of this, most dermatologists have to face patients with this challenging entity [35–38]. The reason for this rising incidence is unknown. The occurrence of FFA in men is rare [39–43].

Graham-Little–Piccardi–Lassueur syndrome is a very rare condition that predominantly affects female adults. It is characterized by LPP of the scalp; noncicatricial of the eyebrows, axilla, and groin; and keratosis pilaris.

Lichenoid drug eruptions can be triggered by many drugs and might present as LPP.

Some of the most common drugs causing lichenoid drug eruption are gold, antimalarials, and captopril. Actinic lichenoid drug eruption is confined to sun-exposed sites. The most likely drugs to cause this are quinine and thiazide diuretics [44,45]. A higher incidence of hepatitis C in patients with lichen planus has been described [46]. Hepatitis C testing should be considered in patients with extensive LPP lesions. Scalp injury has also been suggested to play an etiological role in some cases of LPP [47–49]. Higher incidences of hypothyroidism, androgenetic alopecia, and vitiligo have been found in FFA [37,38,50].

Clinical features

In classic LPP, the affected areas are mostly located at the crown and vertex area and usually show perifollicular erythema and follicular hyperkeratosis (Figure 6.5). The alopecic areas of LPP are often smaller, irregularly

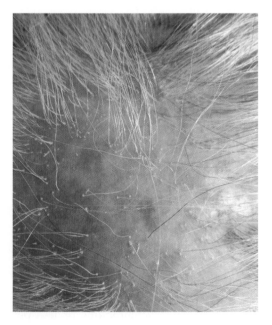

Figure 6.5
Patch of lichen planopilaris on the crown; note the lack of follicular ostia and marked follicular hyperkeratosis.

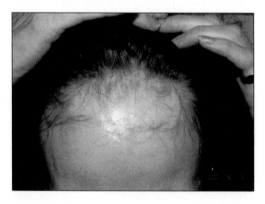

Figure 6.4
Lupus erythematosus: the patient showed marked improvement after 1 year of hydroxychloroquine 200 mg twice daily, monthly intralesional corticosteroid injections, and topical superpotent corticosteroid ointment twice daily.

shaped, and interconnected which can lead to a reticulated clinical pattern as compared to DLE. However, overlapping clinical features with those of DLE are frequently seen. Patients complain about itching, burning sensations, and sensitivity of the scalp [51,52] (Figure 6.6).

FFA is characterized by a frontal, band-like, or circumferential scarring alopecia with perifollicular erythema and follicular hyperkeratosis (Figure 6.7) [4]. In some cases, a few hairs are spared in the original frontal hairline. Alopecia of the eyebrows is also frequently seen and may be the first sign of FFA [38] (Figure 6.8).

Graham-Little–Piccardi–Lassueur syndrome is characterized by the triad of patchy cicatricial alopecia of the scalp, noncicatricial alopecia of the axilla and groin, and a follicular spinous papule on the body, scalp, or both [53] (Figure 6.9).

Histology

The three subgroups of LPP share basically the same histopathological features. A lymphocytic infiltrate and interface dermatitis are predominantly found in and around the upper permanent part of the hair follicle. LPP typically presents with a loss of elastic fibers only in the area of the follicular infundibulum [54]. Sebaceous glands are often destroyed in an early stage of the disease. Unlike DLE, the vascular plexus is not affected by inflammation and mucin deposits are absent [4]. DIF typically shows globular cytoid depositions of IgM, and rarely IgA, IgG, or C3 in the dermis around the infundibulum [55] (Figure 6.10).

Management

First-line treatment for moderately active classic LPP lesions is intralesional triamcinolone acetonide at a concentration of 10 mg/cc every 4–6 weeks or in combination with topical class I or II corticosteroids [10,26]. Literature on the efficacy of oral medication is limited. Options for systemic treatment include anti-inflammatory agents such as hydroxychloroquine, tetracyclines, pioglitazones, retinoids, griseofulvine, and immunosuppressive medications such as cyclosporine, mycophenolate mofetil, and systemic corticosteroids [5,6,56–61]. Oral corticosteroids in the first week of treatment as bridge therapy might be considered in very active cases. Systemic therapy should always be considered in the management of Graham-Little–Piccardi–Lassueur syndrome since the lesions are not limited to the scalp and local, topical, and intralesional therapy is less practicable.

In FFA, topical therapy alone has shown limited effectiveness. Intralesional triamcinolone acetonide at a dose of 2.5–5 mg/cc can be combined with topical corticosteroids, tacrolimus, or pimecrolimus. A concomitant therapy with topical minoxidil, systemic dustesteride, or finesteride has shown some beneficial effects [36,38,62–64]. In rapidly progressive disease the same systemic treatment options as in LPP should be considered (Figure 6.11).

Patients should be advised about camouflage techniques, hairpieces, and wigs. Women with extensive LPP lesions on the crown and vertex benefit highly from a well-designed hairpiece, which can look very natural, particularly if the frontal hairline is preserved, and is usually more comfortable to wear compared to a full wig.

Hair restoration surgery is an option if no disease activity occurs on the scalp for at least 1 year without therapy. The patient has to be warned about a possible disease recurrence and limited graft survival. Patients with clinically very obvious lesions might be very grateful for the cosmetic improvement and might accept lower hair density and even a mild flare of their LPP after surgery.

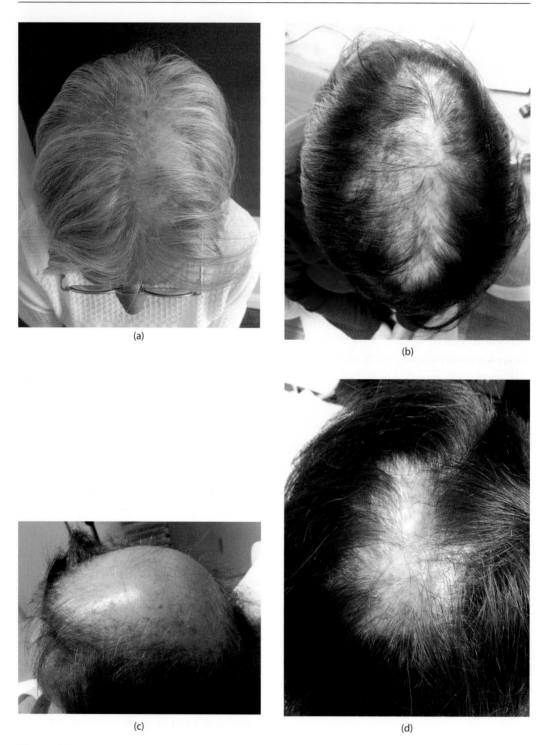

(a)

(b)

(c)

(d)

Figure 6.6
(a–c) Female patients with extensive lichen planopilaris (LPP) on the crown; (d) female
patients with patches of LPP on the crown.

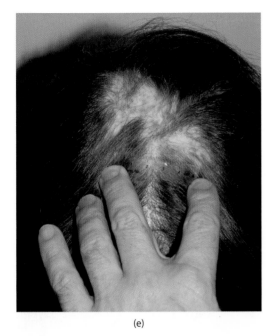
(e)

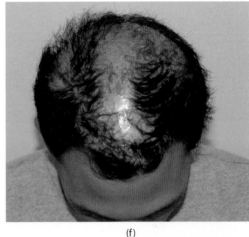
(f)

Figure 6.6 (*Continued*)
(e) Female patients with patches of LPP on the crown; (f) a 27-year-old male patient with extensive LPP.

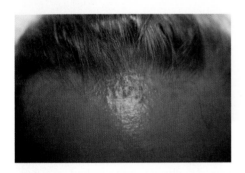

Figure 6.7
Frontal fibrosing alopecia with a band-like scarring alopecia displaying perifollicular erythema and follicular hyperkeratosis.

Classic Pseudopelade of Brocq

Pseudopelade of Brocq (PPB) is classified as an idiopathic lymphocytic primary cicatricial alopecia that predominantly affects the scalp [29]. Women between 30 and 50 years of age are most frequently affected.

Clinical features

PPB usually affects the vertex and occipital area of the scalp. It presents with small flesh-toned alopecic patches with irregular margins. This pattern has been described as "foot-prints in the snow" [65] (Figure 6.12). PPB can also present as a noninflammatory centrifugally spreading patch of alopecia, which might be seen as a variant of central centrifugal cicatricial alopecia (CCCA) in Caucasians. Follicular hyperkeratosis and perifollicular or diffuse erythema are mostly absent [6]. Clinically, the features may overlap with LPP (Figure 6.13).

Histology

Early PPB lesions typically show a sparse to moderate lymphocytic infiltrate around the follicular infundibulum with a complete destruction of the sebaceous glands [66]. In later disease stages, hair follicles are completely replaced by fibrous tracts. Unlike DLE

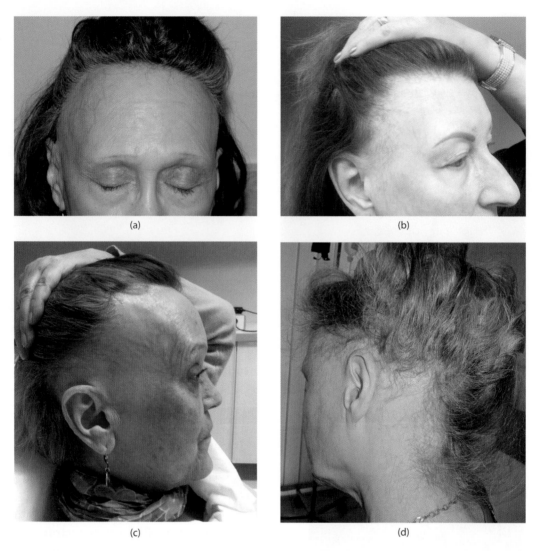

Figure 6.8

(a, b) Frontal fibrosing alopecia in a band-like pattern, loss of eyebrows, and marked atrophy; (c, d) extensive frontal fibrosing alopecia in a circumferential pattern.

and LPP, interface dermatitis is usually absent and the elastic fibers are preserved and thickened in PPB [54].

Management

Without clinical signs and symptoms of inflammation, activity of the disease is sometimes difficult to appreciate. Patient's history, a pull test, and measurements of the size of the lesions help to identify active areas. Intralesional triamcinolone acetonide at a concentration of 10 mg/cc × 2 cc every 4–6 weeks in combination with topical corticosteroids is the treatment of first choice. Hydroxychloroquine, oral prednisone, and isotretinoin have shown some effectiveness in treating PPB [6,29,67].

Hair restoration surgery is an option for PPB if the condition is stable without

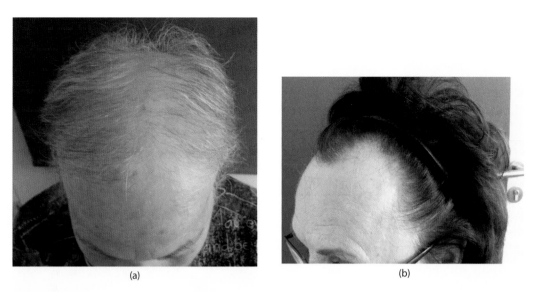

(a)   (b)

Figure 6.9
(a) Patient with extensive lichen planopilaris mimicking female pattern hair loss; this patient also suffered from extensive mucosal lichen planus; (b) patient with frontal fibrosing alopecia (FFA) mimicking androgenetic alopecia in a male pattern. FFA was misdiagnosed as androgenetic alopecia for over 5 years.

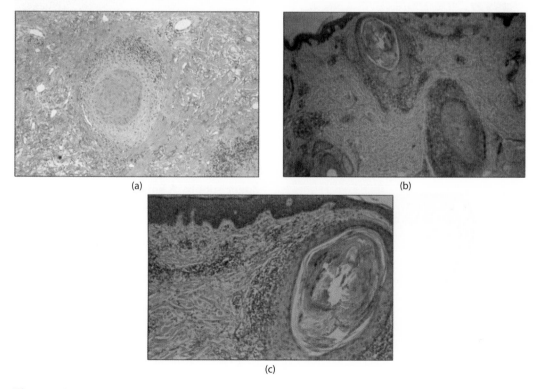

(a)   (b)

(c)

Figure 6.10
(a–c) Pathology of lichen planopilaris displaying the characteristic follicular lymphocytic interface dermatitis. (Courtesy of Dr. Magdalena Martinka.)

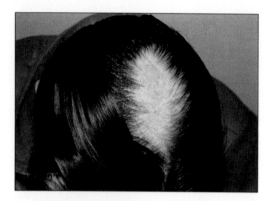

Figure 6.11
Lichen planopilaris with previously ulcerative lichen planopilaris improved markedly with hydroxychloroquine, intralesional corticosteroid, and topical corticosteroid.

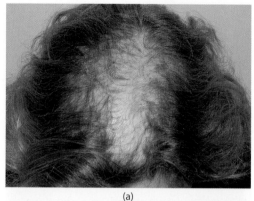

(a)

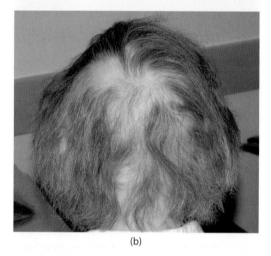

(b)

Figure 6.13
Pseudopelade of Brocq (a) on the crown and (b) vertex.

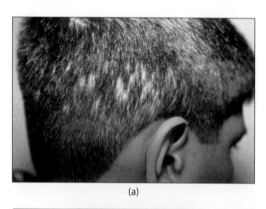

(a)

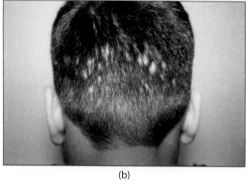

(b)

Figure 6.12
(a, b) An 8-year-old boy with scattered pseudopelade of Brocq.

treatment and the patient has a suitable donor supply. A small test area with a limited number of grafts (20–30 grafts/cm^2 with a maximum total of 100 grafts) 6 months to 1 year before a larger session is helpful to minimize the risk of disease progression and assure the success of a hair transplant procedure.

Central centrifugal cicatricial alopecia

CCCA is a primary lymphocytic cicatricial alopecia of the central scalp seen primarily in women of color. It remains unclear exactly which of the following most contribute to its formation: chemical processing, heat, traction, or other traumas [21,68]. CCCA can rarely be seen in Caucasians (sometimes called "central elliptical pseudopelade") and African American men. Due to clinical and histopathological similarities, it has been debated whether CCCA is a variant of PPB.

Clinical features

CCCA presents with a skin-colored patch of scarring alopecia on the crown, gradually progressing centrifugally to the parietal areas. Perifollicular hyperpigmentation and polytrichia might be present [69]. Patients may complain about itching, tenderness, and "pins and needle" sensations [70] (Figure 6.14).

Histology

Limited studies suggest that histopathological features of CCCA seem to be similar to those of PPB [5,21].

Management

Topical corticosteroids and tetracycline have shown to be effective in active progressive cases [21]. Since a multifactoral etiology is debated for CCCA, some dermatologists recommend a switch to more natural, less traumatizing, hair care practices [6,12,71]. Wigs and hairpieces can help camouflage the alopecia and are frequently used by women with CCCA. Hair transplant surgery is possible in a "burnt-out" stage and might provide a good cosmetic outcome in patients with very curly hair even with lower hair density.

Alopecia mucinosa

Alopecia mucinosa (AM), also known as follicular mucinosis (FM), presents in two forms: a primary idiopathical mucinosis and as a secondary form in association with cutaneous T-cell lymphoma or mycosis fungoides [72–74]. AM presents as indurated,

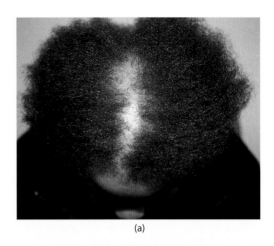

(a)

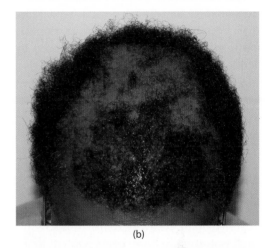

(b)

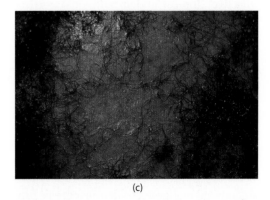

(c)

Figure 6.14
Central centrifugal scarring alopecia (follicular degeneration syndrome): (a, b) African American woman with significant alopecia; (c) close-up of patient illustrating lack of follicular ostia.

well-demarcated erythematosus or skin-colored patches of scarring or nonscarring alopecia that can be accompanied by diffuse hair loss [75] and alopecia of the eyebrows [76]. AM can clinically be mistaken for alopecia areata or other cicatricial hair loss conditions. Grouped follicular papules, follicular cysts, and follicular hyperkeratosis might be present in some cases. Lesions on the neck, the trunk, and the extremities have been described [76]. Early lesions of AM show mucin deposition in the outer root sheath and replacement of the entire pilosebaceous unit by pools of mucin in more advanced lesions [4,76]. Strictly speaking, AM is not a primary cicatricial alopecia because the hair follicle is not replaced by a true scar [4].

Cell atypia and monoclonal populations of T lymphocytes can be present in the idiopathic form of AM as well as in the latter form [72].

Management

Several therapeutic modalities have been reported: oral corticosteroids, minocycline, and isotretinoin have been shown to be effective. Topical and intralesional corticosteroids, low-dose intralesional interferon alpha, dapsone, indomethacin, cyclophosphamide, methotrexate, and light therapy have also been used with variable outcomes, but no drug has a consistent result and the evaluation is difficult since there may be spontaneous involution [77–80]. Treatment of the secondary form is the treatment of the associated disorder. A complete workup is necessary in all cases of AM to rule out an underlying malignancy such as mycosis fungoides and Sézary syndrome, its advanced endpoint. Annual follow-ups for the early detection of alteration signs secondary to malignancies in patients with idiopathic FM are mandatory, and should be performed at least for a period of 5 years [81].

Excision of stable lesions is a possible treatment approach. Hair transplant surgery should only be considered in patients without underlying lymphoproliferative disease or cell atypia and should be reserved for exceptional cases if an excision is not possible or alone does not supply an acceptable cosmetic result.

Keratosis follicularis spinulosa decalvans

Keratosis follicularis spinulosa decalvans (KFSD) together with keratosis atrophicans faciei (also called ulerythema oophrygenes or keratosis pilaris rubra atrophicans faciei) and atrophodermia vermiculata belong to a heterogeneous group of congenital follicular keratinizing disorders. KFSD is X-linked and usually develops during adolescence and mostly presents with scarring alopecic patches, follicular hyperkeratosis, and rarely pustules [4]. Eyebrow and eyelash involvement can also be present [82–84].

KFSD shows an inflammatory infiltrate consisting of lymphocytes and neutrophils in the infundibular area in early lesions. Later, the infiltrate is predominantly lymphocytic and the follicle is eventually replaced by fibrous tissue (Figure 6.15).

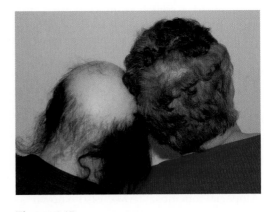

Figure 6.15
Keratosis follicularis spinulosa decalvans: mother with moderate patch of scarring alopecia on the vertex, daughter with extensive scarring alopecia.

The condition might improve with age. Careful calculation of risks and benefits in the treatment of children, teenagers, and young adults is important. Topical and intralesional corticosteroids as well as oral retinoids have shown some effectiveness [85]. Hair restoration surgery can be considered in adult patients with long-standing stable disease (Figures 6.16 and 6.17).

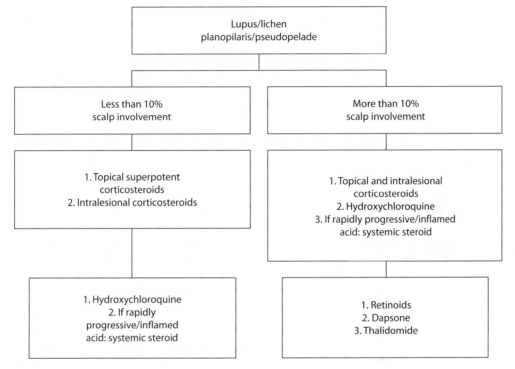

Figure 6.16
Algorithmic approach to treatment of lymphocytic-mediated scarring alopecias.

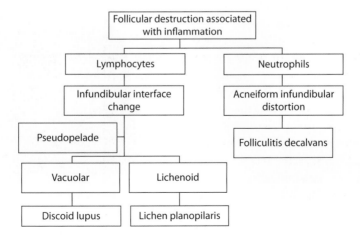

Figure 6.17
Algorithm for diagnosis of major noninfectious scarring alopecias.

Neutrophilic primary cicatricial alopecia

Folliculitis decalvans

Folliculitis decalvans (FD) predominantly occurs in young and middle-aged adults with a slight preference for the male gender. FD seems to occur more frequently in African Americans compared to Caucasians [5,29]. Approximately 11% of all primary cicatricial alopecia cases are diagnosed with FD [5,29].

A bacterial infection involving *Staphylococcus aureus* (*S. aureus*) in combination with hypersensitivity reaction to "superantigens" and a defect in host cell–mediated immunity have all been suspected as possible pathogenetic factors [5,86,87]. *S. aureus* can be cultured from the scalp skin of most patients with FD. The occurrence of FD in identical twins suggests a possible genetic component in this disease [88]. Scalp trauma and surgery has also been assumed as an etiological factor in the development in FD [89].

Clinical features

FD frequently starts at the vertex area of the scalp. The primary lesions are painful or pruritic and present with erythematous alopecic patches, follicular pustules, and follicular hyperkeratosis [86,90,91]. Patients frequently complain about pain, itching dysaesthesia, and/or burning sensations of the entire scalp. With progression, more pustules, papules, crusts, and nodules can be seen. The inflammatory process is followed by the formation of one or more round to irregular patches of scarring alopecia. The patches look like ivory pseudopelade skin centrally with surrounding follicular pustules, crusts, and flaking [12,92]. For severe cases, multiple site involvement as well as coalescence of lesions may be a presenting sign. Although the inflammatory severity fluctuates, the disease course is prolonged and progressive [93].

Tufted folliculitis is typically found in FD but can also occur in other cicatricial inflammatory alopecias. Tufted folliculitis is characterized by multiple hairs (5–15) emerging from one single dilated follicular orifice. In older lesions pustules might be absent but progressive scarring may still continue. An overlap with acne keloidalis is possible since some patients with acne keloidalis not only develop cicatricial lesions on the nape of the neck but also develop progressive cicatricial alopecia that resembles FD in other areas of the scalp (Figure 6.18).

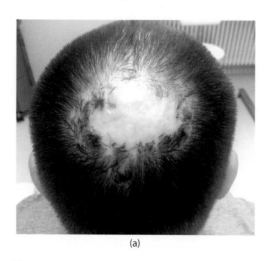

(a)

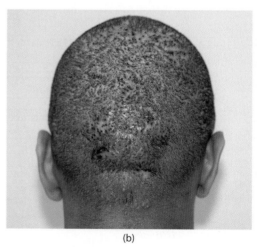

(b)

Figure 6.18

(a, b) Folliculitis decalvans with extensive tufted folliculitis in two young men.

(Continued)

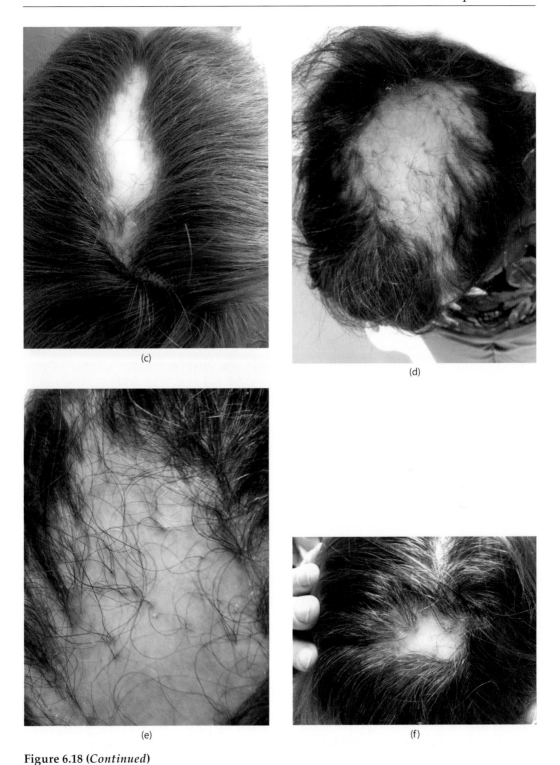

Figure 6.18 (*Continued*)
(c) A 29-year-old male patient with folliculitis decalvans (FD) on the crown; (d) a 49-year-old female patient with extensive FD; (e) close-up illustration of lack of ostia, erythema, and scaling; (f) a 55-year-old female patient with one patch of FD on the vertex.

Histology

Early lesions are characterized by keratin aggregation in the infundibulum with numerous neutrophils, as well as an intrafollicular and perifollicular neutrophilic infiltrate [4–6]. Sebaceous glands are destroyed early. In advanced lesions, the infiltrate may consist of neutrophils, lymphocytes, and plasma cells and extend into the dermis [6,10]. Hair shaft granulomas with foreign body giant cells can frequently be found [5,6]. In end-stage lesions, follicular and interstitial dermal fibrosis as well as hypertrophic scarring can be observed [6] (Figures 6.19 and 6.20).

Management

Bacterial cultures with the testing of antibiotic sensitivities are recommended [94]. Eradication of *S. aureus* with minocycline, erythromycin, cephalosporines, and sulfamethoxazole-trimethoprim has shown some effectiveness. Relapse can often be observed after the antibiotics are discontinued [11,86,95]. If so, the patient might have to stay on low dose antibiotics for many years. Rifampin in combination with clindamycin has shown good response; however, this combination shows a higher incidence of side effects [86,96]. Oral fucidic acid alone or in combination with other agents as well as a systemic therapy with adalimumab has also shown to be effective in some patients [97,98].

Oral therapy should be combined with topical antibiotics such as mupirocin, 1.5% fusidic acid, and 2% erythromycin [96,97] and antibacterial cleansers. Topical tacrolimus has also shown some effectiveness [99]. Intralesional triamcinolone acetonide at a concentration of 10 mg/cc every 4–6 weeks might help to reduce the inflammation and reduces symptoms such as itching, burning, and pain [11,29]. Intranasal eradication of *S. aureus* with topical antibacterial agents has been described to be useful [6].

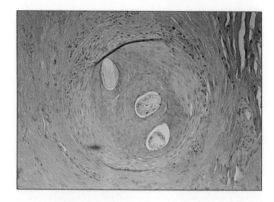

Figure 6.19
Numerous hairs exiting from one infundibulum which clinically appears as polytrichia or tufted folliculitis. (Courtesy of Dr. Magdalena Martinka.)

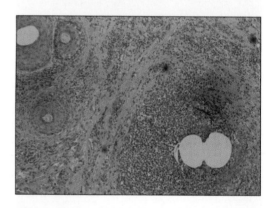

Figure 6.20
Neutrophilic infiltrate in folliculitis decalvans. (Courtesy of Dr. Magdalena Martinka.)

Treatment of FD in general is difficult and disease activity can be noted over many years. Both flare-ups of the condition as well as initial manifestations of FD have occurred after scalp and hair restoration surgery. Therefore, hair transplant surgery should only be considered for exceptional cases in which the patient did not show any signs of inflammation for several years without any treatment. The risk of reactivation after surgery might be much higher in FD compared to other inflammatory cicatricial alopecias (Figure 6.21).

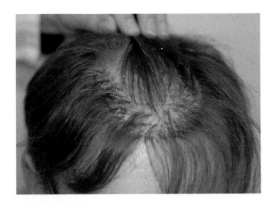

Figure 6.21
This patient developed folliculitis decalvans 20 years after hair restoration surgery with punch graft technique; the disease was restricted to the transplanted punches.

Dissecting folliculitis

Dissecting folliculitis (DF) (or dissecting cellulites or perifolliculitis capitis abscedens et suffodiens of Hoffman) is related to acne conglobata and hidradenitis suppurativa. These three diseases have been described as the follicular occlusion triad. DF predominantly occurs in young men between 18 and 40 years of age [10]. African American men seem to be more commonly affected compared to Caucasian men. The pathogenesis of DF may include follicular occlusion, seborrhea, androgens, and secondary bacterial overpopulation, as well as an abnormal host response to bacterial antigens [100–107].

Clinical features

DF typically presents with fluctuating nodules, abscesses, and sinuses, which frequently show spontaneous discharge of pus, as well as with erythematous, follicular papules, and pustules. Initial lesions are mostly found on the vertex and occipital scalp. Multifocal lesions can form an intercommunicating ridge and

seropurulent exudates can be discharged when pressure is applied to one region of the scalp. The lesions can be pruritic and tender. Chronic and relapsing courses may result in cicatricial alopecia, which can occur as hypertrophic or keloidal scars [107] (Figure 6.22).

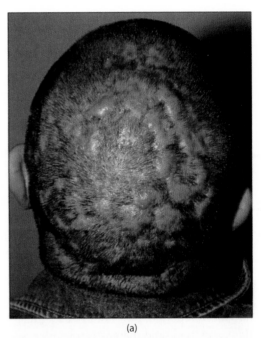

(a)

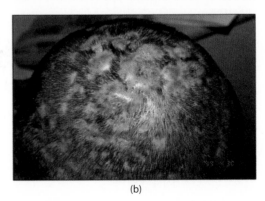

(b)

Figure 6.22
(a) Dissecting cellulitis of the scalp with characteristic boggy cysts; (b) close-up of boggy cysts.

Histology

A deep intrafollicular and perifollicular neutrophilic infiltrate with follicular occlusion are typical features of early lesions [4]. In more advanced stages, interconnecting sinus tracts lined by squamous epithelium, follicular perforation, perifollicular, and deep dermal abscesses are typical findings [4,6,23].

Management

Isotretinoin at a dose of 0.5–1 mg/kg/day has shown prolonged remission and should be considered as a first-line treatment in patients with more than one lesion [108,109]. Multimodal treatment has been reported with successful results, such as systemic antibiotics (minocycline, tetracycline, cloxacillin, erythromycin, cephalosporin, or clindamycin), intralesional corticosteroids, and oral prednisolone [110,111]. The benefits of systemic antibiotics are most likely due to their anti-inflammatory effects rather than to their antibacterial action. Incision and drainage of therapy resistant, painful nodules, marsupialization with curettage of the cyst wall, and complete scalp extirpation with skin grafting have been reported, but should be an exception for extreme and therapy refractory cases [109,112].

Scalp reduction can be considered for smaller burnt-out areas. Hair restoration surgery might be especially difficult because of hypertrophic or keloidal scar tissue. A small test area can help to estimate graft survival.

Mixed primary cicatricial alopecias

Acne keloidalis nuchae

Acne keloidalis nuchae (AKN) predominantly occurs in young men aged from 14 to 25. This idiopathic primary cicatricial alopecia might be triggered by trauma (shirt collars) or infection (demodex or bacteria). Clinically, AKN presents with skin-colored follicular papules, pustules, and plaques as well as keloid-like scarred lesions in the occipital scalp (Figure 6.23a and b). Histologically, acne keloidalis is characterized by an acute inflammation with neutrophilic or lymphocytic infiltration and chronic granulomatous inflammation around the isthmus and the lower infundibulum.

Treatment is usually difficult and protracted. Monthly intralesional triamcinolone acetonide (10–40 mg/mL) alone or combined with topical 2% clindamycin or oral (tetracyclines) antibiotics is the treatment of first choice [5,12,21,113,114]. Class I or II topical steroids alone or in combination with topical antibiotics for mild cases of AKN as well as cryotherapy and laser therapy have shown some success. Surgical excision of extensive keloidal lesions may be considered but should be reserved for therapy refractory, extensive, and symptomatic cases. Hair transplantation is not recommended for AKN because any surgical procedure on the scalp may aggravate the disease and low graft survival can be expected when transplanting into hypertrophic scars. However, excision of the affected area may be an option in some cases.

Acne necrotica (varioliformis)

Acne necrotica varioliformis is a very rare, chronic condition that predominantly occurs in adults. Frontal and parietal scalp, as well as seborrheic areas of the face, are most commonly affected. Acne necrotica presents with umbilicated, pruritic, or painful papules that undergo central necrosis. The condition leaves varioliform or smallpox-like scars [115,116]. Histology shows a suppurative, necrotic, infundibular folliculitis with lymphocytic or mixed inflammatory infiltrate [116].

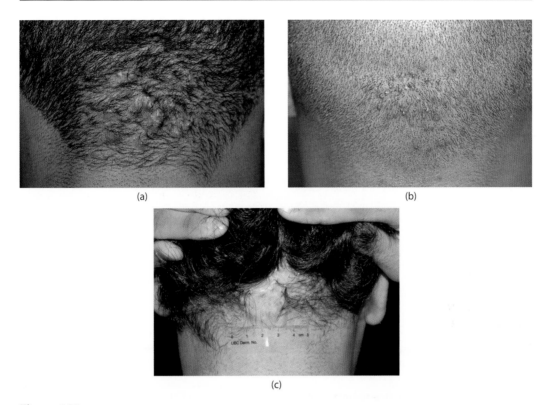

Figure 6.23
(a) Patient with moderate, (b) mild, and (c) more severe acne keloidalis nuchae.

Oral antibiotics, isotretinoin, intralesional, or topical corticosteroids have shown success [117]. Excision of larger scarred areas can be considered. Hair transplantation is not recommended.

Erosive pustular dermatosis

Erosive pustular dermatosis is an uncommon disorder predominantly occurring in elderly women [118,119]. The characteristic lesion is a suppurative, necrotic, erosive papule, or plaque [118,120]. Histology of early lesions is nonspecific, but older lesions show an extensive, chronic mixed inflammatory infiltrate in the dermis as well as dermal fibrosis. Treatment includes class I or II topical steroids with or without topical antibiotics, systemic antibiotics, and oral isotretinoin [118,120]. Hair restoration surgery can be considered for burnt-out lesions.

Differential diagnosis

Scalp psoriasis has the presence of follicular ostia and the lack of follicular plugging and atrophy. However, there are reported cases of scarring alopecia in severe scalp psoriasis [121]. Inflammatory changes in the infundibular area of the follicle in psoriasis may disrupt follicular stem cells and result in scarring alopecia. Tinea capitis can be scarring, but again there is no follicular plugging or atrophy. A potassium hydroxide (KOH) preparation and/or culture will help confirm the diagnosis. Keratoacanthomas and squamous cell carcinomas can mimic hypertrophic lupus erythematosus.

The lymphocytic scarring alopecias can certainly be difficult to tell apart from each other (Figure 6.24). Early CCLE and LLP can look quite similar. In addition, the coexistence of LPP and CCLE has been reported [122].

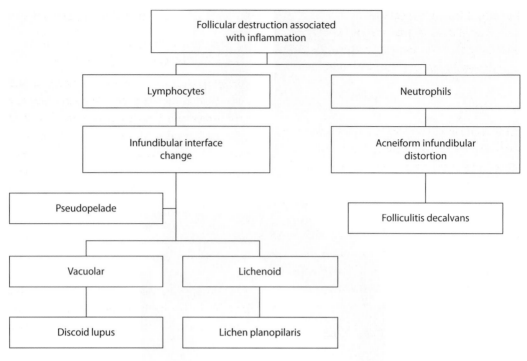

Figure 6.24
Algorithm for pathological assessment of major noninfectious scarring alopecias.

Trichotillomania can mimic different types of alopecia. It can be mistaken for a primary cicatricial alopecia, especially if the condition is long-standing and accompanied by secondary scarring.

A thorough detailed history and clinical examination helps to identify the underlying cause. A scalp biopsy may be necessary to confirm the diagnosis.

Secondary cicatricial alopecias

Secondary cicatricial alopecias are caused by any inflammation or event that results in a scar. The hair follicle is not the primary target of the process, but will be subsequently destroyed together with the interfollicular skin. Various conditions can lead to secondary cicatricial alopecia: (1) genodermatoses and developmental defects with permanent alopecia, (2) physical and chemical injury, (3) infections, (4) inflammatory dermatoses, or (5) tumors.

Developmental defects

Aplasia cutis congenita

Aplasia cutis congenita (ACC) is a localized congenital absence of epidermis and dermis, often including the subcutis. The lesions can involve any location, but most common are scalp defects (60%–85% of cases). In 70% of cases, ACC presents as a single lesion. The skull bone is affected in 20%–30%. Larger, irregular lesions may also involve the dura and leptomeninges. Dilated scalp veins may also be present. Associated ectodermal dysplasias and malformations can be present and should be ruled out. Surgical treatment can be very difficult, especially if dural and lep-tomenigeal defects are present. A scalp x-ray and magnetic resonance imaging (MRI) is mandatory before any surgical intervention.

Cleft lip

Although cleft lip repair has seen revolution-ary changes and subtle technical refinements in the past centuries, every type of surgical reconstruction leaves a scar in the mous-tache area [123]. Moustache reconstruction in patients with a cleft lip with transplantation of micrografts can be a very rewarding pro-cedure to cover the scar, especially in men where a moustache is culturally and socially highly desirable [124] (Figure 6.25).

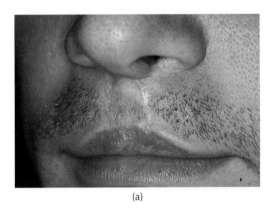
(a)

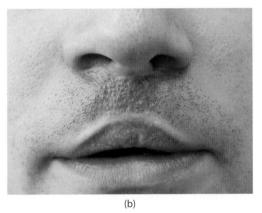
(b)

Figure 6.25
(a) A 24-year-old man with cleft lip; (b) after transplantation of 105 follicular unit grafts. (Courtesy of David Zloty.)

Physical and chemical injury

Mechanical trauma, burns, radiation, chemical injury, and surgical scars

Iatrogenic cicatricial alopecia is usually caused by radiation or surgery. Radiation therapy with x-rays and ionizing rays is used to treat intracranial and skull tumors as well as scalp neoplasms. Depending on the administered dose, chronic radiation dermatitis with per-manent alopecia can develop. Oftentimes, hair follicles are not completely lost but the hair appears finer and sparser. Depending on field size, the areas can be circumscribed or even mimic pattern hair loss (Figure 6.26). Any kind of scalp surgery leaves a scar. Scars from cos-metic surgery such as facelifts (rhytidoplasty), may be visible in the frontal hairline or may lead to a partial or complete loss of sideburns in men (Figure 6.27).

Prolonged traction may lead to transient or, if continued over time, follicular atrophy, resulting in permanent alopecia. Chronic trac-tion can be caused by tight ponytails, braids, heavy dreadlocks, or extensive use of rollers. Due to ethnic differences in hair fragility and cultural differences in hair styling practices, marginal traction alopecia is more commonly seen in women of color due to hair braiding and weaving procedures [125]. Patchy traction

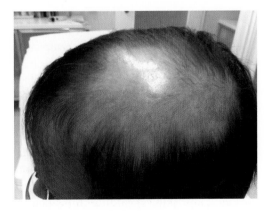

Figure 6.26
A 52-year-old female patient after radiation of a bone metastasis in the skull.

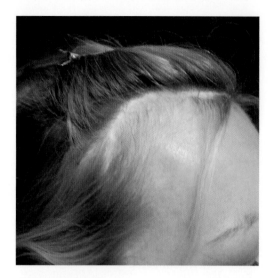

Figure 6.27
A 39-year-old female patient after brow lift.

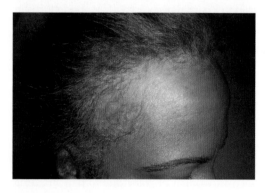

Figure 6.28
A 34-year-old female patient with traction alopecia secondary to tight pony tails.

alopecia in the frontal hairline or temples is commonly seen in Sikh boys, whose hair is usually tied up in a "topknot" [126]. The patient has to be advised to discontinue the injuring hairstyles (Figure 6.28).

Besides prolonged traction, the most common form of mechanically induced cicatricial alopecia results from scalp injuries, such as accidents with pulling of hair and trauma to the scalp skin, including third-degree burns and chemical injury. Burn injuries often involve eyebrows and eyelashes as well as other body parts. Burn injuries are often extremely disfiguring and hair restoration of the entire burned areas may not be possible because of insufficient donor supply. However, partial reconstruction, for example of the hairline and eyebrows, can be very rewarding.

Chemical injuries can be caused by acids, alkalis, and metallic salts and may lead to irreversible scalp damage, depending on their concentration and the duration of exposure. Once scarred areas have developed, they are usually well demarcated and irregular in shape. Cicatricial alopecia can also be caused by birth traumas or postoperative pressure-induced alopecia. The latter usually presents as an oval hairless patch on the occipital scalp.

Trichotillomania (Greek: *tricho* = hair, *tillo* = pull, *mania* = excessive excitement) is a form of traumatic alopecia caused by an irresistible compulsion to pull out, twist, or break off one's own hair. Trichotillomania is relatively common with an estimated incidence of 1 million Americans [127]. Infantile or early onset trichotillomania is typically of short duration and may resolve spontaneously or with simple interventions [128,129]. Trichotillomania that starts around or after puberty shows a more chronic course and is usually a sign of a more severe underlying psychopathology. It is classified as an impulse control disorder [130–132]. Women are far more often affected than men.

The clinical presentation is usually quite distinctive with a single or multiple asymmetrical, occasionally geometrically shaped areas of hair loss on the scalp or other areas of the body. The areas are not smoothly devoid of hairs, as seen in alopecia areata, but display short or bristly anagen hair. Telogen hair in the involved area is usually plugged out easily; anagen hair may be plucked out, twisted, and broken at various lengths. If the diagnosis is in doubt, a scalp biopsy should be performed. The histology usually shows a characteristic increase in catagen hair, trichomalacia, and pigment casts within the follicular canal secondary to traumatic hair removal. Most important in the therapy of trichotillomania is the education of patient and/or parents and in late onset trichotillomania the treatment of the underlying psychopathology with the help of a psychiatrist or psychologist. It is sometime helpful for the patient to wear a tied-in hairpiece or wig.

Infectious and inflammatory disorders

Fungal infection

Infections of the scalp, especially fungal infections, can be highly inflammatory and therefore may lead to cicatricial alopecia. Favus is a specific type of tinea capitis characterized by patelliform scales (scutula), which are sulfuric-yellow concretions of hyphae and skin debris in the follicular orifices and exhibit a distinct malodorant smell. A kerion is a deep, highly inflammatory fungal infection of the scalp. It presents as a highly suppurative, boggy, nodular, deep folliculitis with fistulas and pus secretion. To establish a diagnosis, hair shafts should be plugged out and cultured, as well as examined after KOH preparation. Favus and kerion may lead to scarring hair loss and should therefore be treated aggressively [133–136]. *Microsporum canis* can be diagnosed with the help of Wood's lamp examination and shows green fluorescence (Figure 6.29).

Morphea, lichen sclerosus et atrophicus, cicatricial pemphigoid

Morphea, lichen sclerosus et atrophicus, and cicatricial pemphigoid are considered autoimmune diseases of the skin. Atrophic patches can occur on any body site. Scalp involvement of these inflammatory skin disorders leads to cicatricial alopecia.

Morphea is a localized form of scleroderma. A linear form of morphea affecting the frontal scalp has been termed linear scleroderma en coup de sabre (Figure 6.30). Ocular and neurological abnormalities can

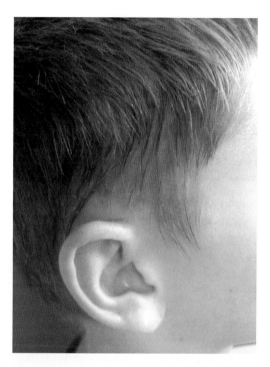

Figure 6.29
A 7-year-old boy with tinea capitis caused by *Microsporum canis*; the hair slowly regrew after successful treatment.

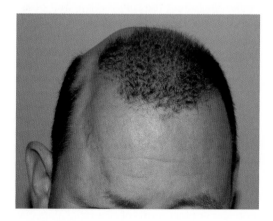

Figure 6.30
Patient with severe linear morphea.

be associated. Linear scleroderma represents the most common cause of cicatricial alopecia in early childhood. It may also be a milder presentation of the rare hemifacial atrophy (Parry–Romberg syndrome), and overlaps have been observed. In this condition,

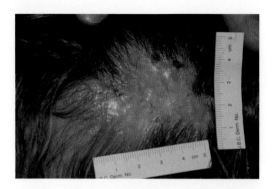

Figure 6.31
Large basal cell carcinoma of the scalp.

subcutaneous fat, muscle, and bone can be affected and the skin is only secondarily affected without prominent sclerosis.

Lichen sclerosus et atrophicus is a chronic inflammatory dermatosis that results in white plaques with epidermal atrophy. In rare cases, it presents with bullae, erosions, and scarring, including scarring alopecia [137,138].

Cicatricial pemphigoid refers to a group of rare chronic autoimmune blistering diseases that predominantly affects the mucous membranes, including the conjunctiva, and occasionally the skin. Patients with cutaneous involvement present with tense blisters and erosions, often on the head and the neck or at sites of trauma [139,140].

Neoplastic

Various tumors can affect the scalp, either primarily or as metastases. It is important to keep in mind that some sclerosing tumors, especially basal cell carcinoma, may mimic a common scar or other forms of cicatricial alopecia. A scalp biopsy is mandatory (Figure 6.31).

Hair restoration surgery in scarring alopecia

General rules apply to hair restoration surgery in scarring alopecia. Scalp biopsies are important to make a definitive diagnosis and

should show absolutely no disease activity before hair restoration surgery is considered. There should be careful preoperative evaluation of scalp thickness and blood supply. A test procedure in a small area (1.5–2 cm^2) to assess potential graft survival 8–12 months before a bigger session should be performed. Hair transplantation can be combined with scalp reduction, sometimes with the use of expanders.

In the first procedure, hairs should be placed at lower densities (10–20 FU/cm^2). More hairs can be added in subsequent sessions with longer intervals (8–12 months minimum). The use of epinephrine should be minimized, because it might decrease the already-limited blood supply and therefore graft survival. Some surgeons even use 2%–5% topical minoxidil solution 1 week preoperatively or pentoxyphylline 400 mg t.i.d. for 2 weeks before surgery to increase blood supply and tissue oxygenation [141]. Pretreatment with carbon dioxide laser has been used to induce blood vessel formation and to achieve a better graft survival [142]. Although some authors recommend larger grafts, others state that small follicular unit grafts have the highest chance of survival. Patients with cicatricial alopecia usually accept less than full growth and are very grateful for any cosmetic improvement.

In secondary cicatricial alopecias, permanent hair loss is caused by various other scalp conditions not related to the hair follicle. In these conditions, the primary event develops outside the follicular unit, which leads to incidental destruction of the follicle. Permanent, chronic traction alopecia and scars from surgery can be considered secondary scarring alopecias as well.

Once the initiating cause of secondary cicatricial alopecia is stopped, hair restoration surgery becomes a treatment option. Small areas may be excised or micrografting can be performed. For larger areas, full thickness scalp rotation flaps and/or split-thickness skin grafts are surgical options [143]. The latter can be followed by hair transplantation, although graft survival in split-grafted skin may be limited. Even partial reconstruction, for example of the hairline and eyebrows, can be very rewarding in patients with extensive secondary cicatricial alopecia. Development of nonmelanoma skin cancer in burn and radiation scars has been reported; therefore, a thorough follow up of the areas is mandatory.

References

1. Cotsarelis G, Sun TT, and Lavker RM, Label-retaining cells reside in the bulge area of pilosebaceous unit: Implications for follicular stem cells, hair cycle, and skin carcinogenesis. *Cell*, 1990. **61**(7): 1329–37.

2. Taylor G et al, Involvement of follicular stem cells in forming not only the follicle but also the epidermis. *Cell*, 2000. **102**(4): 451–61.

3. Stenn KS, Sundberg JP, and Sperling LC, Hair follicle biology, the sebaceous gland, and scarring alopecias. *Arch Dermatol*, 1999. **135**(8): 973–4.

4. Sellheyer K and Bergfeld WF, Histopathologic evaluation of alopecias. *Am J Dermatopathol*, 2006. **28**(3): 236–59.

5. Whiting DA, Cicatricial alopecia: Clinico-pathological findings and treatment. *Clin Dermatol*, 2001. **19**(2): 211–5.

6. Headington JT, Cicatricial alopecia. *Dermatol Clin*, 1996. **14**(4): 773–82.

7. Kossard S, Diffuse alopecia with stem cell folliculitis: Chronic diffuse alopecia areata or a distinct entity? *Am J Dermatopathol*, 1999. **21**(1): 46–50.

8. Newton RC et al., Scarring alopecia. *Dermatol Clin*, 1987. **5**(3): 603–18.

9. Olsen EA et al., Summary of North American Hair Research Society (NAHRS)-sponsored workshop on cicatricial alopecia, Duke University Medical Center, February 10 and 11, 2001. *J Am Acad Dermatol*, 2003. **48**(1): 103–10.

10. Ross EK, Tan E, and Shapiro J, Update on primary cicatricial alopecias. *J Am Acad Dermatol*, 2005. **53**(3): 1–37.

11. Shapiro J, *Hair Loss: Principles of Diagnosis and Management of Alopecia*. Vol. 1. 2002. London: Martin Dunitz. p. 155–74.

12. Olsen EA, Cicatricial alopecia. In *Disorders of Hair Growth: Diagnosis and Treatment*, Bergfeld WF, Editor. 2003. New York: McGraw-Hill. p. 363–98.

13. Callen JP, Chronic cutaneous lupus erythematosus. Clinical, laboratory, therapeutic, and prognostic examination of 62 patients. *Arch Dermatol*, 1982. **118**(6): 412–6.

14. Wilson CL et al., Scarring alopecia in discoid lupus erythematosus. *Br J Dermatol*, 1992. **126**(4): 307–14.

15. George PM and Tunnessen WW Jr, Childhood discoid lupus erythematosus. *Arch Dermatol*, 1993. **129**(5): 613–7.

16. Moises-Alfaro C et al., Discoid lupus erythematosus in children: Clinical, histopathologic, and follow-up features in 27 cases. *Pediatr Dermatol*, 2003. **20**(2): 103–7.

17. Meyers DC, Woosley JT, and Reddick RL, Verruciform xanthoma in association with discoid lupus erythematosus. *J Cutan Pathol*, 1992. **19**(2): 156–8.

18. Garrett AB, Multiple squamous cell carcinomas in lesions of discoid lupus erythematosus. *Cutis*, 1985. **36**(4): 313–4.

19. Sulica VI and Kao GF, Squamous-cell carcinoma of the scalp arising in lesions of discoid lupus erythematosus. *Am J Dermatopathol*, 1988. **10**(2): 137–41.

20. Kossard S, Lymphocytic mediated alopecia: Histological classification by pattern analysis. *Clin Dermatol*, 2001. **19**(2): 201–10.

21. Sperling LC, Solomon AR, and Whiting DA, A new look at scarring alopecia. *Arch Dermatol*, 2000. **136**(2): 235–42.

22. Solomon AR, The transversely sectioned scalp biopsy specimen: The technique and an algorithm for its use in the diagnosis of alopecia. *Adv Dermatol*, 1994. **9**: 127–57.

23. Templeton SF and Solomon AR, Scarring alopecia: A classification based on microscopic criteria. *J Cutan Pathol*, 1994. **21**(2): 97–109.

24. Marmor M et al., Revised recommendations on screening for chloroquine and hydroxychloroquine retinopathy. *Ophthalmology*, 2011. **118**(2): 415–22.

25. Ruzicka T et al., Treatment of cutaneous lupus erythematosus with acitretin and hydroxychloroquine. *Br J Dermatol*, 1992. **127**(5): 513–8.

26. Newton RC et al., Mechanism-oriented assessment of isotretinoin in chronic or subacute cutaneous lupus erythematosus. *Arch Dermatol*, 1986. **122**(2): 170–6.

27. Pringle J, Lichen pilaris spinulosus. *Br J Dermatol*, 1905. **17**: 77–102.

28. Eisen D, The evaluation of cutaneous, genital, scalp, nail, esophageal, and ocular involvement in patients with oral lichen planus. *Oral Surg Oral Med Oral Pathol Oral Radiol Endod*, 1999. **88**(4): 431–6.

29. Tan E et al., Primary cicatricial alopecias: Clinicopathology of 112 cases. *J Am Acad Dermatol*, 2004. **50**(1): 25–32.

30. Chieregato C et al., Lichen planopilaris: Report of 30 cases and review of the literature. *Int J Dermatol*, 2003. **74**(6): 784–6.

31. Feldmann R, Harms M, and Saurat JH, Postmenopausal frontal fibrosing alopecia. *Hautarzt*, 1996. **47**(7): 533–6.

32. Kossard S, Postmenopausal frontal fibrosing alopecia. Scarring alopecia in a pattern distribution. *Arch Dermatol*, 1994. **130**(6): 770–4.

33. Kossard S, Lee MS, and Wilkinson B, Postmenopausal frontal fibrosing alopecia: A frontal variant of lichen planopilaris. *J Am Acad Dermatol*, 1997. **36**(1): 59–66.

34. Meinhard J et al., Lichen planopilaris: Epidemiology and prevalence of subtypes – a retrospective analysis in 104 patients. *J Dtsch Dermatol Ges*, 2014. **12**(3): 229–36.

35. Chew AL et al., Expanding the spectrum of frontal fibrosing alopecia: A unifying concept. *J Am Acad Dermatol*, 2010. **63**(4): 653–60.

36. Ladizinski B et al., Frontal fibrosing alopecia: A retrospective review of 19 patients seen at Duke University. *J Am Acad Dermatol*, 2013. **68**: 749–55.

37. MacDonald A, Clark C, and Holmes S, Frontal fibrosing alopecia: A review of 60 cases. *J Am Acad Dermatol*, 2012. **67**: 955–61.

38. Vañó-Galván S et al., Frontal fibrosing alopecia: A multicenter review of 355 patients. *J Am Acad Dermatol*, 2014. **70**(4): 670–8.

39. Dlova NC and Goh CL, Frontal fibrosing alopecia in an African man. *Int J Dermatol*, 2013. Aug 22. doi: 10.1111/j.1365-4632.2012.05821.

40. Nusbaum BP and Nusbaum AG, Frontal fibrosing alopecia in a man: Results of follicular unit test grafting. *Dermatol Surg*, 2010. **36**: 959–62.

41. Ramaswamy P, Mendese G, and Goldberg LJ, Scarring alopecia of the sideburns: A unique presentation of frontal fibrosing alopecia in men. *Arch Dermatol*, 2012. **148**: 1095–6.

42. Stockmeier M et al., Kossard frontal fibrosing alopecia in a man. *Hautarzt*, 2002. **53**: 409–11.

43. Khan S, Fenton DA, and Stefanato CM, Frontal fibrosing alopecia and lupus overlap in a man: Guilt by association? *Int J Trichology*, 2013. **5**(4): 217–9.

44. Phillips WG et al., Captopril-induced lichenoid eruption. *Clin Exp Dermatol*, 1994. **19**(3): 17–20.

45. Katta R, Lichen planus. *Am Fam Physician*, 2000. **61**(11): 3319–24, 3327–8.

46. Gimenez-Garcia R and Perez-Castrillon JL, Lichen planus and hepatitis C virus infection. *J Eur Acad Dermatol Venereol*, 2003. **17**(3): 291–5.

47. Donovan J, Lichen planopilaris after hair transplantation: Report of 17 cases. *Dermatol Surg*, 2012. **38**(12): 1998–2004.

48. Montpellier RA and Donovan JC, Scalp trauma: A risk factor for lichen planopilaris? *J Cutan Med Surg*, 2014. **18**(3): 214–6.

49. Perrin AJ and Donovan JC, Lichen planopilaris following whole brain irradiation. *Int J Dermatol*, 2014. Jun 5. doi: 10.1111/ijd.12576.

50. Miteva M et al., Frontal fibrosing alopecia occurring on scalp vitiligo: Report of four cases. *Br J Dermatol*, 2011. **165**: 445–7.

51. Kang H et al., Lichen planopilaris. *Dermatol Ther*, 2008. **21**(4): 249–56.

52. Otberg N et al., Diagnosis and management of primary cicatricial alopecia: Part I. *Skinmed*, 2008. **7**(1): 19–26.

53. Pai VV et al., Graham-Little–Piccardi–Lassueur syndrome: An unusual variant of follicular lichen planus. *Int J Trichology*, 2011. **3**(1): 28–30.

54. Elston DM et al., Elastic tissue in scars and alopecia. *J Cutan Pathol*, 2000. **27**(3): 147–52.

55. Mehregan DA, Van Hale HM, and Muller SA, Lichen planopilaris: Clinical and pathologic study of forty-five patients. *J Am Acad Dermatol*, 1992. **27**(6): 935–42.

56. Ott F, Bollag W, and Geiger JM, Efficacy of oral low-dose tretinoin (all-trans-retinoic acid) in lichen planus. *Dermatology*, 1997. **192**(4): 334–6.

57. Mirmirani P, Willey A, and Price VH, Short course of oral cyclosporine in lichen planopilaris. *J Am Acad Dermatol*, 2003. **49**(4): 667–71.

58. Massa MC and Rogers RS 3rd, Griseofulvin therapy of lichen planus. *Acta Derm Venereol*, 1981. **61**(6): 547–50.

59. Baibergenova A and Walsh S, Use of pioglitazone in patients with lichen planopilaris. *J Cutan Med Surg*, 2012. **16**(2): 97–100.

60. Cho BK et al., Efficacy and safety of mycophenolate mofetil for lichen planopilaris. *J Am Acad Dermatol*, 2010. **62**(3): 393–7.

61. Tursen U et al., Treatment of lichen planopilaris with mycophenolate mofetil. *Dermatol Online J*, 2004. **10**(1): 24.

62. Georgala S et al., Treatment of postmenopausal frontal fibrosing alopecia with oral dutasteride. *J Am Acad Dermatol*, 2009. **61**(1): 157–8.

63. Katoulis A et al., Frontal fibrosing alopecia: Treatment with oral dutasteride and topical pimecrolimus. *J Eur Acad Dermatol Venereol*, 2009. **23**(5): 580–2.

64. Tosti A et al., Frontal fibrosing alopecia in postmenopausal women. *J Am Acad Dermatol*, 2005. **52**: 55–60.

65. Ronchese F, Pseudopelade. *Arch Dermatol*, 1960. **82**: 336–43.

66. Braun-Falco O et al., Pseudopelade of Brocq. *Dermatologica*, 1986. **172**(1): 18–23.

67. Bulengo-Ransby SM and Headington JT, Pseudopelade of Brocq in a child. *J Am Acad Dermatol*, 1990. **23**(5): 944–5.

68. Olsen EA et al., Update on cicatricial alopecia. *J Investig Dermatol Symp Proc*, 2003. **8**(1): 18–19.

69. Ross EK and Shapiro J, Management of hair loss. *Dermatol Clin*, 2005. **23**(2): 227–43.

70. Sperling LC and Sau P, The follicular degeneration syndrome in black patients. "Hot comb alopecia" revisited and revised. *Arch Dermatol*, 1992. **128**(1): 68–74.

71. Callender VD, McMichael AJ, and Cohen GF, Medical and surgical therapies for alopecias in black women. *Dermatol Ther*, 2004. **17**(2): 164–76.

72. Boer A, Guo Y, and Ackerman AB, Alopecia mucinosa is mycosis fungoides. *Am J Dermatopathol*, 2004. **26**(1): 33–52.

73. Passos PC et al., Follicular mucinosis – case report. *An Bras Dermatol*, 2014. **89**(2): 337–9.

74. Ingen-Housz-Oro S et al., Folliculotropic T-cell infiltrates associated with B-cell chronic lymphocytic leukaemia or MALT lymphoma may reveal either true mycosis fungoides or pseudolymphomatous reaction: Seven cases and review of the literature. *J Eur Acad Dermatol Venereol*, 2014. Mar 19. doi: 10.1111/jdv.12454.

75. Gibson LE, Muller SA, and Peters MS, Follicular mucinosis of childhood and adolescence. *Pediatr Dermatol*, 1988. **5**(4): 231–5.

76. van Doorn R, Scheffer E, and Willemze R, Follicular mycosis fungoides, a distinct disease entity with or without associated follicular mucinosis: A clinicopathologic and follow-up study of 51 patients. *Arch Dermatol*, 2002. **138**(2): 191–8.

77. Emmerson RW, Follicular mucinosis. A study of 47 patients. *Br J Dermatol*, 1969. **81**(6): 395.

78. Kim KR et al., Successful treatment of recalcitrant primary follicular mucinosis with indomethacin and low-dose intralesional interferon alpha. *Ann Dermatol*, 2009. **21**: 285–7.

79. Parker SR and Murad E, Follicular mucinosis: Clinical, histologic, and molecular remission with minocycline. *J Am Acad Dermatol*, 2010. **62**: 139–41.

80. Schneider SW, Metze D, and Bonsmann G, Treatment of so-called idiopathic follicular mucinosis with hydroxychloroquine. *Br J Dermatol*, 2010. **163**: 420–3.

81. Brown HA et al., Primary follicular mucinosis: Long-term follow up of patients younger than 40 years with and without clonal T-cell receptor gene rearrangement. *J Am Acad Dermatol*, 2002. **47**: 856–62.

82. Aten E et al., Keratosis Follicularis Spinulosa Decalvans is caused by mutations in MBTPS2. *Hum Mutat*, 2010. **31**(10): 1125–33.

83. Castori M et al., Clinical and genetic hetero-geneity in keratosis follicularis spinulosa decalvans. *Eur J Med Genet*, 2009. **52**(1): 53–8.

84. Maheswari UG, Chaitra V, and Mohan SS, Keratosis follicularis spinulosa decalvans: A rare cause of scarring alopecia in two young Indian girls. *Int J Trichology*, 2013. **5**(1): 29–31.

85. Baden HP and Byers HR, Clinical find-ings, cutaneous pathology, and response to therapy in 21 patients with keratosis pilaris atrophicans. *Arch Dermatol*, 1994. **130**(4): 469–75.

86. Powell JJ, Dawber RP, and Gatter K, Folliculitis decalvans including tufted fol-liculitis: Clinical, histological and therapeutic findings. *Br J Dermatol*, 1999. **140**(2): 328–33.

87. Powell J and Dawber RP, Successful treat-ment regime for folliculitis decalvans despite uncertainty of all aetiological factors. *Br J Dermatol*, 2001. **144**: 428–9.

88. Douwes KE, Landthaler M, and Szeimies RM, Simultaneous occurrence of folliculitis decalvans capillitii in identical twins. *Br J Dermatol*, 2000. **143**(1): 195–7.

89. Otberg N et al., Folliculitis decalvans devel-oping 20 years after hair restoration surgery in punch grafts: Case report. *Dermatol Surg*, 2009. **35**(11): 1852–6.

90. Matard B et al., First evidence of bacterial biofilms in the anaerobe part of scalp hair fol-licles: A pilot comparative study in folliculitis decalvans. *J Eur Acad Dermatol Venereol*, 2013. **27**(7): 853–60.

91. Otberg N et al., Folliculitis decalvans. *Dermatol Ther*, 2008. **21**(4): 238–44.

92. Sullivan JR and Kossard S, Acquired scalp alopecia. Part 2: A review. *Australas J Dermatol*, 1999. **40**: 61–70.

93. Templeton SF, Santa Cruz DJ, and Solomon AR, Alopecia: Histologic diagnosis by transverse sections. *Semin Diagn Pathol*, 1996. **13**(1): 2–18.

94. Sillani C et al., Effective treatment of folliculitis decalvans using selected antimicrobial agents. *Int J Trichology*, 2010. **2**(1): 20–3.

95. Brooke RCC and Griffiths CE, Folliculitis decalvans. *Clin Exp Dermatol*, 2001. **26**(1): 20–22.

96. Brozena SJ, Cohen LE, and Fenske NA, Folliculitis decalvans: Response to rifampin. *Cutis*, 1988. **42**: 512–5.

97. Abeck D, Korting HC, and Braun-Falco O, Folliculitis decalvans. Long-lasting response to combined therapy with fusidic acid and zinc. *Acta Derm Venereol*, 1992. **72**(2): 143–5.

98. Kreutzer K and Effendy I, Therapy-resistant folliculitis decalvans and lichen planopilaris successfully treated with adalimumab. *J Dtsch Dermatol Ges*, 2014. **12**(1): 74–6.

99. Bastida J et al., Treatment of folliculitis decalvans with tacrolimus ointment. *Int J Dermatol*, 2012. **51**(2): 216–20.

100. Sivakumaran S, Meyer P, and Burrows NP, Dissecting folliculitis of the scalp with mar-ginal keratitis. *Clin Exp Dermatol*, 2001. **26**: 490–2.

101. Ramasastry SS et al., Severe perifolliculitis capitis with osteomyelitis. *Ann Plast Surg*, 1987. **18**: 241–4.

102. Ongchi DR, Fleming MG, and Harris CA, Sternocostoclavicular hyperostosis: Two cases with differing dermatologic syn-dromes. *J Rheumatol*, 1990. **17**: 1415–8.

103. Libow L and Friar DA, Arthropathy associ-ated with cystic acne, hidradenitis suppu-rativa, and perifolliculitis capitis abscedens et suffodiens: Treatment with isotretinoin. *Cutis*, 1999. **64**: 87–90.

104. Curry SS, Gaither DH, and King LEJ, Squamous cell carcinoma arising in dis-secting perifolliculitis of the scalp. A case report and review of secondary squamous cell carcinomas. *J Am Acad Dermatol*, 1981. **4**: 673–8.

105. Boyd AS and Zemtsov A, A case of pyoderma vegetans and the follicular occlusion triad. *J Dermatol*, 1992. **19**(1): 61–3.

106. Bergeron JR and Stone OJ, Follicular occlu-sion triad in a follicular blocking disease (pityriasis rubra pilaris). *Dermatologica*, 1968. **136**(5): 362–7.

107. Scheinfeld NS, A case of dissecting celluli-tis and a review of the literature. *Dermatol Online J*, 2003. **9**(1): 8.

108. Scerri L, Williams HC, and Allen BR, Dissecting cellulitis of the scalp: Response to isotretinoin. *Br J Dermatol*, 1996. **134**: 1105–8.

109. Koca R et al., Dissecting cellulitis in a white male: Response to isotretinoin. *Int J Dermatol*, 2002. **41**: 509–13.

110. Goldsmith PC and Dowd PM, Successful therapy of the follicular occlusion triad in a young woman with high dose oral antiandrogens and minocycline. *J R Soc Med*, 1993. **86**: 729–30.

111. Adrian RM and Arndt KA, Perifolliculitis capitis: Successful control with alternate-day corticosteroids. *Ann Plast Surg*, 1980.**4**: 166–9.

112. Stites PC and Boyd AS, Dissecting cellulitis in a white male: A case report and review of the literature. *Cutis*, 2001. **67**: 37–40.

113. Halder RM, Pseudofolliculitis barbae and related disorders. *Dermatol Clin*, 1988. **6**: 407–12.

114. Dinehart SM et al., Acne keloidalis: A review. *J Dermatol Surg Oncol*, 1989. **15**: 642–7.

115. Stritzler C, Friedman R, and Loveman AB, Acne necrotica; relation to acne necrotica miliaris and response to penicillin and other antibiotics. *Arch Derm Syphilol*, 1951. **64**: 464–9.

116. Kossard S, Collins A, and McCrossin I, Necrotizing lymphocytic folliculitis: The early lesion of acne necrotica (varioliformis). *J Am Acad Dermatol*, 1987. **16**: 1007–14.

117. Maibach HI, Acne necroticans (varioliformis) versus Propionibacterium acnes folliculitis. *J Am Acad Dermatol*, 1989. **21**: 323.

118. Grattan CE, Peachey RD, and Boon A, Evidence for a role of local trauma in the pathogenesis of erosive pustular dermatosis of the scalp. *Clin Exp Dermatol*, 1988. **13**: 7–10.

119. Ena P et al., Erosive pustular dermatosis of the scalp in skin grafts: Report of three cases. *Dermatology*, 1997. **194**: 80–4.

120. Pye RJ, Peachey RD, and Burton JL, Erosive pustular dermatosis of the scalp. *Br J Dermatol*, 1979. **100**: 559–66.

121. Wright AL and Messenger AG, Scarring alopecia in psoriasis. *Acta Derm Venereol*, 1990. **70**(2): 156–9.

122. Vanderhorst J, Mixed lichen planus-lupus erythematosus disease: A distinct entity: Clinical, histopathological and immunopathological studies in six patients. *Clin Exp Dermatol*, 1983. **8**: 631–40.

123. Liao YF et al., Two-stage palate repair with delayed hard palate closure is related to favorable maxillary growth in unilateral cleft lip and palate. *Plast Reconstr Surg*, 2010. **125**(5): 1503–10.

124. Reed ML and Grayson BH, Single-follicular-unit hair transplantation to correct cleft lip moustache alopecia. *Cleft Palate Craniofac J*, 2001. **38**(5): 538–40.

125. Olsen EA, Disorders of hair growth in African-Americans. In *Disorders of Hair Growth: Diagnosis and Treatment*, Wilborn WS, Editor. Vol. 1. 2003. New York: McGraw-Hill. p. 98.

126. Singh G, Traction alopecia in Sikh boys. *Br J Dermatol*, 1975. **92**: 232.

127. Olsen EA, Infectious, and physical, and inflammatory causes of hair and scalp abnormalities. In *Disorders of Hair Growth: Diagnosis and Treatment*, 2nd edition, Roberts JL and De Villez R, Editors. Vol. 1. 2003. New York: McGraw-Hill. p. 98.

128. Swedo SE and Leonard HL, Trichotillomania. An obsessive compulsive spectrum disorder? *Psychiatr Clin North Am*, 1992. **15**(4): 777–90.

129. Winchel RM et al., Clinical characteristics of trichotillomania and its response to fluoxetine. *J Clin Psychiatry*, 1992. **53**(9): 304–8.

130. Dell'Osso B et al., Epidemiologic and clinical updates on impulse control disorders: A critical review. *Eur Arch Psychiatry Clin Neurosci*, 2006. **256**(8): 464–75.

131. Rothbaum BO and Ninan PT, The assessment of trichotillomania. *Behav Res Ther*, 1994. **32**: 651.

132. Stein DJ et al., Trichotillomania and obsessive-compulsive disorder. *J Clin Psychiatry*, 1995. **56** (Suppl 4): 28–34.

133. Fiedler L et al., Surgical and ketoconazole treatment of a Kerion Celsi caused by Trichophyton mentagrophytes and Candida tropicalis. *Mycoses*, 1988. **Suppl 1**: 81–7.

134. Kron C et al., Bulky superinfected tinea capitis of the scalp. Treatment by surgical resection and reconstruction by cutaneous expansion. *Arch Pediatr*, 1998. **5**: 992–5.

135. Otberg N et al., Kerion due to Trichophyton mentagrophytes: Responsiveness to fluconazole versus terbinafine in a child. *Acta Derm Venereol*, 2001. **81**(6): 444–5.

136. Thoma-Greber E et al., Surgical treatment of tinea capitis in childhood. *Mycoses*, 2003. **46**(8): 351–4.

137. Madan V and Cox NH, Extensive bullous lichen sclerosus with scarring alopecia. *Clin Exp Dermatol*, 2009. **34**(3): 360–2.

138. Foulds IS, Lichen sclerosus et atrophicus of the scalp. *Br J Dermatol*, 1980. **103**(2): 197–200.

139. Elston GE and Harman KE, Recurrent blistering of the scalp with scarring. *Clin Exp Dermatol*, 2006. **31**(4): 605–6.

140. Liew V et al., Complex scalp defects from cicatricial pemphigoid and ionizing radiation. *Burns*, 2004. **30**(5): 495–8.

141. Rose PT, Shapiro R, Transplantation into scar tissue and areas of cicatricial alopecia. In *Hair Transplantation*, Walter RS, Unger P, Editors. Vol. 4. 2004. New York: Marcel Dekker.

142. Kwon OS et al., Staged hair transplantation in cicatricial alopecia after carbon dioxide laser-assisted scar tissue remodeling. *Arch Dermatol*, 2007. **143**(4): 457–460.

143. Schnabl SM et al., Aplasia cutis congenita—plastic reconstruction of three scalp and skull defects with two opposed scalp rotation flaps and split thickness skin grafting. *Neuropediatrics*, 2009. **40**(3): 134–6.

7   Hair restoration surgery

History of hair restoration surgery

Hair restoration surgery has come a long way in the past decades. However, the idea of transplanting hair has been around for a long time. Attempts at hair restoration are found in the earliest ancient Egyptian medical document, the Ebers Papyrus, which was written about 1500 BC [1].

In the nineteenth century, a German Professor, Dom Unger, and his student, Johann Friedrich Dieffenbach, experimented with hair grafts in animals and humans. In 1822, Dieffenbach published the results in his dissertation; he planted six of his scalp hairs on his own arm and two hairs continued to grow. As early as 1908, Tilghman suggested the rotation of scalp flaps in the treatment of alopecia [1]. In 1919, Passot described a flap technique for the treatment of scars [1]. The first study that intentionally focused on the development of a surgical procedure to treat scalp alopecia was most likely reported by Sasagawa in 1930 [2]. In 1939, Okuda, a Japanese dermatologist, described the use of cylindrical punches of hair from a donor site to correct alopecia of the scalp, eyebrows, and moustache [3]. Tamura in 1943 used single hair transplantation to the pubic area [4] and Fujita in 1953 reported single hair transplants to eyebrows in patients with leprosy and used free skin grafts with two to four hairs to correct various defects [5]. This technique was very similar to our modern follicular unit hair transplantation. Unfortunately the Japanese achievements in hair restoration were not recognized outside of Japan until Fujita published his work in English for a book published in the United States in 1976.

Hair restoration as a treatment to hide scars on the scalp was used by Barsky in 1950 with the implantation of small grafts and by Lamont in 1957 by using flap techniques [6,7]. Norman Orentreich, a dermatologist from New York, performed hair transplant surgery for male pattern baldness for the first time in 1952. His achievements were first rejected by the medical community and it took until 1959 for his paper to finally be published [8]. Orentreich created the term "donor dominance" to explain that transplanted hair continues to display the same characteristics of the hair from where it was taken; meaning that scalp hair from the back or sides of the scalp that is transplanted to a thinning area will continue to grow and will keep its original growth patterns. Orentreich performed punch graft techniques by using 4-mm-sized grafts.

Through the 1970s, all hair transplantation procedures involved the transplantation of large grafts, commonly known as plugs [9–12]. The cosmetic results were not always satisfying since it often created a doll-like appearance and cosmetically acceptable hair growth direction was difficult to create with punch grafts (Figure 7.1). Different flap techniques also became popular in the 1970s and 1980s. Jose Juri, an Argentinean surgeon, developed the Juri flap technique that uses two long flaps of hair-bearing scalp brought forward to cover the bald regions and create a new hairline [13]. Ohmori, Stough et al., Bouhanna, Nordstrom, Frechet, and others

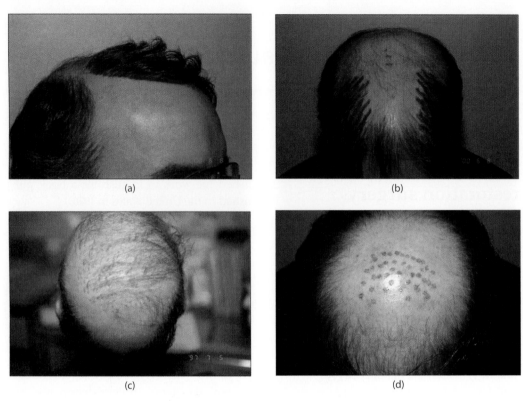

Figure 7.1

(a–c) Hair transplantation three decades ago: Note the unnatural corn-row tufting of hair surgery performed in the 1960s and 1970s. (d) This patient requested laser hair removal to remove his grafts from 30 years ago.

introduced microsurgically anastomosed free flaps in different variations [14–18]. The use of smaller punch grafts (2 mm) or small slit grafts (3 mm) cut from a strip of donor tissue became popular in the mid-1980s [19–22]. Mini grafts containing one to two hairs were first used to soften the frontal hairline to give it a more natural look [20,23]. These mini-grafting procedures gradually replaced the plug technique completely and became the main form of hair restoration surgery. Dr. Carlos Uebel of Brazil transplanted up to 1000 small grafts in one session already in 1983. This was the beginning of the so-called mega session. In the early 1990s, a typical hair transplant procedure involved around 1000 transplanted grafts and took around 12 hours of work. In 1992, the Moser group from Austria demonstrated a large transplant session using

videotapes; in 1994, Dr. William Rassmann introduced single session transplants of over 3600 grafts.

Dr. Robert Limmer started to use stereoscopic microscopes to dissect grafts and to reduce the damage done to the hair follicles in the dissection process [24]. They also identified desiccation as an important cause for graft damage and failure of transplanted hair follicles to grow. Limmer recognized that normal scalp hair naturally grows in groupings of one to four ("follicular units"). Limmer developed the methodology of follicular unit transplantation (FUT), where the donor strip of hair follicles was microdissected by a team of technicians into follicular units under magnification [24]. This was another step to improve the outcome of the mini-graft procedures and the cornerstone to modern follicular unit hair transplantation. FUT soon became the state-of-the-art hair transplant procedure [25–29].

Follicular unit transplantation

Hair transplant surgery is basically a redistribution of hair in one individual. Hair is taken from a hair-bearing area (usually on the scalp) that is not affected by the miniaturization process of androgenetic alopecia. A strip of skin, containing intact follicles, is usually removed from the occipital area and carefully dissected under magnification into small slivers and then into follicular units (FU). The follicular unit grafts have to be kept moist and cool as desiccation will cause damage and a failure to grow. The follicular units are than carefully placed under magnification into small slits or holes in the bald or balding areas. Slits are prepared according to graft size and desired growth direction. Hair restoration surgery is performed under local anesthesia. One session takes, depending on the number of grafts and technique, from a few hours up to a whole day (Figure 7.2).

Single follicular units can also be extracted with small micropunches from the occiput (follicular unit extraction [FUE]) (Figure 7.3). Harvesting follicular unit grafts by removing them directly from the donor area

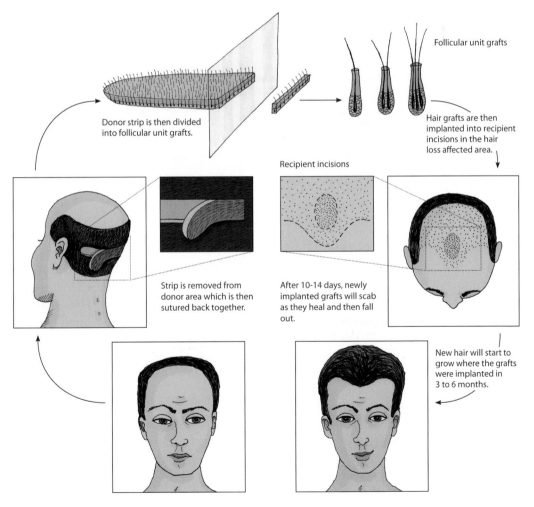

Donor strip is then divided into follicular unit grafts.

Follicular unit grafts

Hair grafts are then implanted into recipient incisions in the hair loss affected area.

Recipient incisions

Strip is removed from donor area which is then sutured back together.

After 10-14 days, newly implanted grafts will scab as they heal and then fall out.

New hair will start to grow where the grafts were implanted in 3 to 6 months.

Figure 7.2
Principle of follicular unit transplantation with strip removal.

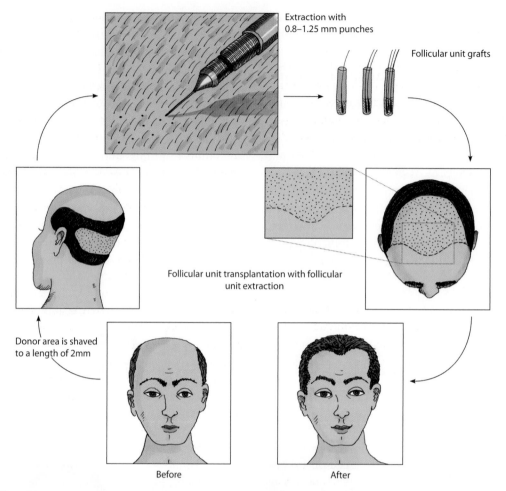

Extraction with
0.8–1.25 mm punches

Follicular unit grafts

Follicular unit transplantation with follicular
unit extraction

Donor area is shaved
to a length of 2mm

Before

After

Figure 7.3
Principle of follicular unit transplantation with follicular unit extraction.

gained popularity in the United States in 2002 with the work of Rassman et al. [30] and gained further popularity with Harris' paper in 2004 [31]. FUE is also an FUT technique since it involves the transplantation of follicular units. However, the term "FUT" is sometimes used synonymously with strip harvesting. Although the FUE technique has some limitations, it has become more and more popular in the past decade. FUE leaves small confetti-like scars, in contrast to strip harvesting, which leaves the patient with a linear scar. FUE is therefore attractive for patients who are planning to wear a very short haircut. In general, FUE sessions are

more time-consuming compared to strip harvesting. However, it is less staff-intensive and the training curve for the performing doctor and staff is much lower.

Donor harvesting

Strip harvesting

The first step is the selection of the donor area. Scalp laxity has to be checked to plan the width of the strip. For an optimal donor scar, the wound closure should be performed with no tension. Scalp laxity is usually checked manually with index and thumb or by using both hands. For a more objective way to measure the laxity of the scalp, a scalp laxometer may be a useful device. In a patient with normal scaly laxity, a strip width of 1 cm is usually safe to take. After the strip width is determined, the strip length has to be calculated according to the desired number of grafts. Therefore, donor hair density should be measured under magnification. A handheld illuminated magnifier, a trichoscope, the Rassman densitometer, or digital imaging devices are useful tools to measure the number of follicular units (FU) per square centimeter. Strip size is now determined by the following formula:

$$\text{Desired number of FUs/donor density} \ (\text{FU/cm}^2) = \text{Strip area (cm}^2) \ [32]$$

The selected donor area is now trimmed and anesthetized using the tumescent technique (Figure 7.4). The tumescent technique involves the injection of large volumes of very dilute local anesthetics and epinephrine. The injected volume helps to keep the scalpel tip away from significant nerves and vessels. The tumescence should be given around 20 minutes to work efficiently; as a result there will be almost no bleeding from smaller vessels.

A single blade (No. 10 or 15) elliptical excision is preferred for the strip removal over multibladed knives to minimize marginal transection of follicles. The incisions have to be placed parallel to the hair follicles and should be no deeper than the hair bulb in the subcutaneous fat. Once the skin has been cut, the strip has to be removed from its subcutaneous attachment. Either the scalpel or undermining scissors can be used to loosen the strip (Figure 7.5) [33]. Some surgeons like to undermine the wound edges. Undermining is usually not necessary if a safe strip width is calculated according to the scalp laxity. It may be useful when wider strips are taken or in subsequent procedures when scalp laxity is decreased.

Before closing the donor defect, 1–2 mm of the overlapping top wound edge should be trimmed off with a small sharp scissor. This is called a trichophytic wound closure. It allows one or two rows of hair to grow through the scar and helps to make the scar less visible (Figures 7.6 and 7.7). The closure can be performed as one layered or two layered. In our clinic, we prefer a two-layered wound closure with buried dissolvable 3-0 or 4-0 monocryl and superficial continuous 3-0 prolene sutures. The prolene sutures are removed after 7–14 days. In subsequent hair transplant procedures, the

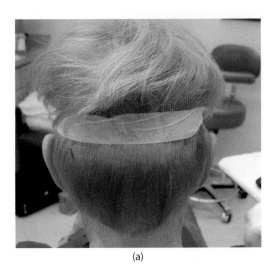

(a)

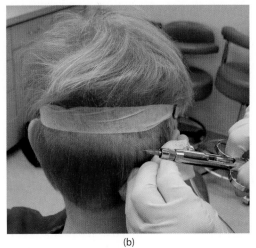

(b)

Figure 7.4
(a) Clipped donor area; (b) donor area anesthesia.

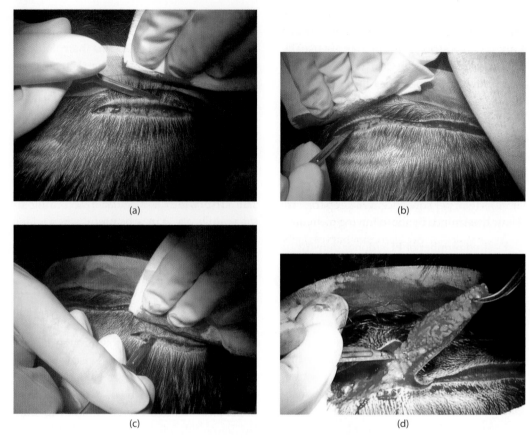

(a)

(b)

(c)

(d)

Figure 7.5
(a–c) Donor strip removal, incisions parallel to the hair follicles to the depth of the hair bulb.
(d) The strip is removed from its subcutaneous attachment with a scalpel.

old scar should always be removed, leaving the patient with only one scar. The graft's yield will be less, since the hair density is slightly decreased; the new strip will contain the old scar and the scalp laxity may only allow the doctor to take a narrower strip. Subsequent hair transplants may be considered not earlier than 6–12 months after the first session.

Almost invisible scars can be created by sessions sized up to 2000 grafts and a strip width of not more than 1 cm and a trichophytic wound closure. Larger sessions require longer strips that may extend into the temporal area and make the removal of a wider strip necessary [33].

A wound dressing of the donor site can be applied for the night after the surgery.

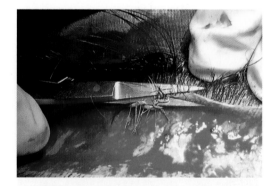

Figure 7.6
Trichophytic wound closure at the overlapping top wound edge is trimmed off with a small sharp scissor.

Wound dressing of the recipient site is not necessary. In our clinic, the patient is advised to remove the wound dressing the following day after the surgery and to wear a cotton bandana during the day time for the first 3 days and a light surgical cap during the first 3 nights after the procedure.

Follicular unit extraction

FUE became more and more popular since it was first described in 2002 [3,10,11]. Instead of removing a strip of full thickness skin from the donor area, in FUE, individual units are removed from the scalp and prepared for direct transplantation into the recipient area.

The first step of an FUE donor harvest is the shaving of the donor area to a length of around 2 mm to allow the detection of the hair growth angle. The donor area is usually fully shaved.

In patients with longer hair who wish for a less noticeable donor site but refuse strip harvesting, rows of 3–5 mm may be shaved with intersections of long hair in between the rows. The donor area is then anaesthetized with tumescence anesthesia. Nerve blocks may also be used. The anesthesia should be given at least 20 minutes to work and to minimize bleeding. The patient is then ideally placed on a comfortable massage stool or bed. To minimize transection, the physician should work with the punch device toward himself. The physician ideally should sit at the top end of the bed. FUE is performed under 2.5- to 5-fold magnification. Good lighting is very important. Use of a headlamp may be helpful in addition to overhead lighting [34] (Figures 7.8 and 7.9).

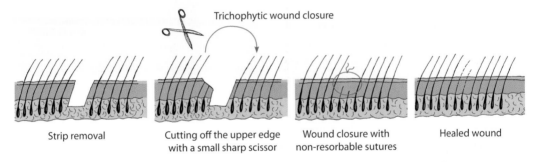

Trichophytic wound closure

Strip removal · Cutting off the upper edge with a small sharp scissor · Wound closure with non-resorbable sutures · Healed wound

Figure 7.7
Trichophytic wound closure.

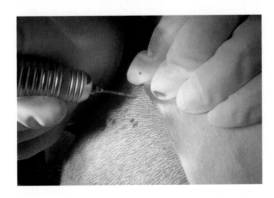

Figure 7.8
Follicular unit extraction two-step procedure with a rotation punch.

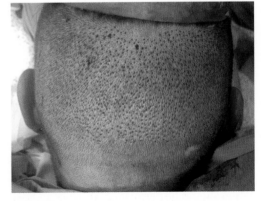

Figure 7.9
Donor area directly after follicular unit extraction.

Manual punches as well as electrical rotating punch devices are available. For bigger sessions, electrical devices are preferred since manual punches may be very hard on the physician's wrist. Usual punch sizes range from 1.2 to 0.75 mm. The punch size is chosen based on follicular unit size and density. A high density usually requires a smaller punch to minimize scalp trauma and damage to the surrounding follicles.

FUEs can be performed in a two-step or three-step procedure. The two-step procedure is less time-consuming and is most frequently used with a sharp punch and an electrical rotating punch device (Figure 7.10). The incision reaches down to the depth of the mid to lower dermis which is around 3–4 mm deep. The three-step technique utilizes a sharp punch to score the area around the FU to approximately 0.5 mm deep, followed by a blunt punch pushed in a unidirectional twisting motion to the level of the lower dermis. The three-step technique is much more time-consuming, but transection rates are usually lower [34].

The FUs are removed from the donor site with special small, curved forceps (Figure 7.11); sometimes the use of a needle helps to remove the grafts. The grafts are then kept moist and cool in normal saline or a holding solution until they are planted into the recipient site.

For wound dressing, nonstick gauze in combination with an antibacterial ointment should be used. Our patients are advised to remove the dressing on the day after the procedure and to carefully wash the donor area.

Graft preparation and handling

After strip harvesting, the strip is immediately placed in chilled saline. All graft preparation should be performed under binocular stereomicroscopes with approximately 4- to 10-fold magnification to avoid unnecessary transection (Figure 7.12). The skin is then

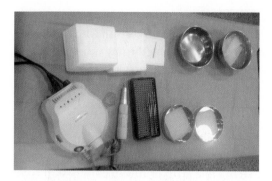

Figure 7.10
Operating table for follicular unit extraction with a rotation punch (two-step procedure).

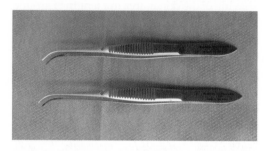

Figure 7.11
Small, curved forceps for follicular unit removal.

subsequently subdivided in thin slivers. These small slices of tissue contain one or two rows of FU. It takes a well-trained, precise technician to perform this very critical step to assure minimal transection of follicles. The slivers are then carefully cut into follicular unit grafts. This meticulous dissection requires well-trained staff and can be done with a no. 10 Personna blade, or a scalpel with a no. 10 blade and fine jewelers' forceps. Excessive amounts of fat, hair without matrices, and any scar tissue (especially from a previous transplant) is removed.

During preparation, grafts are grouped according to size and density on petri dishes on ice (Figures 7.13). It is essential that during this whole process strips and grafts are not permitted to dry out and are well moistened with saline.

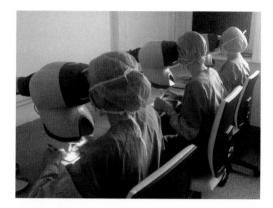

Figure 7.12
Hair transplant assistants with binocular stereomicroscopes.

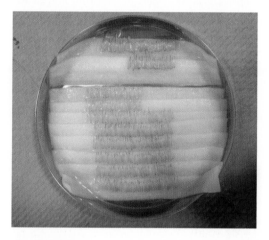

Figure 7.13
Lined up grafts in a metal petri dish in chilled normal saline.

There are a variety of solutions that grafts can be stored in during the hair transplant procedure. Normal saline or Ringer's Lactate are most commonly used as holding solutions. However, some physicians claim that more expensive solutions such as Hypothermosol, Viaspan, Wisconsin solution, or platelet-rich plasma are superior. To date, there is no ideal temperature or holding solution for hair restoration surgery based on current studies. Hair transplant data at this time suggest that chilled grafts in normal saline or Ringer's Lactate seem to thrive

just as well as when they are placed at room temperature in these solutions. It is uncertain whether it is better to use hypertonic solutions at a cool temperature, as is the case with other organs [35].

Recipient area design and technique

Design

The design of the hair transplant is most crucial for the outcome of the procedure and for patient satisfaction. Various factors have to be taken into consideration when designing the recipient site, such as the extent of balding, the patient's age, facial contours and measurements, and the patient's desire and expectations.

The donor hair supply for one single session has to be taken into consideration as a first step. The patient needs to understand that hair restoration surgery is a redistribution of hair and that the hair can never be restored the way it was in his or her teen years. Once the supply is calculated, the physician needs to negotiate where to place the grafts and find out what bothers the patient the most. Usually, facial framing is what the patient wants most, since framing the face makes the greatest difference in the overall appearance. Positioning the hairline is critical, and must be discussed at length with the patient. This is drawn in at the first consultation and before the surgery.

Men

For a satisfying hair design in men, different landmarks of the scalp have to be determined. First, areas of forthcoming thinning have to be identified. If hair is placed only in bald or very thin areas but balding continues in other zones, areas with transplanted hairs may become isolated and may look unnatural. In young men, it is sometimes difficult to estimate how the ultimate hair loss will emerge. If further thinning is expected (like in most hair transplant patients) the patient should be advised to use additional medical therapy for pattern hair loss.

The scalp is divided into three zones: frontal scalp, mid scalp, and vertex. The first hair transplant session is usually focused on framing the face, and therefore the frontal and mid scalp are most important. For the hairline design the mid-frontal point is determined first. This is the distance from the glabella to the frontal hairline. To find a suitable mid-frontal distance, the face should be divided into three areas: (1) chin to nasal spine, (2) nasal spine to glabella, and (3) glabella to hairline. Each distance should ideally display the same length to give an aesthetic appearance (Figure 7.14). The mid-frontal point is normally located 7–11 cm vertically from the mid glabella. The second point that has to be determined is the apex, which resembles the

frontotemporal junction and is basically the highest point of the frontotemporal recession. The apex is best measured from a vertical line drawn from the lateral epicanthus. We feel that the ideal quotient of mid-frontal point distance and apex height should be 0.7, meaning with a mid-frontal point at 7 cm, the apex is ideally placed at 10 cm.

In our clinic, we mostly create a curved, bell-shaped hairline without a flare or a frontotemporal design with a curve into the temples with or without the additional restoration of the temporal hairline and temporal points. Some surgeons prefer to create a frontotemporal design with a flare. The flare is designed by forming a concave trough medial to the non-flared, bell-shaped line. This design can also give very pleasing results, especially if the upper temporal margin is concave and a reconstruction of the temporal hairline is not desired [36].

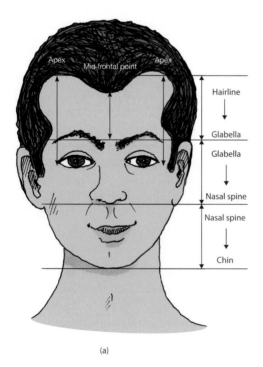

(a)

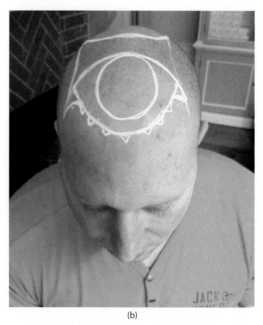

(b)

Figure 7.14

(a) Location and design of the mid-frontal point and the apex, rule of thirds for the measurement of the ideal facial proportions; (b) drawn hairline with mid-scalp design.

If balding is extensive and donor supply limited, the creation of a frontal forelock is an option to achieve a new framing of the face. A variety of designs can be created for the use of a frontal forelock. It can be completely isolated but the connection zone to the temporoparietal fringe is mostly filled in with sparse single hair grafts to give it a more natural look [37].

The reconstruction of temporal points and temple hairline should always be taken into consideration when planning the frontal hairline design. The absence of temporal point or severely recessed temples can create the impression of an unnaturally wide forehead and a "lid"-like appearance of the frontal hairline. The optimal location of the temporal point can be found in the intersection of two lines: (1) nasal tip to pupil, which should cross the lateral third of the eyebrow and merge into the parietal hump and (2) mid-temporal point (as created) to the top of the antitragus [36] (Figure 7.15). For a natural look, the frontal hairline should always be created as a transition zone (6–10 mm wide) of gradually increasing density toward the center.

It is also important to create irregularities. A natural hairline always has restrained or pronounced peaks and microclusters. Around 50% of men and women have at least one or more peaks in their frontal hairline. These macro-irregularities shape the general contour of the hairline and can be seen from several feet away [36]. In contrast to clusters are subtle irregularities. They can be created as 3–6 mm triangles in the frontal hairline and to mimic nature these clusters can be surrounded by randomly scattered single hairs (sentinel hairs) [36] (Figure 7.16). If there is limited donor hair, a reconstruction of the mid-scalp bridge in combination with a small frontal forelock may be the best and most natural solution.

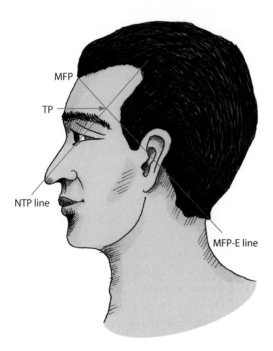

Figure 7.15
Temporal point location at the intersection of two lines: one from the mid-frontal point to the top of the antitragus and one from the nasal tip to the pupil/lateral third of the eyebrow.

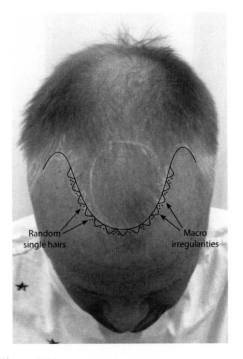

Figure 7.16
Triangular clusters surrounded by randomly scattered single hairs (sentinel hairs).

Even though hair loss in the vertex area has much less impact on a person's appearance compared to the frontal and mid-scalp, many men are very concerned about balding in this area. When transplanting the vertex, one must considerer that the borders are usually not permanent and may migrate more toward the periphery. If hair is only transplanted to the bald or balding areas and hair loss continues, it may leave an island of hair with a halo of thin hair around it. If the entire vertex is transplanted, the first step is to find the center of the whorl or whorls and follow the natural hair direction. The vertex can be transplanted with a uniform density or a graded density (with the lowest density in the center). If the mid-scalp is reconstructed, but the vertex is not transplanted, a transition zone between mid-scalp and vertex has to be created. It can be round, oval, or kidney shaped and should also contain microirregularities to look natural [36].

Ethnic considerations

In Asian and black men, hairline design may differ from the design in Caucasian men. In both Asian and black men, the hairline should be designed in a flatter shape (Figure 7.17).

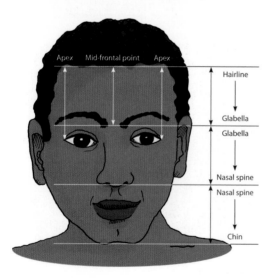

Figure 7.17
Frontal hairline design in black men.

In Asian men, the apex (measured from the lateral epicanthus) should be placed 1–1.5 cm higher than mid-frontal point. In black men usually a flatter hairline is desired; the apex should be placed only slightly higher than the mid-frontal point and lateral to the vertical line drawn from the lateral epicanthus.

The given landmarks and measurements can only be seen as a general benchmark for the design of a hair transplant. Every patient is different and may have different needs and perceptions. The hair transplant surgeon needs to work out the suiting design together with the patient to achieve the best and most satisfying results for each patient.

Women

Women can greatly benefit from hair restoration surgery since the invention of FUT allows the doctor to plant hair between the preexisting hairs in thinning areas. Hairline design in women is different than in men. The ideal female hairline shows no frontotemporal recession. The framing of a female face should be designed as round or heart shaped (with a widows peak). Like in men, the mid-frontal point should be set at about one-third of the vertical length of the face (measured from glabella to hairline). In women, depending on the facial measurements, the ideal height can range from 5 to 8 cm. The apex should be set at the same height or a bit higher than the mid-frontal point measured from the lateral epicanthus.

If a new hairline is created, the reconstruction or enhancement of the temples should always be considered (Figure 7.18). A female temporal hairline shows no peaks or points, but is a soft convex line. Many women with female pattern hair loss have a well-preserved frontal hairline but diffuse frontoparietal thinning. Women with a "Christmas-tree pattern" described by Olsen et al. with a thick donor area with frontal accentuation are ideal candidates for hair restoration surgery.

Hair transplant sessions in women should be limited to around 1500 grafts, because of a frequently occurring shock hair loss after the surgery. This shock loss can be severe and very traumatic for the patient and can last up to 4 months. Women who are planning to undergo hair restoration surgery must be warned and prepared for this side effect.

Transgender

A transgender person identifies with a social gender role opposite to his or her biological sex. The incidence of transsexualism is estimated to be from 1:5,000 to 1:50,000 [38]. Even though male transsexuals receive more medical attention, the incidence in men and women seems to be equal [38]. Transgender men (transwomen) are often seeking a variety of feminizing cosmetic surgeries. Male pattern baldness is specifically regarded as a male stigma and hair restoration is greatly desired.

The first consideration in a male transsexual should be the donor supply. If male pattern baldness is extensive, it may be more satisfying for the patient to first create a new female hairline and cover or enhance mid-scalp and vertex with a good hairpiece. Mid-scalp design in the frontal forelock is not suitable in transgender men. The hairline design should basically follow the same rules as in women. If donor supply is limited, the hairline can be set a bit higher but should still create a round or heart-shaped framing of the face. Older transgender men commonly undergo meloplasty. In this case, valuable hair-bearing areas are removed and can be utilized for FUT.

Scars

Scars on the scalp can be disfiguring and extremely distressing for the patient. Scars can be caused by radiation, burn, injuries, and infections as a secondary alopecia, or by a folliculocentric inflammatory process that ultimately destroys the hair follicle (see Chapter 6). In large scars, blood supply is always a concern. Flap techniques and scalp reduction should be considered first to reduce the scared area. FUT should be performed in a subsequent session with low density. A small test area may be useful to estimate graft survival 6 months before a larger session (Figure 7.19). Large scars

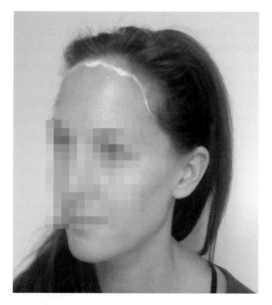

Figure 7.18
Round hairline design in a woman.

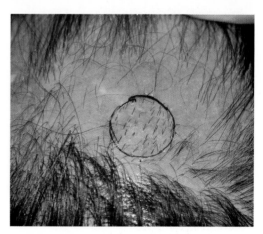

Figure 7.19
Small test area in a patient with burnt-out discoid lupus erythematosus.

should be first transplanted in the periphery to improve vascularization toward the center. Subsequent sessions can then fill the center and increase density.

In primary cicatricial alopecia, hair restoration surgery is an option for burnt-out stages, especially for lymphocytic primary cicatricial alopecia (Figure 7.20). A small test area is always recommended in bigger areas of burnt-out primary cicatricial alopecia to estimate graft survival and reactivation of the disease. The patient has to be educated about the condition and warned about possible disease recurrence and limited graft survival [39]. Neutrophilic cicatricial alopecia even in burnt-out stages seems to be a contraindication for hair restoration surgery of any kind (scalp reduction and FUT) (Figure 7.21).

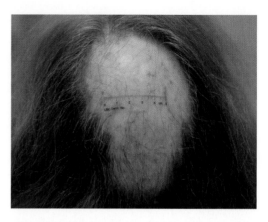

Figure 7.21
Patient with extensive folliculitis decalvans. The patient underwent scalp reduction surgery 10 years prior to her first presentation at UBC hair clinic. The condition got subsequently worse over time. It remains unclear if the scalp surgery aggravated the condition.

Preparation of recipient site

Many different instruments are available to create the recipient site. Density in the different scalp areas and graft size have to be taken into consideration before preparing the area. The incisions are made perpendicular to the intended hair direction. The direction changes in different areas of the scalp and should always follow the original growth direction. The size of the instrument must match the size of the graft and incision depth has to be chosen according to the length of the graft. If the slits are too small, planting will be difficult; if the incisions are too wide for the graft, a desired density is difficult to achieve. Shallow incisions may affect graft survival, and in all cases popping of the grafts may occur during the procedure. Excessively deep incisions bring the risk of planting the grafts too deeply, which causes pitting and an unpleasant look.

In our clinic, we like to use needles usually ranging from 18 to 21 gauge (g) (Figure 7.22) or spearpoints ranging from 0.8 to 1.25 mm (Figures 7.23 and 7.24). Sharpoint (Figure 7.25)

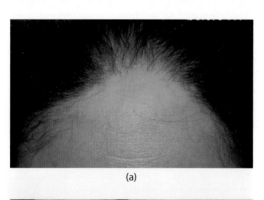
(a)

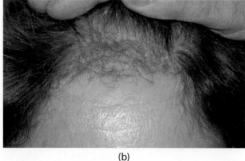
(b)

Figure 7.20
(a) Patient with burnt-out frontal fibrosing alopecia; (b) 5 months after follicular unit transplantation.

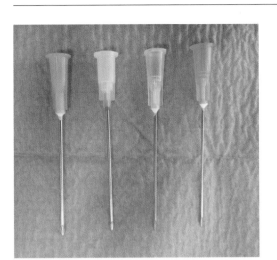

Figure 7.22
Needles for recipient site preparation
18–21 gauge.

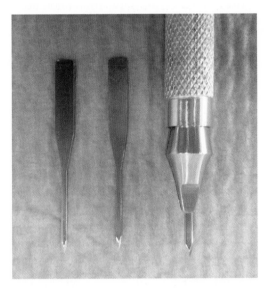

Figure 7.23
Spearpoint metal blades 0.8–1.25 mm.

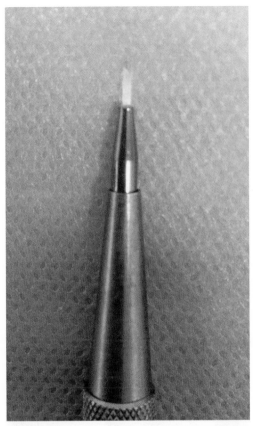

Figure 7.24
Spearpoint diamond blade 0.8 mm.

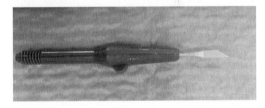

Figure 7.25
Sharpoint blade.

or mindeblades can also be useful, especially for parallel slits. Needles are inexpensive, easily accessible, easy to hold, and therefore gentle to the wrist. Depth control may be a problem, and therefore, doctors who use needles need a bit more experience. Needles are also very useful for the stick and place technique, when the graft is directly placed into the slit. In our clinic, we prefer to create the entire recipient site first before planting the grafts (Figure 7.26).

Graft placing

Planting into the slits is done meticulously with jewelers' forceps (Figure 7.27) with

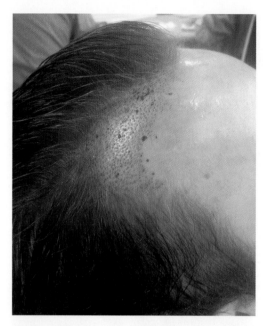

Figure 7.26
Prepared frontal recipient site.

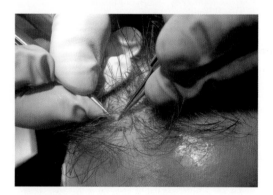

Figure 7.27
Graft planting with two jeweler's forceps.

2.5- to 5-fold magnifying glasses. One or two jewelers' forceps can be used for planting. The technique with two forceps allows the planter to locate and open the slit, but if more than one person is planting the grafts, the technique with only one forceps is preferable. The one-forceps technique allows the planter to have a small amount of grafts on a finger of the non-planting hand and to use the free hand for dabbing.

Special care is taken not to harm any of the grafts. Absolutely no force may be used for placing the grafts and the grafts may not dry out at any time during the process. The hairs in the grafts are aligned with the appropriate angle and direction, fitting directly into the slits. Most hairs, even if they clinically appear straight, have a little bit of a curl or curve. The graft must always be planted with the curve pointing toward the skin, otherwise the hair transplant will result in a tousled look. The grafts can be flush or slightly elevated above the surrounding tissue.

A regular session will usually take 5–6 hours. A mega session may take 6–8 hours to complete. Patients leave the office with a dressing covering only the donor area. The dressing is removed the next day. With appropriate postoperative care and daily shampooing, after 1 week virtually all crusting will have disappeared.

Anesthesia

There are different ways to anesthetize the scalp. Some surgeons prefer nerve blocks, whereas others prefer field blocks by infiltrating the entire treated area.

The principal sensory nerves innervating the scalp are the trigeminal and upper cervical nerves: supratrochlear nerve and the supraorbital nerve from the ophthalmic division (V1) of the trigeminal nerve (V); greater occipital nerve (CII) posteriorly up to the vertex; lesser occipital nerve (C II and III) behind the ear; zygomaticotemporal nerve from the maxillary division (V2) of the trigeminal nerve supplying the hairless temple up to the temporal hair line; and the auriculotemporal nerve from the mandibular division (V3) of the trigeminal nerve supplying the temples (Figure 7.28).

In our clinic, we developed the following regime for anesthetizing the scalp. We usually

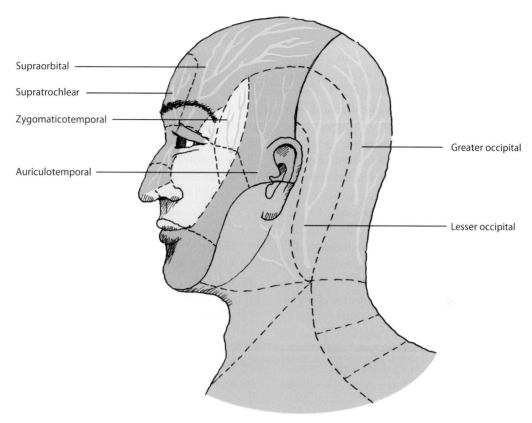

Supraorbital

Supratrochlear

Zygomaticotemporal

Auriculotemporal

Greater occipital

Lesser occipital

Figure 7.28
Sensory supply of the scalp. The area of innervation of the trigeminal nerve and its three branches is shown in red (V1), yellow (V2), and blue (V3). The area of the cervical nerves is shown in green; that of the occipital nerves in orange.

give 10 mg of diazepam before the surgery after the patient has consented to the procedure and to the design. For pain management during or after the surgery, acetaminophen and codeine or 800 mg of ibuprofen can be considered.

After clipping the area (for strip harvesting) or shaving of the donor area to a length of 2 mm (for FUE) we apply an ice pad for 1 minute. Then we infiltrate the occipital area at the height of the external occipital protuberance with lidocaine HCl 2% with epinephrine 1:100,000 while massaging the skin. We use a dental syringe and a 33-g needle to keep the pain at a minimum. Approximately 4–6 mL

is used for this first step. Next we apply a nerve block to the greater occipital and lesser occipital nerves with 2 mL of a longer lasting local anesthetic mixed with epinephrine (25 mL of mepivacain hydrochloride mixed with 1 mL epinephrine 1:1000). Then we infiltrate the entire donor area with tumescence. Our tumescence is mixed as follows: 250 mL normal saline, 50 mL lidocaine HCl 1%, 10 mL bupivacaine hydrochloride 0.5%, 1 mL epinephrine 1:1000.

Before donor harvesting, we wait 20 minutes to maximize vasoconstriction. In strip harvesting procedures we anesthetize the frontal and mid-scalp before taking the strip.

We again apply a cool pad to the frontal hair-line for 1 minute. We then infiltrate the skin along the drawn-in hairline with lidocaine HCl 2% with epinephrine 1:100,000 (approximately 4 mL) while massaging the skin. Next, we additionally infiltrate the area with mepivacain hydrochloride with epinephrine (approximately 4 mL). Tumescence is administered to the entire recipient area once the strip is harvested. Vasoconstriction has then already kicked in and the recipient site can be prepared soon after strip harvesting.

Since donor harvesting with the FUE technique takes several hours, anesthesia of the front and mid-scalp is administered after all grafts are extracted. We sometimes perform nerve blocks of the supratrochlear and supra-orbital nerve or the auriculotemporal nerve (when working on the temporal hairline) using mepivacain or bupivacaine, especially in patients who are known to have a quick release of local anesthetics. Tumescence anesthesia should be given during the day as needed.

4. Allergies to any kind of administered medication, local anesthetic, or topical can occur, even if the patient has not indicated an allergy in the consent process. The surgeon and the entire hair transplant team should be well trained for the case of an allergic shock.

5. Vasovagal syncope can occur, usually after administration of the local anesthesia to the donor area, and is a manifestation of the patient's anxiety. Fainting is far more common in men than in women. Vital signs have to be monitored before, during, and after the procedure in every patient.

6. Infections are very rare. We do not routinely give antibiotics. If folliculitis or cysts occur, an antibiotic may be necessary. In any case, the patient should come to the office for a consultation.

7. Temporary headache may occur, especially when the local anesthesia wears off. We provide Ibuprofen for any kind of pain after the procedure.

Side effects and complications

Every surgical procedure brings the risk of side effects and complications. In general, FUT, if performed with care, has a low complication rate. The following side effects should be discussed with the patient:

1. Facial edema beginning 48 hours after the procedure and lasting for 3–5 days is common and should be expected, especially after mega sessions. Swelling can be reduced by cooling the forehead and neck with ice pads (Figure 7.29).

2. Hematoma or even a bilateral black eye is very rare and more frequently seen in women.

3. Nausea and emesis due to the sedative drugs. We advise our patients to have a light breakfast before the procedure to reduce the possibility of nausea.

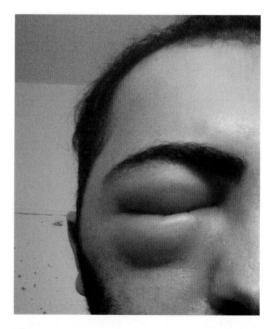

Figure 7.29
Severe edema of the forehead and eye 3 days after hair transplantation.

8. Temporary numbness may occur in the donor as well as in the recipient area. It may last for a few weeks. Massaging the scalp may be useful, but time will solve this problem.

9. Shock loss or telogen effluvium after the surgery can occur in men and women, but is far more common in women. The effluvium can be quite severe and may last for up to 4 months after the surgery. The patient needs to be warned and prepared for this unpleasant and sometimes traumatic side effect.

10. Hypertrophic scarring and keloid formation usually occur in patients with a history of keloids and hypertrophic scars. The patient needs to be asked about wound healing and scarring in the consent process. We consider a history of severe keloids as a contraindication for any kind of aesthetic surgery. In patients with a history of hypertrophic scars, the donor area may be injected with triamcinolone acetonite 5–10 mg/mL after wound closure and at follow-up visits to prevent hypertrophic scarring (Figure 7.30).

11. Several authors and surgeons have found a negative impact of cigarette smoke on wound healing and graft survival. Patients should be advised to keep their cigarette consumption to a minimum. However, in our clinic, we could not find a significant difference in wound healing and graft survival in nonsmokers versus moderate smokers.

Very rare complications are as follows:

1. Persistent or prolonged pain or numbness: Persistent pain in the donor scar may be a result of inadequate suture removal, when nonabsorbable suture material is buried in the scar. Scalp massages may help to solve or weaken this problem.

2. If poor growth occurs, every step of the procedure, including staff involved, protocols followed, and postoperative care, must be evaluated carefully. The surgeon should share his or her own disappointment about the result and should discuss every postoperative finding and practice with the patient. The final result should be evaluated after 12 months. If after 12 months graft survival and growth rates are indeed low, the surgeon may offer a free of charge session where every step of the procedure is extra closely monitored. If after the second procedure growth is still poor, this may be what has been described as the X-Factor [40].

3. Scars and keloids around the grafts: Patients with predisposition for severe keloid formation should be excluded from a hair transplant procedure. If a procedure is considered, a small test area may be useful to estimate the risk.

4. Hair loss of the transplanted hair: If the grafts are taken from a safe donor area, that is not affected by the process of androgenetic alopecia, and the transplanted hair should continue to grow for life, unless the patient develops a scalp disease other than androgenetic alopecia, such as alopecia areata, cicatricial alopecia, or telogen effluvium. These

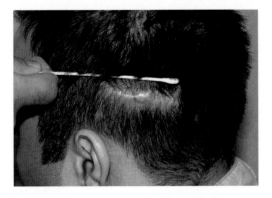

Figure 7.30
Hypertrophic scar 1 year after follicular unit transplantation with strip removal.

scalp disorders affect transplanted and nontransplanted hairs alike.

5. Undesirable scars and necrosis in the donor area: Temporary and permanent effluvium as well as necrosis and infections in the donor area can occur after too-tight wound closure, especially after subsequent procedures (Figure 7.31). Bad donor scars can later be treated with FUEs or camouflaged with micropigmentation.

Consultation and consent

The consultation process is the key to a good relationship between the physician and the patient, to a successful hair restoration procedure, and to patient satisfaction. First of all, the doctor has to evaluate the patients' concerns and goals. The patient needs to understand the nature of the hair loss and the ongoing nature of androgenetic alopecia and the need for medical therapy and/or subsequent sessions. Facial framing has usually the greatest impact on a person's appearance and should be encouraged for the first hair transplant procedure. The goal of every hair transplant procedure is a short- and long-term natural appearance [41].

A thorough medical history has to be taken, including prescription drugs, vitamin and herbal supplements, allergies, and bleeding problems. Blood thinners have to be stopped before transplantation (aspirin for 2 weeks, clopidogrel for 1 week, and warfarin, according to the Partial thromboplastin time, at least 24 hours) [41].

In our clinic, every patient is tested for HIV, hepatitis C, and coagulopathy before the procedure. Patients with cardiovascular problems or a history of a heart attack or arrhythmia are asked to perform an ECG and to get clearance from their cardiologist.

A written informed consent has to be obtained from every patient at least 24 hours before the surgery. International standards for the consent process have been developed and are available via the International Society of Hair Restoration Surgery (ISHRS) (www.ishrs.org). In Germany, consent forms according to the international guidelines are available at www.diomed.de.

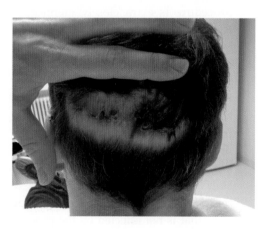

Figure 7.31
Closure under maximum tension after removing 2 donor scars in a third session. Necrosis and effluvium in the donor area 2 weeks after surgery.

Conclusion

Hair transplant surgery has become very popular in both men and women. FUT has made the procedure an efficient technique for increasing hair density in specific areas affected by androgenetic alopecia with cosmetically very natural and pleasing results. Combining medical therapy with systemic finasteride or topical minoxidil solution may certainly add to the cosmetic result.

Before and after

(Figures 7.32 through 7.38)

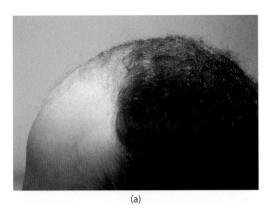
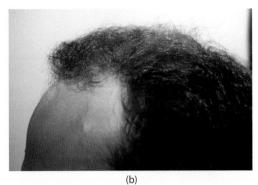

Figure 7.32
(a) Before and (b) after 1345 follicular unit grafts.

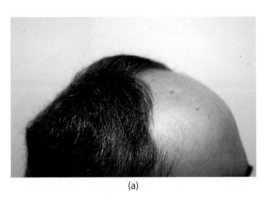
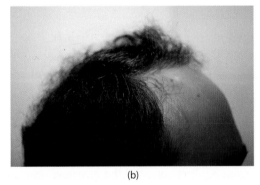

Figure 7.33
(a) Before and (b) after 1234 follicular unit grafts.

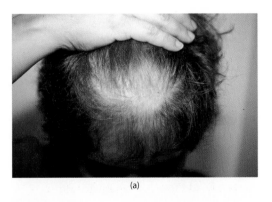
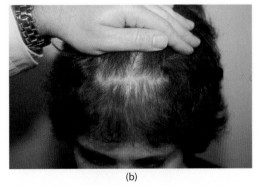

Figure 7.34
(a) Before and (b) after patient with female pattern hair loss, 1367 follicular unit grafts.

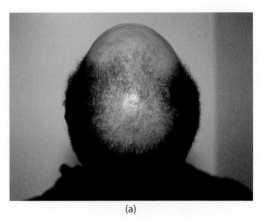
(a)

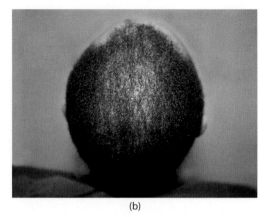
(b)

Figure 7.35
(a) Before and (b) after 2652 follicular unit grafts.

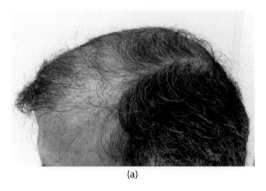
(a)

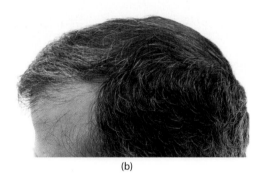
(b)

Figure 7.36
(a) Before and (b) after 1788 follicular unit grafts.

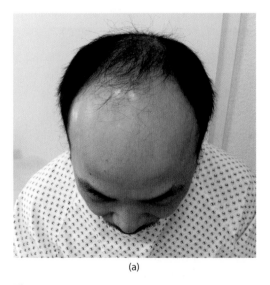
(a)

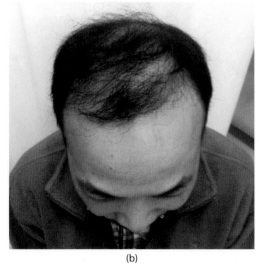
(b)

Figure 7.37
(a) Before and (b) after creation of a frontal forelock, 1139 follicular unit grafts.

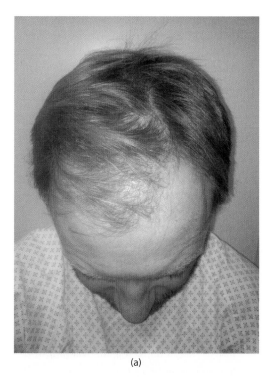
(a)

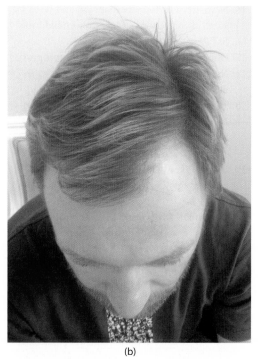
(b)

Figure 7.38
(a) Before and (b) after 812 follicular unit grafts.

References

1. The history of hair transplants. http://www. keratin.com/aw/aw001.shtml.

2. Sasagawa M, Hair transplantation. *Jpn J Dermatol*, 1930. **30**: 493.

3. Okuda S, The study of clinical experiments of hair transplantations. *Jpn J Dermatol*, 1939. **46**: 135–8.

4. Tamura H, Pubic hair transplantation. *Jpn J Dermatol*, 1943. **53**: 76.

5. Fujita K, Brow plasty. *J Lepra*, 1953. **22**(4): 218.

6. Barsky AJ, *Principles and Practice of Plastic Surgery*. 1950. Baltimore, MD: Williams & Wilkins. p. 137–140.

7. Lamont ES, A plastic surgical transformation. Report of a case. *West J Surg Obstet Gynecol*, 1957. **65**: 164–5.

8. Orentreich N, Autografts in alopecias and other selected dermatological conditions. *Ann N Y Acad Sci*, 1959. **20**(83): 463–79.

9. Orentreich N, Hair transplantation. *N Y State J Med*, 1972. **72**(5): 578–82.

10. Selmanowitz VJ and Orentreich N, Hair transplantation in blacks. *J Natl Med Assoc*, 1973. **65**(6): 471–82.

11. Orentreich DS and Orentreich N, Hair transplantation. *J Dermatol Surg Oncol*, 1985. **11**(3): 319–24.

12. Orentreich N, Hair transplantation: The punch graft technique. *Surg Clin North Am*, 1971. **51**(2): 511–8.

13. Juri J, Use of parieto-occipital flaps in the surgical treatment of baldness. *Plast Reconstr Surg*, 1975. **55**(4): 456–60.

14. Bouhanna P, The postauricular vertical hair-bearing transposition flap. *J Dermatol Surg Oncol*, 1984. **10**(7): 551–4.

15. Frechet P, A new method for correction of the vertical scar observed following scalp reduction for extensive alopecia. *J Dermatol Surg Oncol*, 1990. **16**(7): 640–4.

16. Nordström R, Tissue expansion and flaps for surgical correction of male pattern baldness. *Br J Plast Surg*, 1988. **41**(2): 154–9.

17. Ohmori K, Microsurgical free temporoparietal flaps in surgery for male pattern baldness. *Clin Plast Surg*, 1991. **18**(4): 791.

18. Stough DB 3rd and Cates JA, Transposition flaps for the correction of baldness: A practical office procedure. *J Dermatol Surg Oncol*, 1980. **6**(4): 286–9.

19. Unger WP, A new method of donor site harvesting. *J Dermatol Surg Oncol*, 1984. **10**(7): 524–9.

20. Stough DB 4th, Nelson BR, and Stough DB 3rd, Incisional slit grafting. *J Dermatol Surg Oncol*, 1991. **17**(1): 53–60.

21. Swinehart JM and Griffin EI, Slit grafting: The use of serrated island grafts in male and female-pattern alopecia. *J Dermatol Surg Oncol*, 1991. **17**(3): 243–53.

22. Nelson BR et al., Hair transplantation in advanced male pattern alopecia. The role of incisional slit grafting. *J Dermatol Surg Oncol*, 1991. **17**(7): 567–73.

23. Uebel CO, Micrografts and minigrafts: A new approach for baldness surgery. *Ann Plast Surg*, 1991. **27**(5): 476–87.

24. Limmer R, Elliptical donor stereoscopically assisted micrografting as an approach to further refinement in hair transplantation. *Dermatol Surg*, 1994. **20**: 789–93.

25. Bernstein RM and Rassman WR, Follicular transplantation. Patient evaluation and surgical planning. *Dermatol Surg*, 1997. **23**(9): 771–84.

26. Bernstein RM et al., Standardizing the classification and description of follicular unit transplantation and mini-micrografting techniques. The American Society for Dermatologic Surgery, Inc. *Dermatol Surg*, 1998. **24**(9): 957–63.

27. Epstein JS, Follicular-unit hair grafting: State-of-the-art surgical technique. *Arch Facial Plast Surg*, 2003. **5**(5): 439–44.

28. Stough D and Whitworth JM, Methodology of follicular unit hair transplantation. *Dermatol Clin*, 1999. **17**(2): 297–306.

29. Unger WP, Follicular unit hair transplanting—End of the evolution or a good thing taken too far? *Dermatol Surg*, 2000. **26**(2): 158–60.

30. Rassman WR et al., Follicular unit extraction: minimally invasive surgery for hair transplantation. *Dermatol Surg*, 2002. **28**(8): 720–8.

31. Harris JA, The SAFE System: New instrumentation and methodology to improve follicular unit extraction (FUE). *Hair Transplant Forum Int*, 2004. **14**: 163–4.

32. Parsley WM, Management of the postoperative period. In *Hair Transplantation*, Unger WP and Shapiro R, Editors. 2004. New York: Marcel Dekker, Inc. p. 565–566.

33. Marzola M, Single-scar harvesting technique. In *Hair Transplantation*, Stough D, Haber R, Dover JS, Alam M, Editors. 2006. Philadelphia, PA: Elsevier. p. 83–6.

34. Bicknell LM et al., Follicular unit extraction hair transplant harvest: a review of current recommendations and future considerations. *Dermatol Online J*, 2014. **20**(3): p. pii: doj_21754.

35. Cole JP, *The Optimal Holding Solution and Temperature for Hair Follicle*. http://www.forhair.com/optimal-holding-solution-and-temperature-for-hair-follicle/.

36. Rose PT and Parsley WM, Science of hair line design. In *Hair Transplantation*, Stough DB, Haber R, Dover JS, Alam M, Editors. 2006. Philadelphia, PA: Elsevier. p. 55–71.

37. Beehner M, Terminology in hair transplant surgery. In *Hair Transplantation*, Haber RS, et al., Editors. 2006. Philadelphia, PA: Elsevier Inc. p. 27–34.

38. Shiell R, Hair transplantation in the genetically male transsexual. In *Hair Transplantation*, Stough DB, Haber RS, Dover JS, Alam M, Editors. 2006. Philadelphia, PA: Elsevier. p. 169–172.

39. Rose PT and Shapiro R, Transplantation into scar tissue and areas of cicatricial alopecia. In *Hair Transplantation*, Shapiro R, Unger WP, Editors. Vol. 4. 2004. New York: Marcel Dekker.

40. Marzola M and Vogel JE, Complications. In *Hair Transplantation*, Stough DB, Haber R, Dover JS, Alam M, Editors. 2006. Philadelphia, PA: Elsevier. p. 173–85.

41. Stough DB, The consultation. In *Hair Transplantation*, Stough DB, Haber RS, Dover JS, Alam M, Editors. 2006. Philadelphia, PA: Elsevier. p. 43–8.

8 Nonmedical approaches to hair loss: What is available?

Medical and surgical therapies for hair loss may sometimes not be enough to achieve a cosmetically acceptable result for the patient. Every physician dealing with hair loss should be able to give advice on different camouflage techniques and help the patient to find the best and most suitable solution.

Scalp prostheses

Scalp prostheses comprise not only wigs but also hairpieces. Wigs and hairpieces are available in different qualities with different mounting possibilities. Wigs can either be wefted or knotted, or both techniques may be used. A wefted foundation usually consists of rows of synthetic hair and is held on the scalp with an elastic band in the back and sometimes clips in the front (Figure 8.1).

A knotted wig has a very fine mesh as a foundation in which synthetic and/or human hair is knotted in by hand. Knotted wigs can be attached with tapes, glue, or barrette combs. They can be premade or custommade. A custom-made wig assures a perfect fit and involves making a custom plaster mold of the patient's scalp. From the mold, a custom-made foundation can be formed. The foundation can be made out of a very fine mesh or different types of film tulle. The quality of a custom-made wig depends on the type of foundation, the hair and knot density, and the hair quality (Figure 8.2).

The types of fibers used in synthetic wigs have improved considerably over the past few decades to better approximate the look and feel of human hair [1]. Real hair, as opposed to synthetic hair, usually gives a more natural look but generally needs more care and maintenance. Different hair types are available, including animal hair such as angora hair or yak tail. Human hair is categorized as Chinese, Indian, or European hair. The quality of human hair should ideally match the original hair type of the patient (Figure 8.3). Indian and Chinese hair is widely used but is usually processed for Caucasian wigs where the hair needs to have a finer caliber to create a natural look (Figure 8.4).

Another type of custom-made wig is the vacuum wig, which consists of a silicone or polyurethane base. Vacuum wigs are pushed down on the scalp to expel air and form a seal. This type of wig remains tightly attached to the scalp and allows an individual to swim and engage in any physical activities [1]. However, vacuum wigs may be uncomfortable, especially in hot weather since they do not allow air to circulate.

Hairpieces are used for patients with partial hair loss and are created to blend into the natural hair. Patients with cicatricial alopecia or alopecia areata can greatly benefit from custom-made hairpieces since they are usually more comfortable to wear and create a more natural look (Figures 8.5 and 8.6). A variety of hair systems for men are available on and the market. Hair systems need to be custom-made, and the quality depends on the type of foundation, quality

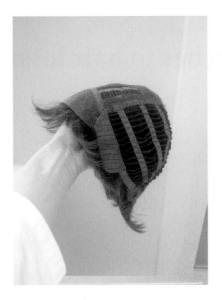

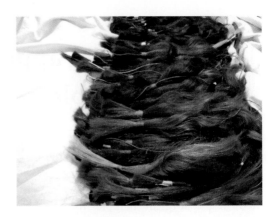

Figure 8.3
High-quality untreated European hair.
(Courtesy of Marc Rieke, mr*.)

Figure 8.1
Wefted foundation of a synthetic wig.

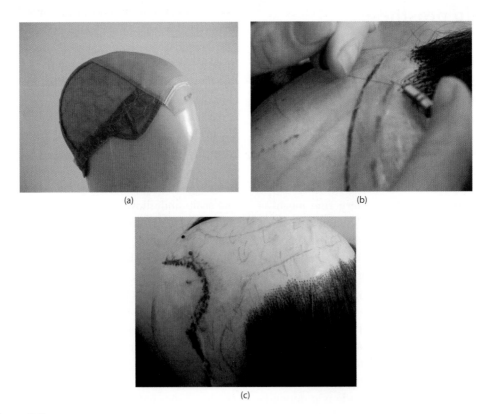

(a)

(b)

(c)

Figure 8.2
(a) Wig foundation made out of different types of gauze and film tulle; (b) human hair knotted by hand into the wig foundation; (c) high-quality custom-made wig with dense knots and natural hair direction. (Courtesy of Marc Rieke, mr*.)

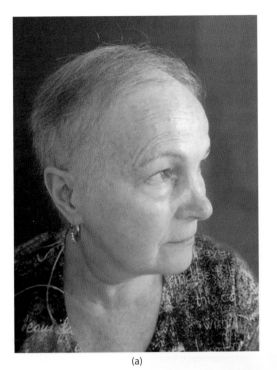

(a)

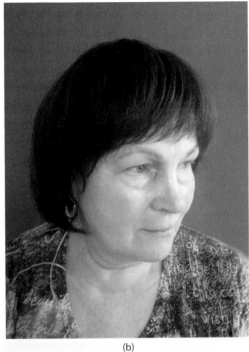

(b)

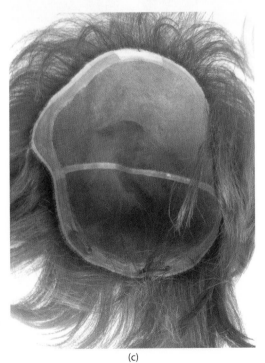

(c)

Figure 8.4
(a) Patient with extensive lichen planopilaris; (b) with a custom-made human hair wig;
(c) with a light gauze foundation and barrette combs. (Courtesy of Marc Rieke, mr*.)

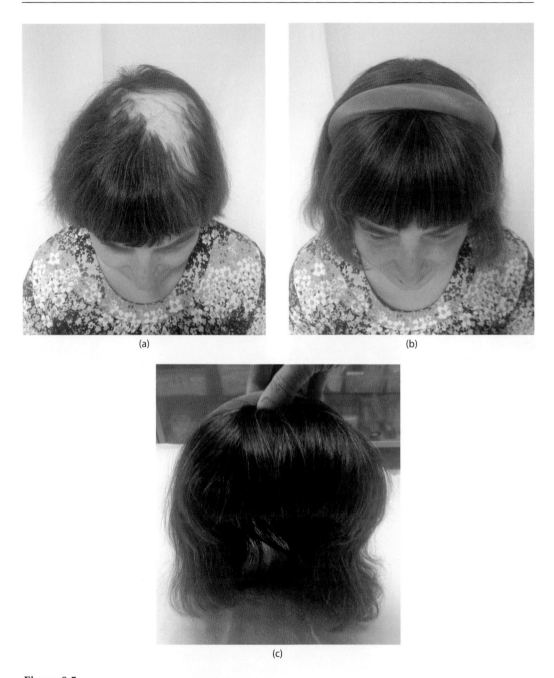

(a)

(b)

(c)

Figure 8.5
(a) Patient with extensive folliculitis decalvans; (b) with a custom-made human hairpiece; (c) the hairpiece is simply fixed with a hair band. (Courtesy of Marc Rieke, mr*.)

of hair, and the expertise of the wig maker. Hair systems for men can be glued, taped, or wefted. Hairpieces can create a great density for patients with extensive male pattern baldness. Hair systems can contribute greatly to a patient's self-esteem, but the level of comfort depends on expert care and maintenance (Figure 8.7).

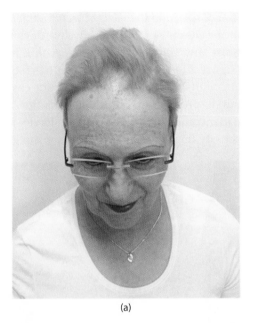
(a)

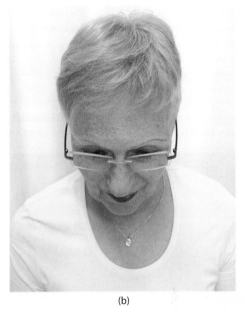
(b)

Figure 8.6
(a) Patient with extensive androgenetic alopecia, frontal fibrosing alopecia, and additional mechanical alopecia in the frontal hairline from a wig fixated with large barrette combs; (b) patient wearing a light custom-made hairpiece.

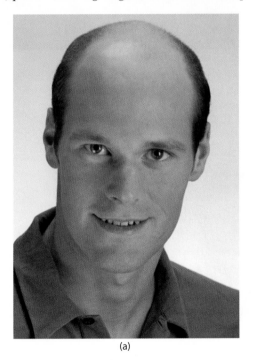
(a)

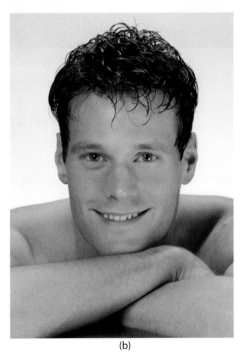
(b)

Figure 8.7
(a) Patient with extensive androgenetic alopecia; (b) with a glued custom-made hairpiece. (Courtesy of Svenson® Hair Institute.)

Instead of a hairpiece that is fixed with weaving, a technique called Intralace™ provides another style choice and may give the patient a more confident feeling. Intralace™ involves a mesh or lattice tulle that is placed on the scalp; the preexisting hair is lifted through the mesh and plaited with miniscule braids/plaits on the outside of the foundation, and then a light weft is attached to the mesh. This way, the weave does not cause any traction on the preexisting hair (Figure 8.8). The technique, like hairpieces and wefts, needs maintenance and is costly, but it provides a natural feeling for the patient and allows the patient to do any activity (Figure 8.9). This technique can give

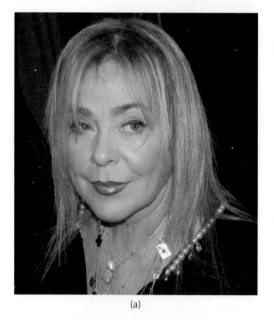

(a)

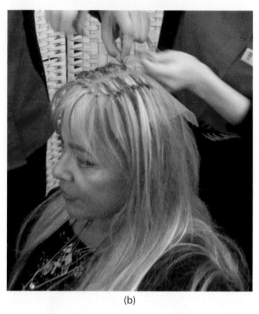

(b)

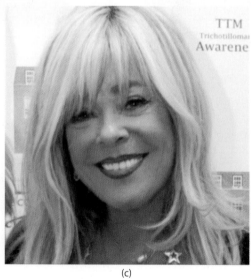

(c)

Figure 8.8
(a) Patient with thin hair and moderate female pattern hair loss; (b) process of the Intralace™ technique; (c) patient after the procedure. (Courtesy of Lucinda Ellery™.)

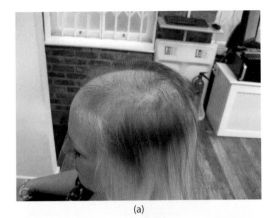

(a)

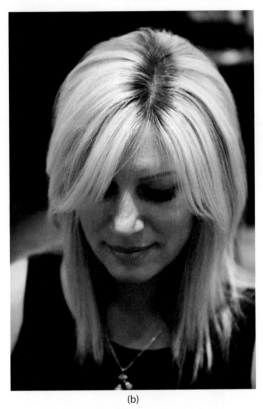

(b)

Figure 8.9
(a) Patient with extensive female pattern hair loss; (b) patient after Intralace™ procedure. (Courtesy of Lucinda Ellery™.)

very pleasing results for women with extensive androgenetic alopecia, women with sparse hair after chemotherapy or scalp radiation, or can even support therapy in patients with trichotillomania.

Hair extensions

Hair extensions have become very popular in the last decade. Extensions are strands or laces of synthetic or human hair that are glued, braided, twisted, sewn, clipped, or fused onto the preexisting hair [1]. Clip-on extensions can be taken out at any time and can be useful if the patient only occasionally desires fuller or longer hair for certain hair styles or occasions. Any type of extension can be problematic if the weight of the hair is too high. Heavy hair extensions can cause tension on existing hair and can result in traction alopecia. Tension can be limited by using light lace extensions, carefully sewn into the preexisting hair (Figures 8.10 and 8.11). Glue can damage the hair shaft, which can ultimately lead to hair breakage.

Scalp camouflage with color and topical hair fibers

Topical hair fibers consist of positively charged keratin fiber particles usually made of wool keratin that clings by electrostatic forces to a negatively charged terminal and vellus hair fibers on the scalp and function to make hair look thicker and fuller [1,2]. Hair fibers are available in different hair colors, which can also be mixed to match the patient's hair color. They are sprinkled onto the preexisting, thinning hair and can additionally be fixed with hairspray (Figure 8.12). Topical hair fibers require a minimal density of existing hair to bind. They are not effective in areas totally devoid of hair, such as patches of cicatricial alopecia or alopecia areata. Hair fibers can still be helpful in these diseases, when the pattern of hair loss is more reticulated and the individual patches are small, by thickening the surrounding hair.

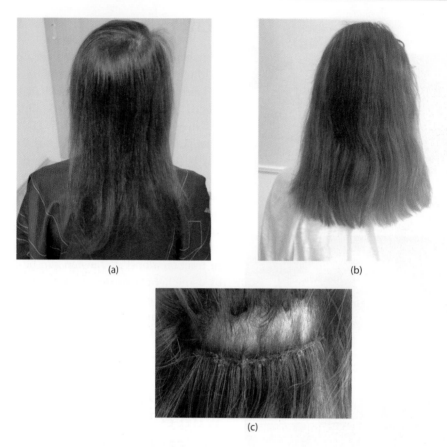

Figure 8.10
(a) Patient with female pattern hair loss; (b) wearing light lace extensions; (c) sewn into the preexisting hair with the support of minimal use of glue. (Courtesy of Marc Rieke, mr*.)

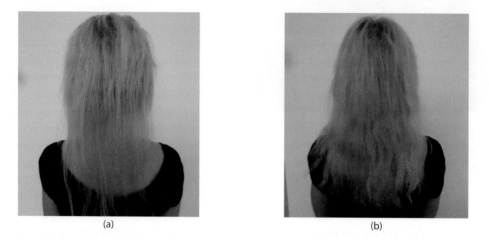

Figure 8.11
(a) Patient with resolved massive telogen effluvium; the hair had already grown back nicely for 9 months but the length was still very sparse; (b) with light lace extensions. (Courtesy of Marc Rieke, mr*.)

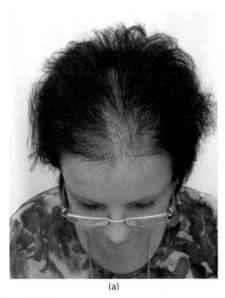
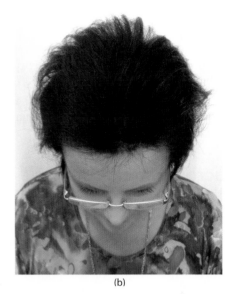

Figure 8.12
(a) Patient with female pattern hair loss and frontal accentuation; (b) after using hair fiber.

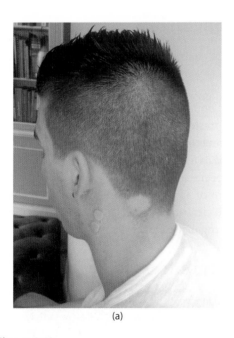
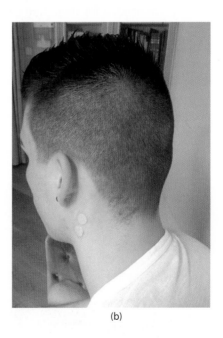

Figure 8.13
(a) Patient with a patch of alopecia areata; (b) after using simple waterproof mascara.

Scalp paint can be very useful for camouflaging hair loss by eliminating the color contrast between normal hair and scalp. Several products are available in different application forms such as powders, lotions, and sprays (Figure 8.13).

If the patient is using any topical medical therapy, such as minoxidil or topical corticosteroids, the scalp needs to be dry before any of the camouflaging agents are applied [1,2]. Hair fibers and scalp paint can also be useful to camouflage temporary shock loss after hair restoration surgery. The products can be applied 7–10 days postsurgery [3].

Micropigmentation

Permanent makeup is a form of permanent or semipermanent tattoo. It is frequently used to produce artificial eyebrows in patients who have lost them completely or to enhance sparse eyebrows. The eyebrow should always be placed in its natural location. It takes an experienced permanent makeup artist to create a cosmetically pleasing result. Permanent makeup of the eyebrows may create excellent results in women (Figures 8.14 and 8.15). It is not recommended for men. Individuals seeking advice on permanent tattooing should be aware of the possibility of the tattoo changing color over time [1].

Micropigmentation of the scalp continues to gain more popularity as a more permanent option to camouflage hair loss. Small dots, resembling hair follicles are tattooed on the scalp. Tattooing can be used for men

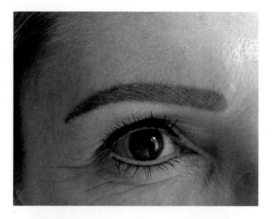

Figure 8.15
Micropigmentation of the eyebrows in a patient with sparse overplucked eyebrows.

as well as women [1]. Pleasing results can be achieved when carried out by experienced tattoo artists, especially in black men with very short (1–2 mm) hair styles.

Conclusion

Wigs, hairpieces, and camouflaging techniques can provide nice cosmetic outcomes, can have a great impact on a patient's physical appearance, and may contribute to the restoration of a patient's self-esteem. Nonmedical approaches to hair loss can be used as a temporary solution in patients with alopecia areata or anagen and telogen effluvium or as a permanent solution in patients with cicatricial alopecia, alopecia areata, and androgenetic alopecia.

References

1. Donovan JCH et al., A review of scalp camouflaging agents and prostheses for individuals with hair loss. *Dermatol Online J*, 2012. **18**(8): 1.
2. Kobren SD, *The Truth about Women's Hair Loss*. 2000. New York: McGraw-Hill.
3. Parsley WM, Management of the postoperative period. In *Hair Transplantation*, Unger WP and Shapiro R, Editors. 2004. New York: Marcel Dekker. p. 565–6.

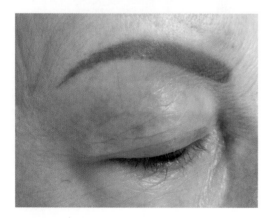

Figure 8.14
Micropigmentation of the eyebrows in a patient with frontal fibrosing alopecia.

Index

Note: References to figures are indicated by 'f' and references to tables by 't'.